Disaster and Development:
An Occupational Perspective

DEDICATION

To the planet, and all its living beings...

To the people who have lost their battles with disastrous events, and those currently engaged in struggles to survive and recover from traumatic experiences, and to future generations in building a wisdom and resilience to manage the challenges we are to face in coming times ...

For Elsevier

Senior Content Strategist: *Rita Demetriou-Swanwick*
Content Development Specialist: *Nicola Lally*
Project Manager: *Julie Taylor*
Designer/Design Direction: *Miles Hitchen*
Illustration Manager: *Amy Faith Naylor*

Disaster and Development: An Occupational Perspective

EDITED BY

NANCY RUSHFORD, PhD, MSc OT Reg (Ont), MA (Counselling Psychology)

Director of Programs & Implementation, Alzheimer Society of Ontario, Canada

KERRY THOMAS, BSc (OT), Grad Dip (Health Management)

interPART, Australia

FOREWORDS BY

VALERIE SCHERRER, MA, OT

Director, Emergency Response Unit, CBM; Co-ordinator, Conflict and Emergency Task Group of the International Disability and Development Consortium, Germany

MARILYN PATTISON, B App Sc (OT), MBA, FWFOT

President, World Federation of Occupational Therapists (WFOT); Managing Principal, MPOT Pty Ltd, Australia

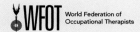 World Federation of Occupational Therapists

ELSEVIER   Edinburgh   London   New York   Oxford   Philadelphia   St Louis   Sydney   Toronto 2015

ELSEVIER

ISBN 978-0-7020-4047-4

Notices

Knowledge and best practice in this field are constantly changing. As new research and experience broaden our understanding, changes in research methods, professional practices, or medical treatment may become necessary.

Practitioners and researchers must always rely on their own experience and knowledge in evaluating and using any information, methods, compounds, or experiments described herein. In using such information or methods they should be mindful of their own safety and the safety of others, including parties for whom they have a professional responsibility.

With respect to any drug or pharmaceutical products identified, readers are advised to check the most current information provided (i) on procedures featured or (ii) by the manufacturer of each product to be administered, to verify the recommended dose or formula, the method and duration of administration, and contraindications. It is the responsibility of practitioners, relying on their own experience and knowledge of their patients, to make diagnoses, to determine dosages and the best treatment for each individual patient, and to take all appropriate safety precautions.

To the fullest extent of the law, neither the Publisher nor the authors, contributors, or editors, assume any liability for any injury and/or damage to persons or property as a matter of products liability, negligence or otherwise, or from any use or operation of any methods, products, instructions, or ideas contained in the material herein.

your source for books,
journals and multimedia
in the health sciences

www.elsevierhealth.com

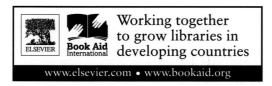

Working together
to grow libraries in
developing countries

www.elsevier.com • www.bookaid.org

The
publisher's
policy is to use
**paper manufactured
from sustainable forests**

Printed in China

CONTENTS

RECOVERY

DEVELOPMENT

ENTERING THE FIELD

PREFACE

Our home, planet Earth, is finite; all life shares its resources and the energy from the sun, and therefore has limits to growth. For the first time, we have touched those limits. When we compromise the air, the water, the soil and the variety of life, we steal from the endless future to serve the fleeting present.

The Universal Declaration of Interdependence,
David Suzuki Foundation

Disaster has become a part of everyday discourse – a kind of global narrative that speaks largely about people and their relationship to each other and the environment around them, and less about the events themselves. Climate change and extreme weather events, earthquakes, wildfires and tsunamis, epidemics, technological and complex emergencies… The escalation of these events around the globe renders disaster a global social and ecological crisis, and arguably one of the most pressing issues of the twenty-first century. Compounded by the economic and environmental costs of providing for an ever-increasing population and consumption-driven growth, there is an urgent need for a collective and integrated response that effectively engages communities and individual citizens, as well as a diverse mix of experts and practitioners representing disciplines, sectors and perspectives. The occupational therapy profession is only just beginning to forge a path into the field of disaster and development. As such, it is an auspicious time to explore the relevance of 'occupation' and an occupational perspective to the field in order to illuminate new possibilities for interdisciplinary collaboration and engagement.

Disaster and Development: An Occupational Perspective aims to articulate an occupational perspective in the field through the stories of people who have survived disaster and practitioners, as well as others who endeavour to help. Personal narratives provide a gateway into experience and therefore an opportunity to explore how occupation relates to resilience and the process of building communities that are equitable, supportive and sustainable into the future. Njelasani et al (2012) defines an occupational perspective as 'a way of looking and thinking about human doing' (p. 8). As editors of this book, we hold the view that occupation acts as the medium through which people relate to each other and the world around them. Occupation gives shape to the choices of everyday life and gives rise to the habits and routines upon which social structures and relationships are based. More broadly, we believe that occupation forms a nexus between society and the natural world, and therefore holds the potential to influence much needed social and ecological change. The stories captured within the pages of this book reveal some of the challenges and complexities associated with disaster and development. They also illustrate the power of human connection, the importance of hope, and tremendous opportunities for change and transformation. Through these stories of personal experience, the concept of occupation is linked to the global narrative of disaster, and the tremendous potential of occupation and collaborative engagement is illuminated.

Disaster and Development: An Occupational Perspective is written primarily for an audience within the profession of occupational therapists, but broadly aims to have cross-disciplinary relevance and utility for humanitarian aid and development practitioners from other disciplines whose work ultimately aims to enable positive social change as it involves the lives of individuals and communities most at risk and affected by disaster. As such, the book is well aligned with primary care and health promotion approaches in disaster contexts including wellness and preventative medicine, community development, social justice and ecological sustainability as an emerging holistic approach to development.

The disasters included in this book are mostly classified as 'natural' disasters, such as earthquakes, hurricanes, wildfires and drought. Not all types of disasters could be addressed and explored to our satisfaction within the limits of this book. Epidemics, including HIV and AIDS, and technological disasters such as nuclear events, for example, are not examined; neither is the topic of complex emergency explored in depth or from the perspective of occupational therapists working in military contexts.

OUTLINE OF THE BOOK

Part I provides a general introduction to the field of disaster including key concepts, principles and issues related to humanitarianism, human rights, sustainable development and inclusive approaches to managing disasters and reducing risk. The field is extensive, crossing many disciplines and areas of focus. As such, it is beyond the scope of this book to provide a comprehensive historical account or in-depth critical analysis of the field. Rather, our aim is to provide a basic outline and introduction that lays the foundation for an occupational perspective to emerge.

Part II represents a collection of case stories based on experiences in the field. Most, but not all contributors are occupational therapists who have worked closely with survivors on individual and collective levels. Some contributors have themselves survived disaster; all have been affected and even transformed in some way by their experiences and their connection to others. The practitioners share their insights and lessons learned.

Part III draws upon the collective knowledge and experience contained in the case series against the backdrop of the literature and contemporary practice in the field. Based on this analysis we have articulated the Disaster and Development Occupational Perspective Framework (DDOP), a framework that conceptually links occupation to the field of disaster and introduces the notion of 'occupational stewardship'. The framework is an evolving construct to be continuously shaped by dialogue, cross-disciplinary debate and developments in the field. DDOP is related to phases of emergency response, recovery and development, all under an umbrella of resilience building and risk reduction. Considerations for policy, practice and professional development are discussed.

It is not the strongest of the species that survives, nor the most intelligent, but the one most responsive to change.

Charles Darwin

NANCY RUSHFORD

KERRY THOMAS

REFERENCE

Njelesani, J., Tang, A., Jonsson, H., Polatajko, H., 2012. Articulating an occupational perspective. J. Occup. Sci. doi:10.1080/14427591 .2012.717500.

FOREWORDS

VALERIE SCHERRER
Director, Emergency Response Unit, CBM;
Co-ordinator, Conflict and Emergency Task Group
of the International Disability and Development
Consortium, Germany

When talking about disasters, we often refer to major events which we become more aware of as media reporting and communication technology has improved. Yet there are large numbers of disasters that remain unreported as they are only affecting small numbers of people in poor communities. The impacts of those everyday disasters are destructive to the lives of people and often drive them into the poorest living conditions. Persons with disabilities and ageing populations, as well as other marginalized groups, are usually disproportionately affected by disasters while very little is done to ensure they have access to emergency response services. There will be no hope for sustainable development if disasters are not considered as an element of day to day life and strategy to reduce risk is not addressed systematically by all.

The interconnectedness between disasters and development is complex and requires comprehensive analysis to enable governments, policy makers, international and local organizations, community and individuals to define appropriate measures to address disaster risk reduction at all occupation levels and throughout the disaster management cycle. Disaster is everyone's business.

One expression often used by disaster risk reduction professionals is 'coping mechanisms'. It refers to communities defining strategies and adapting their occupation to decrease the impact of disasters but also to facilitate self-recovery. To me, this resonates with the ultimate goal of occupational therapy: enabling people to function within their environment and independently contribute to the life of their community.

Occupational therapists, through their unique understanding of occupation, are very well positioned to support and facilitate the necessary changes at individual, family and community level to minimize risks and build up resilience to disasters. Occupational therapists are trained in looking at activities/occupation through a multidimensional perspective considering social, emotional and biological factors, among others. Occupational therapists are creative professionals who are used to identifying innovative ways of performing an activity and seeing potential where others don't. Their capacity to comprehensively analyse occupation and adapt it to the specific condition of an individual provides them with the necessary framework to comprehend the complex context of disaster and its relationship with development. Occupational therapists have a role to play in changing patterns for better risk prevention but also in supporting people affected by disaster to adapt to their new environment and life. Together with other professionals, we can work on building a safer, more equitable, and better world.

I would like to welcome this publication as it provides guidance to occupational therapists to engage in this field. Governments, organizations, communities, persons with disabilities, the ageing population and other marginalized groups will most certainly benefit from a stronger commitment of occupational therapy to integrate disaster management and disaster risk reduction in their practices.

M ARILYN PATTISON *B App Sc(OT),*

MBA, FWFOT
President, World Federation of Occupational Therapists;
Managing Principal, MPOT Pty Ltd, Australia

The World Federation of Occupational Therapists' (WFOT) agenda is directly driven by the United Nations (UN) through the World Health Organization (WHO) and underpinned by the Millennium Development Goals (MDGs). These goals set forth a road map for human development that reflect universal human rights and the need to address poverty and protect our common environment and the future of humanity (UNISDR 2005a). Building the resilience of nations and communities to disaster is an integral part of achieving the MDGs and enabling a prosperous, equitable and sustainable global society (UNISDR 2005b). Over the last decade the WFOT has spearheaded a major shift in the focus of practice from the medical model of health to the social model, from health of the individual to population health, from institutionally based practice to community based practice and beyond.

The WFOT has expanded its focus on the realms of occupational therapy practice to embrace:

- Disaster Preparedness and Response
- Environmental Sustainability and Sustainable Practice
- Community Development and Capacity Building
- Community Based Rehabilitation
- Human Rights
- Social Entrepreneurship.

The WFOT Position Statement on Human Rights identifies that occupational therapists have the knowledge and skills to support persons who experience limitations or barriers to participation in occupation. Occupational therapists also have a role and responsibility to develop and synthesize knowledge to support participation within a sustainable development framework as reflected in the WFOT position statement on environmental sustainability; to identify and raise issues of occupational barriers and injustices; and to work with groups, communities and societies to enhance participation in occupation for all persons. Achieving this is to achieve an occupationally just society (WFOT Position Statement on Human Rights 2006).

Occupational therapy, like every other allied health profession, is impacted upon by the changing world and changing health environment. Occupational therapists need to understand what is impacting on the health landscape of the future and be ready to meet the changes. Our expertise lies in the design of creative solutions to complex problems. It is the integration of multi-level variables into workable, effective and sustainable solutions that is the core of occupational therapy practice. If we are to meet these challenges that the future inevitably holds we will need to take occupational therapy beyond its traditional boundaries and we need to strive to move beyond them because that is what they are – boundaries. They fence us in and limit our practice. This book issues that challenge to us all.

Occupational therapists work with individuals, families and communities in all aspects of productive and independent living. As occupational therapists we can and should be involved with every stratum of society including the general population as well as a range of vulnerable populations (e.g. people with disabilities, children, and unaccompanied minors, the aged and women) and including those who have experienced physical and psychosocial trauma.

Occupational therapists' increasing involvement in disaster preparedness and response and community based rehabilitation, among other emerging areas of practice, is underpinned by the concept of social justice. Working directly with communities on projects that are meaningful to each community, having influence on local and higher health and policy makers, and working with nongovernmental organizations (NGOs), positions occupational therapists as having a unique contribution to the goals of a civil society.

However, whilst we may feel pleased with ourselves for our achievements thus far, if we are to continuously grow and develop as a profession we need to keep pushing ourselves, and it is through publications such as this one that this can be achieved. I absolutely commend this book and my colleagues who have been involved in its development as this group of authors has pushed the boundaries, issuing a call to arms to occupational therapy to live up to the social agenda. It supports all of us as we strive to take our rightful place as agents of social change and equity.

REFERENCES

UNISDR, 2005a. The link between Millennium Development Goals (MDGs) and disaster risk reduction. <http://www.unisdr.org/2005/mdgs-drr/link-mdg-drr.htm>.

UNISDR, 2005b. Reducing Disaster Risk: A Challenge for Development. United Nations Development Programme. Bureau for Crisis Prevention and Recovery. <http://www.unisdr.org/2005/mdgs-drr/undp.htm>.

WFOT, 2006. Position Statement on Human Rights. World Federation of Occupational Therapy.

ABOUT THE EDITORS

NANCY RUSHFORD, *PhD, MSc OT Reg (Ont), MA (Counselling Psychology)*

Nancy has worked in the field of health and rehabilitation in various community contexts including Canada, Australia and South East Asia, where she served as a rehabilitation project manager following the 2004 Indian Ocean tsunami. Nancy has recently completed a PhD through the University of Sydney, Australia. Her research linked contemporary occupational therapy theory and practice to the field of disaster and development, and draws upon experiences of disaster from around the globe. Nancy is a member of the WFOT Disaster Preparedness and Response (DP&R) International Advisory Group. She currently works for the Alzheimer Society of Ontario, Canada, as the Director of Programs & Implementation.

KERRY THOMAS, *BSc (OT), Grad Dip (Health Management)*

Kerry has thirty years of experience working in disaster and development contexts globally. She is the director of *inter*PART (International Partners in Action, Research and Training), an Australian-based organization that specializes in promoting resilience and sustainable development with and on behalf of people who are the most vulnerable in society. Kerry is a consultant in capacity building and participatory approaches to planning, monitoring and evaluation. She also teaches at the University of South Australia. Kerry helped shape and facilitate the WFOT Tsunami Response, and establishment of the WFOT DP&R International Advisory Group.

CONTRIBUTORS

SIYAT HILLOW ABDI BEd (Hons), MA, PhD Community Rehabilitation
President of the Western Australian Somali Welfare
  Society (WASSO)
Member of Western Australia Self Advocacy and Peer
  Support (SAPS) Australia

NAZMUL BARI MA
Director, Centre for Disability in Development
  (CDD)
Member, Disability inclusive Disaster Risk Reduction
  Network (DiDRRN)
Bangladesh

MARIE CLAUDE BERNARD MSc OT
Occupational Therapist, The Institute of Physical
  Rehabilitation, Québec
Canada

JENNY BIVEN Diploma in OT (CCHS), Graduate Diploma in Health Counselling (SA)
Member of Occupational Therapy Australia
Member, Partners in Disability and Development
Australia

MARIANA BOFFELLI
Occupational Therapist, The National University of
  the Littoral, Santa Fe
Argentina

CARLA BOGGIO
Occupational Therapist, The National University of
  the Littoral, Santa Fe
Argentina

CATHERINE BRIDGE BAppSc (OT), MCogSc, PhD (Arch)
Director of the Home Modification Information
  Clearinghouse Service
Program Director, the Enabling Built Environment
  Research Program (EBEP), CityFutures Research
  Centre
University of NSW
Australia

DANIELA CHIAPESSONI
Occupational Therapist, The National University of
  the Littoral, Santa Fe
Argentina

MARÍA DEL CARMEN HEIT
Occupational Therapist, The National University of
  the Littoral, Santa Fe
Argentina

MARÍA DE LOS MILAGROS DEMIRYI
Occupational Therapist, The National University of
  the Littoral, Santa Fe
Argentina

MAURO DEMICHELIS
Occupational Therapist, The National University of
  the Littoral, Santa Fe
Argentina

RUTH DUGGAN MScOT (C), OT Reg (NS)
Occupational Therapist, Cornerstone Occupational
  Therapy Consultants
Canada

ZOE EDMONDS BSc (Hons) OT
Occupational Therapist, Goulburn Valley Area
    Mental Health
Australia

CECILIA FARIAS BASADRE
Occupational Therapist, University of Chile
Biology of Cognition Specialist, University of Chile
Sensory Integration Certified
S.I. Academic Committee, I.S. Chile Member
Chilean Society of Occupational Science Member
ISOS Member (International Society of Occupational
    Science)
Chile

**SOLÁNGEL GARCÍA-RUÍZ Magister in
Educational and Social Development**
Research Director, District Secretariat of Health of
    Bogotá
Colombia

**SUE HANISCH British Diploma in
Occupational Therapy, Diploma in Human
Givens Psychotherapy**
Health Professions Council/ College of Occupational
    Therapy, Human Givens Institute
UK

REBECCA JORDAN MScOT
Occupational Therapist, Certified Brain Injury
    Specialist, Case Manager, Neuro Community Care,
    AOTA Member
USA

NATHAN KELLY RN, BScN
Registered Nurse, Niagara Region Public Health
Master's Degree Candidate with specialization in
    Disaster Healthcare
Secretary, Board of Directors, Canadian Medical
    Assistance Teams (CMAT)
Member-at-Large, Socio-Political Affairs, Board of
    Directors, Registered Nurses' Association of
    Ontario (RNAO)
Canada

MIRIAM KOLKER BScOT, MSc Public Health
Complex Discharge Coordinator
Prince of Wales Hospital, Randwick, Sydney
Australia

BRIAN MATTHEWS PhD
Adjunct Senior Lecturer, Disability & Community
    Inclusion, Flinders University
Australia

**MARILYN PATTISON B App Sc (OT),
MBA, FWFOT**
President, World Federation of Occupational
    Therapists (WFOT)
Managing Principal, MPOT Pty Ltd
Australia

SOLOMON PATRAY
Developmental Service Worker-1, Department of
    Mental Health, State of Massachusetts
USA

**ADELE PERRY BAppSc OT, MSc Social Science
(International Development)**
Consultant; previously worked with CBM Australia
    and Handicap International
Australia

EMILY F. PIVEN OTD, MHE, OTR
Health Matters First of Florida, Inc.
Associate Editor of Occupational Therapy
    International
Retired Associate Professor of Occupational Therapy
USA

NICK POLLARD PhD, DipCOT
Senior Lecturer in Occupational Therapy, Sheffield
    Hallam University
UK

CHANTAL RODER BSc (Hons)
Principal at Chantal Roelofs Coaching & Consulting,
    Brisbane
Australia

VALERIE RZEPKA NP, BScN, MSc
Nurse Practitioner, Bridgepoint Active Healthcare-
    Family Health Team
Executive Director, Canadian Medical Assistance
    Teams (CMAT)
Director at Large, Centre for Excellence in
    Emergency Preparedness (CEEP)
Canada

BROJA GOPAL SAHA BCom
Assistant Director, Centre for Disability in
    Development (CDD)
Bangladesh

DIKAIOS SAKELLARIOU MSc, PhD
School of Health Sciences, Cardiff University
UK

VALERIE SCHERRER
Director, Emergency Response Unit, CBM
Co-ordinator, Conflict and Emergency Task Group
    of the International Disability and Development
    Consortium
Germany

PENNY SCOTT MSc
Manager NRM Strategy and Community
    Partnerships, Terrain Natural Resource
    Management
Australia

TANIA SIMMONS
Formerly Environment Recovery Officer, Terrain
    Natural Resource Management
Australia

KIT SINCLAIR BScOT, PhD, FWFOT, FAOTA
Editor, WFOT Bulletin
WFOT Ambassador, World Federation of
    Occupational Therapists
Hong Kong

RACHEL THIBEAULT PhD, MSc, BScOT
Occupational Therapy Programme, University of
    Ottawa
Canada

YVONNE THOMAS PhD, M Ed, DipCOT
Senior Lecturer and Course Lead
Institute of Health and Society, University of
    Worcester
UK

**SUSANN BAEZ ULLBERG PhD Social
Anthropology**
Senior Analyst, CRISMART Crisis Management
    Research & Training, Swedish National Defence
    College
Sweden

**SAMANTHA WHYBROW BAppSc OT,
M Policy Studies**
Occupational Therapist
Australia

LIST OF ABBREVIATIONS

APM	antipersonnel mines
AQANU	Association Québécoise d'Appui aux Nations Unies
CAOT	Canadian Association of Occupational Therapists
CARE	Christian Action Research and Education
CBA	community-based adaptation
CBDM	community-based disaster management
CBDRR	community-based disaster risk reduction
CBR	community-based rehabilitation
CFS	child friendly spaces
COAT	collaborative occupation and transformation
CRDP	Convention on the Rights of Persons with Disabilities
CRED	Centre for Research on the Epidemiology of Disasters
CSC	Coalition to Stop the Use of Child Soldiers
DDOP	disaster and development occupational perspective (framework)
DDR	disarmament, demobilization and reintegration
DPRR	disaster preparedness, response and recovery
DROP	disaster resilience of place (model)
DRR	disaster risk reduction
DSM	Diagnostic and Statistical Manual
ICF	International Classification of Functioning, Disability and Health
IDDC	International Disability and Development Consortium
IDNDR	International Decade for Natural Disaster Reduction
IDP	internally displaced persons
IFRC	International Federation of Red Cross and Red Crescent Societies
INGO	international nongovernmental organization
MDGs	Millennium Development Goals
MOHO	model of human occupation
mOSCE	model of occupational stewardship and collaborative engagement
NGO	nongovernmental organization
OPA	older people's association
OT	occupational therapy/therapist
PAHO	Pan American Health Organization
PEO	person–environment–occupation
PEOP	person–environment–occupation–performance
PME	participatory monitoring and evaluation
PTSD	post-traumatic stress disorder
PWD	persons with disabilities
SHG	self-help group
UN	United Nations
UNCSD	United Nations Conference on Sustainable Development
UNDP	United Nations Development Programme

UNHCR	United Nations High Commissioner for Refugees	USAID	United States Agency for International Development
UNISDR	United Nations International Strategy for Disaster Reduction	UXO	unexploded ordnance
UNOCHA	United Nations Office for the Coordination of Humanitarian Affairs	WFOT	World Federation of Occupational Therapists
		WFP	World Food Programme
		WHO	World Health Organization

PART I   Disaster and Development

Part I frames disaster as a global socio-ecological crisis – one that is embedded in patterns of human activity and interrelationships between people and with the broader environment. Key concepts, viewpoints and practices relevant to the field are explored from the perspective of the spirit of humanitarianism and the evolution of an international system to enable humanitarian action. Particular attention is given to the social construction of disasters and how disaster is experienced individually and through culture and everyday life. Emphasis is placed upon patterns of vulnerability and resilience from the perspective of social inequity and the experiences of particularly vulnerable groups including people with disabilities. Within this, attention is given to the relationship between 'disaster' and 'development', and the way in which they interrelate and influence one another. We argue that the discipline of occupational therapy may be well aligned with efforts to transform everyday patterns of activities (occupations) into more equitable and sustainable choices and social relations; however, substantive research is needed to elucidate an occupational perspective in the field that is based on diverse cultural perspectives and experiences of disaster and occupation.

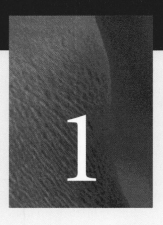

DISASTER AND DEVELOPMENT: A CALL TO ACTION

NANCY RUSHFORD ■ KERRY THOMAS

DISASTER AND ITS CLASSIFICATIONS

Disaster risk is on the rise along with greater complexity (i.e. synchronous or cascading disasters) and consequences. In particular, some climate-related natural hazards (e.g. floods, drought, storms) have increased in frequency and magnitude (Intergovernmental Panel on Climate Change 2012). Driven largely by a global situation of deepening poverty and ecological destruction (Halloway and Boff 2009), disasters threaten the health and wellbeing of humanity and the viability of the planet.

Disaster is defined as:

a serious disruption of the functioning of a community or a society involving widespread human, material, economic or environmental losses and impacts, which exceeds the ability of the affected community or society to cope using its own resources
(the United Nations International Strategy for Disaster Reduction (UNISDR) Secretariat 2009, p. 9)

Disasters are classified in terms of hazards of natural origin (e.g. geological, hydro-meteorological and biological – such as earthquakes, floods and epidemics, respectively) or those induced by human processes (e.g. environmental degradation, technological hazards such as nuclear accidents, and armed conflict (Figure 1-1)) (Guha-Sapir et al 2011). They may occur suddenly or have a slow onset (e.g. drought), and may result from several different hazards or a complex combination of natural and human-made causes (e.g. food insecurity, epidemics, conflicts and displaced

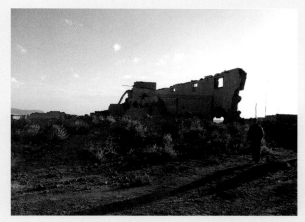

FIGURE 1-1 ■ Aftermath of conflict in Ethiopia.

populations) commonly referred to as 'complex emergencies' (IFRC n.d., para 1).

According to the Centre for Research on the Epidemiology of Disasters (CRED), a hazardous event qualifies as a disaster when one of the following criteria has been met:

- 10 or more people reported killed;
- 100 or more people reported affected;
- declaration of a state of emergency;
- a call for international assistance (Guha-Sapir et al 2011).

NATURAL DISASTER ON A GLOBAL SCALE

The Centre for Research on the Epidemiology of Disasters EM-DAT and international disaster database

3

websites and global assessment reports (e.g. UNISDR 2009, 2011, 2013) document patterns of injuries, mortality profiles and the economic impact of natural disasters on a global scale. Between 2000 and 2012, 2.9 billion people were affected by disaster, 1.2 million people were killed and $1.7 trillion United States dollars (USD) were lost in damages (UNISDR, 2012). In the year 2011, economic damages from natural disasters were the highest ever registered, with an estimated cost of $366.1 billion USD; 30 773 people were killed and there were 244.7 million victims overall, including people physically injured, traumatized, ill and displaced as a direct consequence of disaster (Guha-Sapir et al 2011). The occupational impacts – in terms of the activities of everyday living and the functioning of society – are staggering.

Furthermore, natural hazards (e.g. wildfires (Figure 1-2), tsunamis (Figure 1-3)) can induce sudden, large-scale movements of people to the nearest safe place. In the case of slow onset disasters (e.g. drought) they may result in environmental migration over time to less affected or urban/semiurban areas due to depleted environmental resources and unsustainable livelihoods. Poorly managed displacement and migration can cause instability in host environments due to stretched environmental resources and public services with implications for living standards, health and nutrition (International Organization for Migration, n.d.). In 2012 alone, 15 million people were forced to move due to disaster (IFRC 2012).

Health consequences arising from disaster include outbreaks of infectious disease, death, injuries (e.g. fractures, limb amputations, spinal cord injuries, traumatic brain injuries, crush injuries, burns and peripheral nerve injuries) and related mental health conditions such as post-traumatic stress disorder. There may also be damage to critical infrastructure including hospitals, health facilities, services (including personnel injured or killed) and medical equipment. Additionally, emergencies create a new generation of people who experience disability resulting from their injuries, poor surgical and medical care, emergency-induced mental health and psychological problems, a breakdown in social supports and abandonment (WHO 2013). All of these effects have long-term implications for health, participation, wellbeing and everyday functioning of society (Rathore et al 2012). These impacts are even greater for people displaced, forced to migrate or left behind, people living in poverty, those with pre-existing health issues and other vulnerable groups, notably people with disability and the elderly.

RISK AND INEQUALITY

The United Nations Development Program (2004) reports that 11% of people exposed to disaster live in low human development countries and yet 53% of

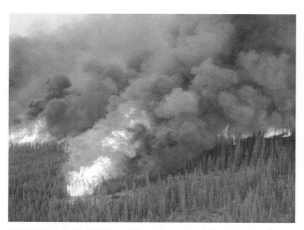

FIGURE 1-2 ■ Wildland fire. *Reproduced from* Auerbach, P., 2011. *(Wilderness Medicine, sixth ed. Elsevier, London. © Elsevier.)*

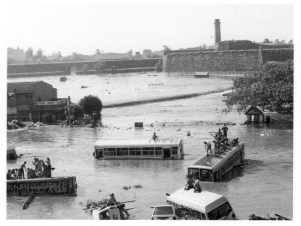

FIGURE 1-3 ■ The city of Galle, Sri Lanka, immediately after the tsunami of 2004. *Reproduced from* Ruwanpura, P.R., Hettiarachchi, M., Vidanapathirana, M., Perera, S., 2009. *(Management of dead and missing: aftermath tsunami in Galle. Legal Medicine 11 (Suppl. 1), S86–S88. © Elsevier.)*

disaster mortality is concentrated in those countries. Globalization and the increasing interconnectedness and interdependence of modern society configure scenarios of risk where the greatest burden is placed upon the poor and threatens to reduce overall economic and human development gains (UNISDR 2009).

Furthermore, climate change is expected to magnify the interactions between disaster risk and poverty resulting in an increase in disaster impacts and poverty outcomes for poorer, less resilient countries and communities (UNDP 2004, UNISDR 2009, 2011, 2013).

Population growth, poor urban infrastructure and governance, vulnerable rural livelihoods and declining ecosystems represent underlying risk drivers that drive poverty and undermine sustainable development in low-income communities and households (UNISDR 2011, xiii).

At every level, be it local communities, nation states, regions or the globe, the relationship between disaster risk, vulnerability and development is complex, contextual and dynamic.

THE INTERNATIONAL HUMANITARIAN SYSTEM

In response to emergencies and disasters occurring around the globe, the international humanitarian system emerged and has continued to evolve and grow in complexity. Ultimately, the responsibility for the provision and coordination of assistance rests with the affected country. However, when an international appeal for assistance is made, the international community channels assistance to people and places most in need through a complex web of relationships and accountabilities. The system comprises various actors operating at local, national and international levels who represent a wide range of organizations (i.e. UN agencies, International Federation of Red Cross and Red Crescent Societies (IFRC), nongovernmental organizations (NGOs) and community-based organizations). These actors ostensibly partner with host states and their ministries to deliver assistance that is oriented to saving lives, protecting dignity and the immediate relief of suffering (Humanitarian Coalition n.d.).

As part of the UN Humanitarian reform process in 2006, many of these organizations now work together in 'clusters' towards common objectives within a particular sector of emergency response (e.g. shelter, health). The cluster approach strengthens partnerships and builds links between the humanitarian and development sectors, paving the way for recovery (UNOCHA n.d.).

Strong links between the humanitarian and development sectors facilitate the management of resources and responsibilities in all aspects of preparing for and responding to disasters, including both pre- and post-disaster activities, as outlined in Table 1-1. This occurs in a phased sequence of action commonly referred to as the 'disaster cycle' or 'disaster management cycle'. (Malalgoda et al 2010; Walker & Maxwell 2009).

THE DISASTER MANAGEMENT CYCLE

The disaster management cycle provides a foundational framework within which to conceptualize and understand the relationship between disaster risk, vulnerability and development, as it relates to key elements of disaster management (Figure 1-4).

Disaster management is comprised of three main components:

- preparedness (encompassing disaster risk reduction: prevention and mitigation of risk) and early warning systems
- humanitarian aid/relief
- recovery (including rehabilitation and reconstruction) and development.

Within the disaster management cycle, development provides the framework and systems to support recovery from disaster in ways that build resilience as well as reduce vulnerability and risk to future shocks.

DISASTER RISK REDUCTION, SUSTAINABLE DEVELOPMENT AND RESILIENCE

Disaster risk reduction (DRR) measures and activities are incorporated into the disaster management cycle as a systematic means to analyse and manage the causal factors of disaster (UNISDR 2009, p. 10). DRR measures include, for example, environmental management, poverty reduction, protection of critical facilities, networking and partnerships that promote a culture of prevention and innovation, and financial

TABLE 1-1

Disaster Management and Risk Reduction Activities

Phase of Cycle	Objectives	Activities
Disaster Preparation	To develop knowledge and capacities at local, national and international levels to anticipate and respond effectively to natural hazardous events or conditions and their potential consequences (social, political, economic and environmental); focus is on imminent threats and future risks.	Risk assessment; vulnerability mapping/hazard analysis; early warning systems; establishing legal and policy frameworks; contingency planning; stockpiling of equipment and supplies; coordination planning; evacuation and public information; training and field exercising; public awareness; sector training.
Disaster Response	To provide emergency services and public assistance during or immediately after a natural hazardous event/disaster in order to save lives, mitigate impacts and ensure public safety; focus is largely on short-term and immediate needs.	Search and rescue; medical assistance; emergency shelter; water and sanitation; food aid; rapid assessment (injuries, losses).
Disaster Recovery	Restoration, reconstruction, rehabilitation and improvement of infrastructure, facilities, livelihoods and quality of life; long-term recovery and sustainable development focus.	Search and rescue; medical assistance; emergency shelter; water and sanitation; food aid; rapid assessment (injuries, losses).
Disaster Mitigation	The lessening or limitation of adverse impacts of hazards and related disasters.	Hazard resistant construction and engineering; improved public awareness and environmental policies; land use plans; building codes.

DISASTER MANAGEMENT CYCLE

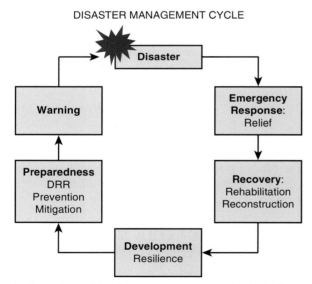

FIGURE 1-4 ■ The disaster management cycle. DRR, disaster risk reduction.

and economic measures to ensure a safety net in case of disasters (UNISDR 2009). In this respect, DRR is both an inherent aspect of development and a distinct component of disaster preparedness.

The Hyogo Framework for Action 2005–2015 guides DRR on a global level with the UNISDR secretariat serving as the focal point within the UN system for the coordination of DRR strategies and programmes (UNISDR n.d.). A key aspect of the role of the secretariat is mainstreaming DRR into relief and development sectors via the post-2015 Development Agenda and a sustainable development foundation (Harris 2000, Sustainable Development Solutions Network 2013). The ultimate goal is a prosperous and equitable world where all people have capabilities and freedoms to avoid or mitigate risk, and live long and healthy lives without undermining the integrity of natural systems and the environment or compromising the ability of future generations to meet their needs.

However, the impact of human-induced climate change, coupled with escalating global population and inequitable resource consumption, has brought the planet to a tipping point beyond which many consider sustainable development, as it is currently defined, to be no longer adequate in assisting policy development fit for today's global challenges and objectives (e.g. Ross 2008). Underpinning this view is a concern that the concept of sustainable development does not take account of the reality of the limits to earth's resilience. The emerging scenario is now stimulating a reconfiguration in our understanding of disaster and development and associated approaches. Principles have been proposed to build resilience and sustainability (Berkes & Folke 1998), with increasing focus on adaptability and transformability within the relational sphere, and particular attention to the interrelationships between human systems and ecosystems (Walker et al 2004).

DISASTER AND DEVELOPMENT: MERGING

In the face of recurrent crises, the ability of people, households, communities, countries and all living systems to mitigate, adapt to and recover from shocks and stresses in a manner that reduces chronic vulnerability and facilitates sustainable development for all is the hallmark and focus of resilience (USAID 2012). Increasingly disaster is being understood and managed within a broader – even integrated – approach to development, that holds the potential to transform how we live on the planet, interact with each other and the environment around us. This opens up the possibility for an occupational perspective on disaster and development to emerge and take shape.

INTRODUCING OCCUPATION

Occupation refers to the activities of everyday living that sustain life and give it meaning and purpose. Occupations include things people need to, want to and are expected to do.

Occupation embraces and serves all humanitarian aid and development functions, to which the case stories and material presented in this book will testify. As illustrated in Figure 1-5, occupation in disaster and development has two main roles. Firstly, occupation is a defining characteristic of both disaster and development contexts – it is the disruption and the later rebuilding and transformation of occupational activities and processes that typify the disaster and development contexts. Secondly, occupation is the medium through which disaster response, recovery, future preparedness and ongoing community, sustainable and resilience development occurs and is achieved. As such, occupational therapists are potentially well placed to respond to disaster and work in humanitarian aid and development contexts.

A CALL TO ACTION

The disproportionate distribution of disaster risk, and the inordinate burden of disaster placed upon the most vulnerable communities and poorest regions of the world, calls for transformative action at the point of activities of everyday life, where natural hazards, social relations and individual choice converge (Blaikie 1994) to equitably and collectively reduce disaster risk, promote sustainable recovery and strengthen resilience. This necessitates ongoing interdisciplinary collaboration to: (1) determine and encourage healthy

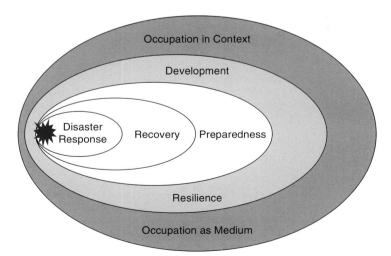

FIGURE 1-5 ■ Disaster and development occupational perspective (DDOP) – an elementary conceptualization.

patterns of life that are equitable, sustainable and/or resilient into the indefinite future, and (2) address the social and political forces that hold existing patterns in place.

Occupational therapy was founded on the humanistic ideal of promoting health and wellbeing through occupation, for all persons (Reitz 1992). Until relatively recently, very little attention was given in the literature to the role of occupational therapy in humanitarian action and disaster resilience and recovery processes. The magnitude of loss and devastation associated with the 2004 Indian Ocean tsunami, followed closely by Hurricane Katrina in 2005, galvanized the profession into action on a global scale in an effort to forge a path in the field and effectively build its capacity to respond to increasing disaster risk and the occurrence of disaster around the globe. Much has been done since the 2004 Indian Ocean tsunami to link the role of occupational therapists to disaster and development, but more is needed. The time to imagine possibilities and escalate our action is now.

Times of crisis can be creative times, times when new visions and new possibilities emerge.
(Hathaway and Boff 2009)

REFERENCES

Auerbach, P., 2011. Wilderness Medicine, sixth ed. Elsevier, London.

Berkes, F., Folke, C., 1998. Linking Social and Ecological Systems: Management Practices and Social Mechanisms for Building Resilience. Cambridge University Press, Cambridge.

Blaikie, P., Cannon, T.I., Davis, I., et al., 1994. At Risk: Natural Hazards, People's Vulnerability, and Disasters. Routledge, London, UK, p. 7.

Guha-Sapir, D., Vos, F., Below, R., Ponserre, S., 2011. Annual disaster statistical review 2010: the numbers and trends. Retrieved from: <http://cip.management.dal.ca/publications/ADSR_2010.pdf>.

Harris, J.M., 2000. Basic principles of sustainable development. (Working paper 00-04). Retrieved from Tufts University, Global Development and Environment Institute: <http://www.ase.tufts.edu/gdae/publications/working_papers/Sustainable%20Development.PDF>.

Hathaway, M., Boff, L., 2009. The Tao of Liberation. Exploring the Ecology of Transformation. ORBIS Books, New York.

Humanitarian Coalition, n.d. <http://www.humanitariancoalition.ca>.

IFRC, 2012. Forced migration: the dynamics of displacement and response. World Disaster Report 2012. Focus on forced migration and displacement. Retrieved from IFRC website: <http://www.ifrcmedia.org/assets/pages/wdr2012/>.

IFRC, n.d. Complex/manmade hazards: complex emergencies. Retrieved from: <http://www.ifrc.org/en/what-we-do/disaster-management/about-disasters/definition-of-hazard/complex-emergencies/>.

Intergovernmental Panel on Climate Change, 2012. Managing the risks of extreme events and disasters to advance climate change adaptation. Special report of working groups I and II of the intergovernmental panel on climate change. Edited by Field, C.B., Barros, V., Stocker, T.F., et al. Retrieved from IPPC website: <http://www.ipcc.ch/publications_and_data/publications_and_data_reports.shtml#2>.

International Organization for Migration, n.d. Disaster risk reduction, climate change adaptation and environmental migration. A policy perspective. Retrieved from IOM website: <http://publications.iom.int/bookstore/index.php?main_page=product_info&cPath=41_7&products_id=664>.

Malalgoda, C., Amaratunga, D.M., Pathirage, C., 2010. Exploring Disaster Risk Reduction in the Built Environment. School of the Built Environment, University of Salford, UK.

Rathore, F.A., Gosney, J.E., Reinhardt, J.D., et al., 2012. Medical rehabilitation after natural disasters: why, when, and how? Arch. Phys. Med. Rehabil. 93, 1875–1881.

Reitz, S.M., 1992. A historical review of occupational therapy's role in preventive health and wellness. Am. J. Occup. Ther. 46 (1), 50–55.

Ross, A., 2008. Modern interpretations of sustainable development. J. Law Soc. 36 (1), 32–54.

Ruwanpura, P.R., Hettiarachchi, M., Vidanapathirana, M., Perera, S., 2009. Management of dead and missing: aftermath tsunami in Galle. Leg. Med. 11 (Suppl. 1), 86–88.

Sustainable Development Solutions Network, 2013. An action agenda for sustainable development. Report for the UN Secretary General. Retrieved from: <http://unsdsn.org/files/2013/11/An-Action-Agenda-for-Sustainable-Development.pdf>.

UNDP, 2004. Reducing disaster risk. A challenge for development. Retrieved from: <http://www.chs.ubc.ca/archives/files/Reducing%20Disaster%20Risk%20A%20Challenge%20for%20Development.pdf>.

UNISDR, 2009. Risk and poverty in a changing climate: invest today for a safer tomorrow. United Nations global assessment report on disaster risk reduction. Retrieved from: <http://www.unisdr.org/we/inform/publications/12163>.

UNISDR, 2011. Revealing risk, redefining development. United Nations global assessment report on disaster risk reduction. Retrieved from: <http://www.preventionweb.net/english/hyogo/gar/2011/en/home/index.html>.

UNISDR, 2012. Disaster data & statistics, 2000–2012 – graphic. Retrieved June 24, 2013 from: <http://www.preventionweb.net/english/professional/statistics/>.

UNISDR, 2013. From shared risk to shared value: the business case for disaster risk reduction. United Nations global assessment report on disaster risk reduction. Retrieved from: <http://www.preventionweb.net/english/hyogo/gar/2013/en/home/index.html>.

UNISDR, n.d. Hyogo Framework for Action (HFA). Building the resilience of nations and communities to disaster. Retrieved from: <http://www.unisdr.org/we/coordinate/hfa>.

UNOCHA, n.d. <http://www.unocha.org/what-we-do/coordination-tools/cluster-coordination>.

USAID, 2012. Building resilience to recurrent crisis. USAID Policy and Program Guidance. Retrieved from: <http://www.usaid.gov/sites/default/files/documents/1870/USAIDResiliencePolicyGuidanceDocument.pdf>.

Walker, B., Holling, C.S., Carpenter, S.R., Kinzig, A., 2004. Resilience, adaptability and transformability in social-ecological systems. Ecol. Soc. 9 (2), 5.

Walker, P., Maxwell, D., 2009. Shaping the Humanitarian World. Routledge, London, UK.

WHO, 2013. Guidance note on disability and emergency risk management for health. Retrieved from: <http://apps.who.int/iris/bitstream/10665/90369/1/9789241506243_eng.pdf>.

2

DISASTER, DEVELOPMENT AND OCCUPATIONAL THERAPY: HISTORICAL PERSPECTIVES AND POSSIBILITIES

NANCY RUSHFORD ■ KERRY THOMAS

INTRODUCTION

The aim of this chapter is to explore key disaster and development concepts from a historical perspective and evolving opportunities. These include humanitarianism, human rights and justice, sustainable development, and disaster risk reduction. Central to this discussion is a general overview of the international humanitarian and development system as it has evolved in response to crises and disasters taking place around the world. 'Occupation' and the discipline of occupational therapy is subsequently located in the disaster and development field, with reference to a review of the occupational therapy literature.

Although the humanitarian aid and development sectors are distinct and are guided by a different but inter-related set of principles, we have chosen to represent and consider these as one system. This reflects the evolution toward an integrated approach to disaster and development.

In addition, it is important to note that our reference to the term 'humanitarianism' is broader than its common association with humanitarian aid. We consider humanitarianism in terms of the characteristics of the human spirit, and use it as the vehicle through which we trace the evolution of the humanitarian aid and development system.

Although the discussion may suggest linearity, there is no simple history that can be sequentially traced to contemporary practice in the field. Rather, the chapter is based on our interpretations of the literature, informed by experience and a process of weaving together the many strands that give shape to its evolution and the activities recognizable in the field today. This involves linking humanitarian aid with sustainable development, and resilience, and comprehensive approaches to managing disasters and reducing disaster risk in the broader context of social inequality and global risk drivers and processes of change.

DISASTER AND THE ORIGINS AND EVOLUTION OF HUMANITARIANISM

From 'All is Well'
Would it console the sad inhabitants
Of these aflame and desolated shores
To say to them: "Lay down your lives in peace;
For the world's good your homes are sacrificed;
Your ruined palaces shall others build,
For other peoples shall your walls arise;
The North grows rich on your unhappy loss;
Your ills are but a link in general law ..."

(Voltaire, 1755)

Disaster is one of the most pressing issues of modern day society, as the current global picture and its stark statistics suggest, yet for centuries it has revealed the complex and emergent relationship between nature and society.

Following the great tragedy of the Lisbon earthquake in 1755, Voltaire illuminated the social dimension of disaster by juxtaposing the wealth of the North with the poverty and suffering of the South (Voltaire 1905). In doing so he revealed how society protectively cloaks some people against the hazards of nature while it exposes others. His criticism of the role that society has played in shaping conditions of vulnerability conflicted with one-dimensional views of disaster that historically have dominated thinking. These views attributed disaster to deliberate and punitive acts of God or, conversely, random forces of nature that had similar impacts on people exposed and were largely out of people's control (Zebrowski 1997, Steinberg 2003). Consistent with these one-dimensional views, humanitarian response has traditionally been event specific, giving rise to rescue efforts aimed at the immediate relief from suffering.

Walker & Maxwell (2009) claim that at the heart of the intention to alleviate suffering is universal altruistic human behaviour based on the principle of humanity, 'that humankind is one family and it is an intrinsic part of our humanity to both seek assistance and wish to provide assistance to those in need' (p. 2).

Humanitarianism features in all major world religions today and is intimately tied up with the evolution of religious ideals (most notably charitable action) and institutions largely associated with Christianity, Judaism, Islam and Buddhism; it is also historically rooted in the powerful states of Europe and North America and the business of the ruling elite from the eighteenth century onwards (Walker & Maxwell 2009, Bornstein & Redfield 2010). Beyond this, Wright (2009, as cited by Bornstein & Redfield, 2010, p. 2) argues that humanitarianism is a part of '15 000 years of cultural evolution where altruism has developed beyond the family, the clan, the tribe, the city-state, the nation and the international community'.

Over time this has given rise to the design of complex institutions and systems to enable humanitarian action, including the Red Cross and Red Crescent movement in 1863, the United Nations (UN) along with its designated offices, and agencies to coordinate humanitarian affairs and administer relief (e.g. Office for the Coordination of Humanitarian Affairs (OCHA), United Nations International Strategy for Disaster Reduction (UNISDR), the World Food Programme (WFP)), coupled with the emergence of non-governmental organizations (NGOs) in the twentieth century (e.g. Christian Action Research and Education (CARE), Oxfam, Save the Children). In particular, the Red Cross marked the beginnings of the global humanitarian system and established some of the fundamental ideals and methodologies of humanitarianism, including impartiality, neutrality and independence (Forsythe 2005).

SYMBOLS OF SUFFERING AND MISFORTUNE

Historically, humanitarianism defined itself through exceptional states of misfortune, and emphasized the physical and psychological condition of suffering above all else. Today, that language is considered 'both moral and broadly medical' (Bornstein & Redfield 2010, p. 6). More specifically, Bornstein and Redfield describe how wellbeing has typically been defined through species-level needs and health, or conversely the care of the soul and one's spiritual duties. Whether motivated by religious faith that is tied to the ideals of charity, or the ethic of care espoused by medical models, the language of humanitarianism has, arguably, placed the balance of power with the 'saviour' or 'expert' who rescues 'the needy' and essentially brings order to chaos. This language portrays people affected by disaster as weak, confused or helpless victims dependent upon external support and professional expertise.

Although rooted in the past, these symbols endure because they evoke pity, stimulate charitable action and inspire public or political support. Bankoff (2001) describes further how Western cultural discourse 'denigrates large regions of the world as disease ridden, poverty stricken and disaster prone' and privileges Western expertise as the magic that can provide security in place of misery (p. 19). Rodriguez et al (2006) argue further that the image of the confused victim suggests that extraordinary measures need to be initiated. This engenders 'command and control' policies and management approaches that potentially undermine local capacities and fail to respond to local realities.

Sociologists and anthropologists that study cultural symbols, framing and collective identity note their significance in the field in terms of how they influence behaviour, perpetuate myths and propel social movements via the media, popular culture and discourse (Furedi 2007, Johnston & Klandermans 1995, Tierney 2003, Webb 2006). Organizations use images of suffering to elicit funds; governments have used the causal language of 'God' (disaster as punishment) or 'nature' (disaster as an unforeseeable act of nature) to abdicate themselves from moral responsibility for death and destruction, to avoid fiscal accountability and to preserve the ad hoc nature of international relief (Alexander 1997). For example, following Hurricane Katrina in the United States in 2005, Stallings (2006) observed how the government and various social groups drew upon a broad repertoire of causal explanations for the disaster from mass culture (e.g. God, nature, human agency) to help them to push their particular religious, environmental and political interests and agendas.

PITY TO EMPOWERMENT: A HUMAN RIGHTS LENS

The development of the UN and the emergence of human rights discourse in the aftermath of the Second World War marked a turning point for humanitarianism and gave shape to a narrative that broadened the cultural repertoire of symbols and associated responses (Bornstein & Redfield 2010). Depictions of disaster as situations of inequality and injustice contrasted with deeply embedded symbols of exceptional misfortune. This shed new light on the relationship between nature, society and the human condition of suffering, in that it exposed social conditions of vulnerability and illuminated the role of human agency in shaping experiences of disaster. Quarantelli et al (2006) point out that people have faced disaster since the beginning of civilization, and that 'the very survival of the human race is testimony to the coping and adjustive social mechanisms of humans as they face such threats' (p. 20). Disaster increasingly came to be viewed as 'crisis with a devastating ending with the potential to be avoided or mitigated' (Boin and 't Hart 2006, p. 42), effectively stirring interests beyond crisis response, towards disaster management and risk reduction, as underpinned by key principles related to humanitarianism, development assistance and risk reduction (refer to Table 2-1) that are largely embedded in Western culture and an ideology that values human rights and individualism and democratic models of governance. These conceptions are continuing to evolve and shift in response to the overarching challenges wrought by a changing climate, and include a focus on repositioning humanity within finite ecological systems (Figure 2-1).

TABLE 2-1	
Key Principles in Disaster, Development and Risk Reduction	
Humanitarian Aid	Humanity
	Human rights (the right to life with dignity and equal opportunity/access to protection and relief)
	Impartiality
	Neutrality
	Independence
	***Protection and Relief**
Development Assistance	Sustainability (economic, environmental, social)
	Human rights (equality, empowerment, participation, access, and full inclusion of all persons in all aspects of development and society)
	***Enabling Environment** (enlarging people's choices)
Risk Reduction	Prevention, mitigation and preparedness
	Environmental protection and sustainable development
	Human rights
	Shared responsibility and cooperation
	Information and knowledge exchange (access to appropriate technology)
	Community involvement and participation
	***Vulnerability and Hazard Reduction**

*Main objective.

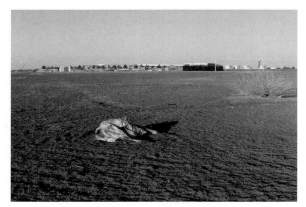

FIGURE 2-1 ■ Rehabilitation centre in Sudan.

A GLOBAL VISION

Collectively the principles that guide activities in the field reflect a global vision of a prosperous and equitable world where all people have dignity, choices, capabilities and freedoms to avoid or mitigate risk and live long and healthy lives without undermining the integrity of natural systems and the environment and, further, without compromising the ability of future generations to meet their needs (Sustainable Development Solutions Network 2013, World Commission on Environment and Development 1987).

This ambitious vision encompasses a sustainable human development approach that is supported by the Millennium Development Goals, along with their accompanying principles of equity, participation, empowerment and accountability (Sen 1995, UNDP 2012). Legal frameworks and standards uphold the vision and serve to guide interventions in the field, including, for example, international humanitarian law, human rights law and, more recently, International Disaster Response Laws, Rules and Principles (GSDRC 2013); the Universal Declaration of Human Rights and its associated conventions; the Humanitarian Charter and minimum standards in humanitarian response (Sphere Project 2011); and the code of conduct of the Red Cross and Red Crescent societies and NGOs in disaster relief as outlined on the IFRC's website.

Through this emergent global vision, images of vulnerable, helpless and confused victims of disaster have transformed into those of empowered and engaged survivors with equal rights, capable of rebuilding their lives and mitigating their vulnerability and risk. Humanitarian action thus extended beyond the gift of charity and relief towards justice, equality and capacity building that would effectively reduce the risk of loss and casualty by enabling vulnerable communities to anticipate, cope with and recover from natural hazardous events.

Several key international events, as outlined in Box 2-1, have reinforced this vision by strengthening the links between humanitarian aid, sustainable development, disaster risk reduction and, more recently, resilience and climate change adaptation. Consequently, many international humanitarian aid agencies that historically focused on crisis response and relief have adopted multiple mandates to more comprehensively 'manage disasters' and 'reduce risk'. These agencies now link humanitarian relief with human rights advocacy, sustainable development practices, disaster mitigation measures and, increasingly, resilience building.

HUMANITARIAN ACTION AND ITS 'SHADOW SIDE'

The evolution of humanitarian action from relief to development with increasing emphasis on risk reduction and global sustainability has enabled agencies to reposition themselves from their role as 'saviour' or 'expert' rescuing the needy to that of external advocate who empowers vulnerable people.

This has led to the development of community-based participatory approaches to disaster management and disaster risk reduction such as community-based disaster management (CBDM) and community-based disaster risk reduction (CBDRR). Communities are rich repositories of knowledge about the local context and possess traditional coping mechanisms and inherent capacities with which to guide efforts to reduce vulnerability and risk. Nolan (2002) argues that for interventions to succeed, humanitarian and development efforts need to connect the diverse cultural worlds involved in ways that acknowledge diversity and produce results that are sustainable and universally seen as fair and satisfactory. CBDM and CBDRR aim to integrate local knowledge with science and technology to produce a more comprehensive and culturally relevant picture of disaster risks and

---

BOX 2-1
DISASTER, DEVELOPMENT AND CLIMATE CHANGE – GLOBAL EVENTS TIMELINE

1990-1999 International Decade for Natural Disaster Reduction (IDNDR) – declared by the UN General Assembly in recognition of the increasing impact of natural hazardous events and the need for knowledge and capacity to respond effectively.

1992 – The 1992 United Nations Conference on Sustainable Development (UNCSD) – also known as the 'Earth Summit', was an important milestone that brought environment and development issues into the public arena.

1992 – UN Framework Convention on Climate Change – countries joined an international treaty to cooperatively consider how to address climate change.

1994 – The Yokohama Strategy and Plan of Action for a Safer World – stresses that every country has the sovereign and primary responsibility to protect its people, infrastructure and national, social and economic assets from the impact of natural hazardous events.

1997 – Kyoto Protocol – adopted following negotiations to strengthen global response to climate change. The protocol legally binds developed countries to emission reduction targets.

2000 – International Strategy for Disaster Reduction – establishes an international agenda for the implementation of disaster risk reduction. Represents a major shift from the traditional focus on disaster response to disaster prevention and in effect seeks to promote a culture of prevention.

2000 – Millennium Summit/Millennium Development Goals – world leaders adopt the United Nations Millennium Declaration committing their nations to a new global partnership to reduce extreme poverty, including a series of time-bound targets (deadline 2015) known as the Millennium Development Goals (MDGs).

2005 – Second World Conference on Disaster, Kobe, Hyogo, Japan – governments and agencies agree on the Hyogo Framework for Action 2005-2015: Building the resilience of nations and communities to disaster.

2007 – The Global Platform for Disaster Reduction – a forum for the exchange of information, ideas and discussions of latest development and knowledge; opportunity for partnership building across sectors; takes place every two years.

2009 – Copenhagen Climate Change Conference – raised climate change to the highest political level; advanced the negotiations on the infrastructure needed for effective global, climate change cooperation; produced the Copenhagen Accord to constrain carbon and respond to climate change.

2012 – Rio + 20 United Nations Conference on Sustainable Development – discussions aimed at the development of an institutional framework for sustainable development with a focus on a 'green economy'; sets a firm foundation for sustainable development and a post-2015 framework to continue guiding nations.

---

vulnerabilities by engaging communities in all aspects of disaster response, recovery, preparedness and mitigation (Abarquez & Murshed 2004, Ishiwatari 2012). The goal is to facilitate the capacity of all segments of a community to participate democratically where the emphasis is on the *actual* needs and capabilities or assets of people, ostensibly leading to locally owned and culturally relevant solutions and practices that create more resilient, equitable and sustainable communities (Hutton 2001, Pierce 2003).

These approaches are based on authentic partnerships (Dupuis et al 2012) that enable the transfer of power from those providing resources and assistance to those affected by disaster and receiving assistance. Globalization and its associated social, political and economic pressures and opportunities complicate good intentions in the field and potentially undermine these participatory approaches and empowerment processes. Humanitarian aid has become an increasingly politicized and competitive humanitarian enterprise, where those engaged in the field are confronted with growing insecurity in regions in which they operate and face ethical dilemmas, particularly in situations of complex emergencies (Minear 2002, Slim 1997).

THE POLITICIZATION AND SECURITIZATION OF AID

Experts and practitioners have argued that the increasing politicization and securitization of aid has enabled moral judgements about the worthiness of recipients and fostered aid conditionality (Fox 2001, Macrae 1998, Pupavac 2005, Slim 1997, Walker & Maxwell 2009, Watson 2011). Adding to complexity in the field is the orientation to disaster management that potentially drives competition. Hilhorst (2002) observes that actors within the system often compete over media exposure, funding and beneficiaries in a climate that is increasingly business oriented and profit driven. These interests potentially overshadow the actual needs and priorities of disaster-affected communities. In addition, well-intentioned organizations and individuals that enter the field lacking sensitivity to the social and political climate or awareness of existing disaster response coordination mechanisms risk undermining local capacities and doing more harm than good. Moreover, humanitarian aid or assistance may inadvertently reinforce social divisions along political and ethnic lines and in doing so contribute to preexisting social conflict and political discontent.

Following the 2004 Indian Ocean tsunami (Figure 2-2), the unprecedented level of donations or 'gifts' that were largely based in good intentions collided with divergent practices, discourses and expectations

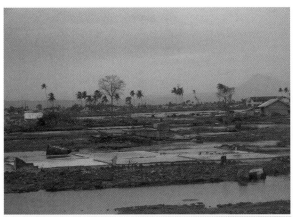

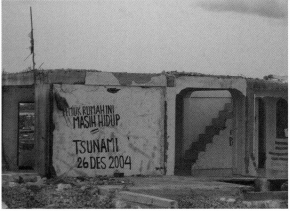

FIGURE 2-2 ■ Aceh, Indonesia, after the 2004 tsunami.

once it entered the local domain. In Sri Lanka, this undermined the peace process (Korf et al., 2010). Anthropologists have explored the idea of the 'altruistic gift' of aid from a cultural perspective in terms of patterns of social exchange. These exchanges are embedded in cultural meaning that centre upon obligations to give, receive and return (Feldman & Ticktin 2010, Korf et al 2010, Wilk & Cliggett 2007). 'Gifts are not just material transfers of "aid" but are also embodiments of cultural symbolism, social power and political affiliations' (Korf et al 2010, p. 60). This is evidenced by the transformation in the humanitarian ethos from compassion and charity (humanitarian aid) to social change (sustainable development) to containment related to the world ordering and security strategies of the North (Collinson et al 2010). Ironically, within this climate it may be the 'beneficiaries' of aid that lose while those giving the gift gain, be it related to profit, politics, power or the self-satisfaction of doing a good deed (Bornstein & Redfield 2010).

SITUATING OCCUPATION AND OCCUPATIONAL THERAPY WITHIN THE FIELD

The position presented thus far is that disaster and disaster risk are consequences of the social conditions of everyday life and, further, that these conditions, in the manner in which they reflect weaknesses in the social structures, relationships and systems, call for social action and change. The discipline of occupational therapy is conceptually well positioned to contribute to efforts to reduce vulnerability and risk disaster from the perspective of the transformation of everyday patterns of activities or occupations, and the social structures and relations that underpin them.

However, occupational therapists are limited in their ability to translate the value of occupation into social action and change (Kronenberg et al 2005, Pollard & Sakellariou 2012). Dominant models of occupation within the occupational therapy literature focus predominantly on the individual sphere of occupation and activity. Consequently, opportunities are limited for occupational therapists to develop the competencies to navigate effectively the complex social, cultural and political terrain. These models are largely embedded in Western culture and ideologies centred upon competitive and possessive forms of individualism and espoused values of independence, empowerment and mastery or control of the environment (Hammell 2009).

Furthermore, occupational therapists typically operate within the constraints of medical rehabilitation models in the health sectors, within hospital and community settings where interventions target individual health, function and wellbeing. They focus on the activities of everyday living and work with people to enhance their ability to engage in the occupations they want to, need to, or are expected to do. They also modify the occupation or the environment to better support a person's occupational engagement (WFOT 2012).

TOWARD A SOCIAL VISION

Relatively recently, the profession has espoused, and reaffirmed, a broader social vision of enabling a just and inclusive society, through occupation, that is largely based on the therapeutic value of occupation and its transformative potential. However, Pollard & Sakellariou (2012) argue that the 'prescription of interventions for specific conditions is different from the development of practices for social change' (p. 8), and further that this has resulted in the use and development of therapeutic activities in what they refer to as a clinical milieu outside of the wider social context. One of the challenges facing the profession as it forges a path into the realm of disaster and development is that there is no substantive evidence on the effectiveness of occupational therapy intervention within, or outside, traditional medico-rehabilitative models/ teams in the field, upon which to advocate deepening the profession's involvement within an interdisciplinary context.

OCCUPATIONAL THERAPY AND DISASTER RESEARCH

Literature that links occupational therapy to disaster is mostly theoretical and is oriented to individual recovery and adaptive processes. Insights drawn from other practice contexts and common assumptions about occupation that are upheld by the profession are applied to the disaster, without a substantive basis in the field itself. These limitations are undoubtedly influenced by the fact that disaster and development are nontraditional practice contexts for occupational therapists, and further, the number of occupational therapists working in the field is unknown. This renders access to research participants a barrier and challenges the effective transfer and development of knowledge. More broadly, there are several additional challenges associated with disaster research, including the lack of standardized, systematic data collection during disasters, study design limitations, and poorly developed medical rehabilitation services in disaster affected regions, coupled with little emphasis on the role and experience of allied rehabilitation professionals (Rathore et al 2012).

Despite these limitations, practical suggestions for occupational therapists' involvement in disaster can be found in the occupational therapy literature based on a combination of practitioners' experiences in the field, insights drawn from other practice contexts largely related to 'stressful situations', and the complex role of occupation in remediating illness and maintaining health (Diamond and Precin 2003, Fine 1991, McColl 2002, Oakly et al 2008, Scaffi et al 2006, Stone 2006). In 1982, Rosenfeld articulated an activity-based model in post-disaster settings that illuminated the therapeutic use of activities to facilitate adaptive responses and hasten individual recovery.

Another more recent study examined changes in occupational performance and emotional responses one year after Hurricane Katrina and found that satisfaction with both improved but did not reach pre-Katrina baseline responses after a year, particularly for women affected by the disaster (Taylor et al 2011). Emotional responses and related losses are linked to occupational disruptions (e.g. in social roles, habits, activities and routines) and concepts of social and occupational justice, and therefore speak to the social dimension of occupation and disaster (Townsend & Wilcock 2004). However, thinking and practice that are oriented to issues of individual occupational performance and engagement do not readily translate into social action and change. This limits the transformative potential of occupation. It also illuminates the need to build the capacity of the profession in order to strengthen and support its involvement in the field.

SUMMARY

This chapter has described the origins and evolution of humanitarianism as it relates to disaster and has provided a snapshot of contemporary practice that links humanitarian aid with sustainable development and risk reduction. Our focal point has been on the social dimension of disaster as it pertains to society's role in shaping patterns of disaster risk and vulnerability. We have outlined the prevailing global vision for an equitable and sustainable global society and its guiding principles. This vision is tempered by the shadow side of humanitarianism and its host of complexities and tensions that threaten the integrity of the system and a coordinated global response. Further to this, we have situated the discipline of occupational therapy in the field based on the profession's social vision of health, wellbeing and justice (through occupation) and have illuminated a practice gap that potentially limits the profession's capacity to realize its vision. The following chapter takes a closer look at the concept of risk as it lies at the interface where natural hazards, social relations and individual choice converge, and further positions the concept of occupation and occupational therapy practice at this critical juncture.

REFERENCES

Abarquez, I., Murshed, Z., 2004. Community based disaster risk management: field practitioners' handbook. Asian Disaster Preparedness Centre. Retrieved January 20, 2014 from: <http://www.adpc.net/pdr-sea/publications/12Handbk.pdf>.

Alexander, D., 1997. The study of natural disasters, 1977–1997: some reflections on a changing field of knowledge. Disasters 21 (4), 284–304.

Bankoff, G., 2001. Rendering the world unsafe. Vulnerability as western discourse. Disasters 25, 19–35.

Boin, A., 't Hart, P., 2006. The crisis approach. In: Rodriguez, H., Quarantelli, E.L., Dynes, R.R. (Eds.), Handbook of Disaster Research. Springer, New York, NY, pp. 42–54.

Bornstein, E., Redfield, P., 2010. Forces of Compassion. Humanitarianism Between Ethics and Politics. School for Advanced Research Press, Santa Fe, CA.

Collinson, S., Elhawary, S., Muggah, R., 2010. States of fragility: stabilisation and its implications for humanitarian action (HPG Working Paper). Retrieved from Overseas Development Institute website: <http://www.odi.org/sites/odi.org.uk/files/odi-assets/publications-opinion-files/5978.pdf>.

Diamond, H., Precin, P., 2003. Disabled and experiencing disaster. Occup. Ther. Ment. Health. 19 (3–4), 27–31.

Dupuis, S.L., Gillies, J., Carson, J., et al., 2012. Moving beyond patient and client approaches: mobilising 'authentic partnerships' in dementia care, support and services. Dementia 11 (4), 427–452.

Feldman, I., Ticktin, M. (Eds.), 2010. The Name of Humanity: The Government of Threat and Care. Duke University Press, Durham, NC.

Fine, S.B., 1991. Resilience and human adaptability: who rises above adversity? 1990 Eleanor Clarke Slagle Lecture. Am. J. Occup. Ther. 45 (6), 493–503.

Forsythe, D.P., 2005. The Humanitarians: The International Committee of the Red Cross. Cambridge University Press, Cambridge.

Fox, F., 2001. New humanitarianism: does it provide a moral banner for the 21st century? Disasters 25 (4), 275–289.

Furedi, F., 2007. The changing meaning of disaster. Area 39 (4), 482–489.

GSDRC, 2013. International legal frameworks for humanitarian action: topic guide. GSDRC, University of Birmingham, Birmingham, UK. Retrieved from: <http://www.gsdrc.org/go/topic-guides/ilfha>.

Hammell, K., 2009. Sacred texts: a sceptical exploration of the assumptions underpinning theories of occupation. CJOT 76 (1), 6–13.

Hilhorst, D., 2002. Being good at doing good? Quality and accountability of humanitarian NGOs. Disasters 26 (3), 193–212.

Hutton, D., 2001. Psychosocial aspects of disaster recovery: integrating communities into disaster planning and policy making. ICLR Research Paper Series – No. 4. Retrieved from Institute for Catastrophic Loss Reduction website: <http://www.iclr.org/healthimpactspsychologic.html>.

Ishiwatari, M., 2012. Government roles in community-based disaster risk reduction. In: Shaw, R. (Ed.), Community-Based Disaster Risk Reduction (Community, Environment and Disaster Risk Management, Volume 10). Emerald Group Publishing Limited, Bingley, UK, pp. 19–33.

Johnston, H., Klandermans, B., 1995. Social Movements and Culture. Springer, Minneapolis, MN.

Korf, B., Habullah, S., Hollenback, P., Klem, B., 2010. The gift of disaster: the commodification of good intentions in post-tsunami Sri Lanka. Disasters 34 (Suppl. 1), S60–S77.

Kronenberg, F., Simo Algado, S., Pollard, N. (Eds.), 2005. Occupational Therapy Without Borders: Learning from the Spirit of Survivors. Elsevier/Churchill Livingstone, Oxford.

Macrae, J., 1998. Purity or political engagement? Issues in food and health security interventions in complex political emergencies. Journal of Humanitarianism Assistance. Retrieved from: <http://sites.tufts.edu/jha/archives/126>.

McColl, M.A., 2002. Occupation in stressful times. Am. J. Occup. Ther. 56, 350–353.

Minear, L., 2002. The Humanitarian Enterprise: Dilemmas and Discoveries. Kumarian Press Inc, Bloomfield, CT.

Nolan, R., 2002. Development Anthropology: Encounters in the Real World. Westview Press, Boulder, CO.

Oakly, F., Caswell, S., Parks, R., 2008. Occupational therapists' role on U.S. Army and U.S. Public Health Service Commissioned Corps disaster mental health response teams. Am. J. Occup. Ther. 62, 361–364.

Pierce, L., 2003. Disaster management and community planning and public participation: how to achieve sustainable hazard mitigation. Nat. Hazards 28, 211–228.

Pollard, N., Sakellariou, D., 2012. Politics of Occupation-Centred Practice. Reflections on Occupational Engagement Across Cultures. Wiley-Blackwell, Oxford, UK.

Pupavac, V., 2005. The demoralized subject of global civil society. In: Baker, G., Chandler, D. (Eds.), Global Civil Society: Contested Futures. Routledge, New York, NY, pp. 45–58.

Quarantelli, E.L., Lagadec, P., Boin, A., 2006. A heuristic approach to future disasters and crises: new, old, and in-between types. In: Rodriguez, H., Quarantelli, E.L., Dynes, R.R. (Eds.), The Handbook of Disaster Research. Springer, New York, NY, pp. 16–41.

Rathore, F.A., Gosney, J.E., Reinhardt, J.D., et al., 2012. Medical rehabilitation after natural disasters: why, when, and how? Arch Phys Med Rehabil 93, 1875–1881.

Rodriguez, H., Quarantelli, E.L., Dynes, R.R., 2006. The Handbook of Disaster Research. Springer, New York.

Rosenfeld, M.S., 1982. A model for activity intervention in disaster-stricken communities. Am. J. Occup. Ther. 36, 229–235.

Scaffi, M.E., Gerardi, S., Herzberg, G., et al., 2006. The role of occupational therapy in disaster preparedness, response, and recovery. Am. J. Occup. Ther. 60 (6), 642–649.

Sen, A., 1995. Inequality Re-examined. Harvard University Press, Cambridge, MA.

Slim, H., 1997. Doing the right thing: relief agencies, moral dilemmas and moral responsibility in political emergencies and war. Disasters 21 (3), 244–257.

Sphere Project, 2011. 2011 edition of the Sphere Handbook: What is New? Retrieved August 6, 2013 from: <http://www.sphereproject.org/silo/files/what-is-new-in-the-sphere-handbook-2011-edition-v2.pdf>.

Stallings, R.A., 2006. Causality and 'natural' disasters. Contemp. Sociol. 35 (3), 223–227.

Steinberg, T., 2003. Acts of God: The Unnatural History of Natural Disaster in America. Oxford University Press, Oxford, UK.

Stone, G.V.M., 2006. Occupational therapy in times of disaster. Am. J. Occup. Ther. 60 (1), 7–8.

Sustainable Development Solutions Network, 2013. An action agenda for sustainable development. Report for the UN Secretary General. Retrieved from: <http://unsdsn.org/files/2013/11/An-Action-Agenda-for-Sustainable-Development.pdf>.

Taylor, E., Jacobs, R., Marsh, E.D., 2011. First year post-Katrina: changes. In: John, O.P., Robins, R.W., Pervin, L.A. (Eds.), Handbook of Personality: Theory and Research, third ed. The Guilford Press, New York, NY.

Tierney, K.J., 2003. Disaster beliefs and institutional interests: recycling disaster myths in the aftermath of 9-11. In: Clarke, L. (Ed.), Terrorism and Disaster: New Threats, New Ideas: Research in Social Problems and Public Policy. Elsevier, New York, pp. 33–51.

Townsend, E., Wilcock, A.A., 2004. Occupational justice and client-centred practice: a dialogue in progress. Can. J. Occup. Ther. 71 (2), 75–87.

UNDP, 2012. The Millennium Development Goals Report 2012. Retrieved from: <http://www.undp.org/content/undp/en/home/librarypage/mdg/the-millennium-development-goals-report-2012/>.

Voltaire, 1905. The Lisbon Earthquake and Other Poems. Kessinger Publishing ILC, Whitefish, MT.

Walker, P., Maxwell, D., 2009. Shaping the Humanitarian World. Routledge, London, UK.

Watson, S., 2011. The 'human' as referent object? Humanitarianism as securitization. Security Dialogue 42 (1), 3–20.

Webb, G.R., 2006. The popular culture of disaster: exploring a new dimension of disaster research. In: Rodriguez, H., Quarantelli, E.L., Dynes, R.R. (Eds.), The Handbook of Disaster Research. Springer, New York, NY, pp. 430–440.

WFOT, 2012. About occupational therapy: definition of occupational therapy. Retrieved from:: <http://www.wfot.org/AboutUs/AboutOccupationalTherapy/DefinitionofOccupationalTherapy.aspx>.

Wilk, R., Cliggett, L.C., 2007. Economies and Cultures: Foundations of Economic Anthropology, second ed. Westview Press, Boulder, CO.

World Commission on Environment and Development, 1987. Brundtland Report. Retrieved from:: <http://en.wikisource.org/wiki/Brundtland_Report>.

Zebrowski, E., 1997. Perils of a Restless Planet: Scientific Perspectives on Natural Disasters. Cambridge University Press, Cambridge, UK.

3

DISASTER RISK, VULNERABILITY AND RESILIENCE: AN EMERGENT SOCIO-ECOLOGICAL PERSPECTIVE

NANCY RUSHFORD ■ KERRY THOMAS

INTRODUCTION

The purpose of this chapter is to examine the interactions between the individual, society and the natural world as they shape the context for disaster risk, vulnerability, resilience and adaptation. Against the backdrop of global risk drivers and processes of change, a socio-ecological perspective emerges that calls into question the resilience of contemporary global society to disaster. This chapter expands upon the idea that disaster is a reflection of inequitable social relations and unsustainable patterns of human activity to embrace an ecologically sustainable perspective. Central to the discussion is the topic of human consumption, environmental degradation and human-induced climate change and its role in exacerbating social inequalities and threatening global sustainability. The concept of occupation and the practice of occupational therapy is considered within a dynamic, emergent and socio-ecological perspective.

RISK AS A REVOLUTIONARY IDEA

Risk is a revolutionary idea in that it defines the boundary between modern times and the past (Bernstein 1996). In the past, ideas of the future were based on the acceptance of uncertainty, 'God's punishment' or one's 'fate' and encouraged passivity of society. In contemporary Western society the emphasis is on human agency, self-determination and control as it involves mastery of the environment and the control and containment of risks. Sociological theorists label

modern Western society as a 'risk society' where the language of risk organizes individual and institutional thinking and behaviour (Beck 1999, Giddens 1990, Hall 2002). According to Giddens (1990), sensitivity to risk is a consequence of modernity and has resulted from the erosion of Western tradition and religion combined with the rise of individualism and globalization with its associated technological, political-economic and social changes.

The concept of reducing disaster risk is multifaceted and has captured the attention of numerous disciplines. These disciplines have collectively contributed a broad constellation of approaches and perspectives to the field. Alexander (1991, 1997) classifies approaches to disaster into several schools of thought involving geography, anthropology, sociology and social psychology, engineering and architecture, medicine and public health, and development studies. These various disciplines have proposed a multitude of definitions of disaster reflecting their particular standpoints in relation to the idea of disaster risk (Perry and Quarantelli 2005, Perry 2006). For example, some attribute disaster risk to failure of technological systems; others consider it a manifestation of weaknesses in social structures or systems (Rodriguez et al 2006, Tarn et al 2008). From a sustainable development perspective, failure is attributed to poor development policies and practices that compromise ecological integrity (Commission on Climate Change and Development 2008).

At present a universally agreed upon definition of disaster to integrate the various perspectives is lacking;

however, disciplines traditionally engaged in hazards and vulnerability research (e.g. geographers, anthropologists, sociologists, psychologists) converge at the point of their shared interest in human–environment interactions and the 'conceptual triumvirate of vulnerability, adaptation and resilience' (Gall 2007, p. 8). Holzmann & Jørgensen (2001) have developed a conceptual framework for measuring risk and vulnerability based on a social risk management perspective. Their framework has been criticized for imposing constraints to practice due to its complexity, but has contributed well-known simplifications in the practice literature as represented by the equation:

$$\text{Risk} = \text{Hazard} \times \text{Vulnerability}/\text{Capacity}$$

A FORMULA FOR DISASTER RISK

The risk equation depicts disaster in terms of the dynamic interplay between the natural hazard, vulnerabilities and capacities, where risk and vulnerability are not simply a function of the natural hazard or physical event itself, but are shaped by the complex interplay between the hazard, conditions of vulnerability and the resources (capacities) available to prevent a crisis from becoming a disaster or mitigate its impact. Consistent with Western society's concern with containing or controlling risk, disaster research has predominantly focused on natural hazards themselves and controlling natural processes. This has given rise to the dominance of technical interventions designed to predict the hazard or modify its impact. These efforts have proved to be insufficient in many parts of the world as social and demographic pressures have disproportionately heightened the rate of exposure of people and places to natural hazards (Cannon 2000). Consequently, research and intervention have expanded to explore the social dimension of vulnerability, balanced by attention to resilience and capacities, as reflected in social science research in North America (Cannon 2000, Rodriguez et al 2006).

VULNERABILITY AND RESILIENCE: KEY CONCEPTS

Social science research has provided great insight into the human condition of suffering and human adaptability in the broader context of social structures and relationships. The systematic study of disaster in the social sciences in North America began in the 1950s and has involved what Perry (2006) categorizes as three focal points over the past several decades: (1) the classic approach, (2) the hazards-disaster tradition approach and (3) the socially-focused tradition. The classic approach focused largely on human behaviour and society, characterizing disaster by a cycle of stability–disruption–adjustment. The hazards-disaster tradition investigated processes associated with the natural hazard itself (e.g. tornado, pollutant, flood), but evolved to examine vulnerability and resiliency to environmental threats. The socially-focused tradition placed people and social relationships within the context of social change at the core of research on disasters. In particular, the focus on vulnerability as a means to better understand disaster and disaster risk emerged in the literature in the 1970s with early definitions of vulnerability largely referring to the quantitative degree of potential loss in the event of the occurrence of a natural hazard (Gaillard 2007).

The concept of vulnerability soon evolved to encompass the wider social context or 'conditions' of society that rendered people and places more susceptible to natural hazards (Alexander 2008, Cannon 2000, Gaillard 2007). This was later balanced by attention to resilience and capacity building approaches in the field. Enarson (2000) defines social vulnerability as 'a function of people's relative exposure to hazards, mitigation efforts and access to key resources needed to anticipate, cope with and recover from the effects of disastrous natural events' (p. 3). Whereas vulnerability looks at the susceptibility of people, systems and places to loss, resilience examines capabilities and coping strategies. Both concepts have a broad theoretical base with roots in psychology, ecology and development, and numerous frameworks, conceptual models and assessment techniques (Cutter et al 2003, 2008).

Some researchers consider resilience to be a paradigm in itself, others view it in close relation to vulnerability, and more recently within the ecological literature it is referred to within the context of adaptive capacity (Manyena 2006), where adaptive capacity extends beyond immediate coping strategies to refer to the ability of ecological, as well as human or social systems, to evolve strategies to respond to the negative effects of natural hazards in the long term (Cutter et al 2008, WorldRiskReport 2012).

From a disaster and development perspective, resilience is considered to be the ability of people, households, communities, countries and systems to mitigate, adapt to and recover from shocks and stresses in a manner that reduces chronic vulnerability and facilitates inclusive growth (USAID 2012). Where shocks and stresses intersect with chronic poverty and marginalization, crises tend to be recurrent and development gains are undermined. This in turn feeds a spiral of increasing vulnerability. It is in these spaces where adaptive capacity and resilience building – the ability to respond quickly and effectively to new circumstances – is most needed, together with improved ability to address and reduce risk.

SOCIAL VULNERABILITY AND ADAPTIVE CAPACITY

Social vulnerability and resiliency perspectives on disaster and disaster risk challenge the assumption that human responses to natural hazards are primarily rooted in the way individuals think, behave and interact in the environment as a reflection of their individual attributes and characteristics or inherent susceptibilities (Fine 1991, Hutton 2001). Research into disaster and patterns of human response has shown that a combination of individual and environmental factors influence the development of personalized adaptive strategies and long-term adjustment, including pre-disaster factors (e.g. gender and age, past history of exposure, preexisting resources such as coping skills and social support), within-disaster factors (e.g. the objective nature of individuals' exposure and their subjective perceptions of the event) and post-disaster factors or secondary stressors (e.g. receipt and nature of assistance) (Kaniasty & Norris 2004, Norris et al 1999).

PERSONALIZED ADAPTIVE STRATEGIES

Psychology, with its many branches of knowledge, contributes to the understanding of the development and use of personalized adaptive strategies to manage life stressors including, for example, the ideas of emotional defences and cognitive strategies. According to psychoanalytic theory, defence mechanisms such as 'avoidance' and 'denial', when used appropriately, act as coping capacities helping individuals to manage stress (Freud 1966). Furthermore, cognitive functions such as attention, perception and memory also help people to appraise situations, solve problems and find meaning, ultimately transforming situations into new realities (Freud 1966, Reisberg 2013). This depends largely upon how a person interprets situations. Individual psychologists suggest interpretation is based on 'personal theories of reality' (idea of self in relation to the world) that are a product of society and relationships in that they are informed by personal experiences and opportunities in life (Ansbacher & Ansbacher 1964, 1979). Essentially, social interactions, institutions and systems of cultural values and practices interact with individual attributes and characteristics and influence the choices and opportunities that people have available to them in situations of disaster or risk. Having access to a strong social fabric facilitates adaptation in that it serves as a buffer against stress by providing the emotional, material and structural support (e.g. social networks, livelihood diversification or savings, political-organizational structures) necessary to anticipate, cope with and recover from disaster (Cannon 2000, Cohen and Wills 1985, Van den Eynde & Veno 1999).

SOCIAL CAPITAL AND RESILIENCE

Research into the long-term psychological effects of disaster shows that the majority of people studied are able to cope and respond adaptively to disaster over time. Symptomatology (e.g. anxiety, post-traumatic stress, depression) peaks during the first year and becomes less prevalent over time, leaving only a minority of communities and people affected by disaster substantially impaired (Norris et al 1999). Furthermore, social capital is linked to positive health outcomes and development following disaster as it involves the mobilization of resources that are embedded within social networks (Beaudoin 2007). Bourdieu (1986) asserts that social capital is the channel through which one form of capital (e.g. economic, cultural, physical, ecological, symbolic) can be interchanged with another, towards a particular goal or benefit (as cited by Schuurman 2003). Lin (2000) stresses that this process is dependent upon the actor's position within the social network and network characteristics. The actor may be an individual in the context of the community, or more broadly societies as they are positioned within the broader global network of international relations.

Social capital has been used as a theory to explore social vulnerability and resilience in contexts of disaster (Beaudoin 2007). Certain groups within society lack access and control over key resources to prepare for disaster or recover, including for example, social protection and power, money and land, information, good health and personal mobility (Blaikie et al 1994, Cutter et al 2003). These groups have been differentiated from others and positioned at the margins of society based on social factors such as income, gender, race, class, age and disability and consequently represent 'particularly vulnerable groups' in situations of disaster and disaster risk. Kaniasty & Norris (2004) note that patterns of neglect have been reported in a number of studies that investigate the distribution of relief following disasters. They describe the pattern of help following disasters as a pyramid with the broad foundation being family, friends and neighbours followed by local religious congregations and finally formal agencies and institutions. This pyramid may be expressed as an altruistic community, however they emphasize that not all survivors are equally involved in these helping communities. Cannon (2000) argues that in order to understand conditions of vulnerability and resilience it is important to decipher how human systems place people in relation to each other and the environment.

MODELS OF VULNERABILITY AND RESILIENCE

Several models of vulnerability and resilience have been developed to map out the relationship between social conditions, hazardous events and the physical or built environment. Blaikie et al (1994) developed the pressure and release model of disaster which depicts a progression of vulnerability that accounts for the influence of social conditions and global forces. The model outlines how unsafe conditions (vulnerability) emerge through dynamic pressures (e.g. urbanization) that are placed upon preexisting conditions (e.g. marginalization) that in combination with natural hazards create the potential for disastrous outcome. The hazards-of-place model of vulnerability (Cutter 1996, Cutter et al 2003) incorporates mitigation efforts into understandings of vulnerability and offers a broader socio-cultural perspective. According to this model, vulnerable places are a function of risk (an objective measure of the likelihood of a hazard event) interacting with mitigation measures (measures to lessen risks or reduce their impact) to produce the hazard potential. The hazard potential is either moderated or enhanced by a geographic filter (site and situation of the place, proximity) as well as the social fabric of the particular place consisting of collective past experience with hazards (Cutter 1996, Cutter et al 2003). This is well captured by Alexander (2008), who states that:

In the lives of people who live through them, disasters are milestones, points of reference and yardsticks by which subsequent experience is measured. For society as a whole, catastrophic events are absorbed into the matrix of history, which forms the background of culture.

The disaster resilience of place (DROP) model (Cutter et al 2008) reflects a shift in emphasis in the disaster literature from vulnerability to resilience. DROP depicts resilience as a dynamic process dependent on the interactions between antecedent conditions, event characteristics and coping capacities where the local impact of a hazardous natural event can be moderated by the ability of the community to absorb the impacts using predetermined coping strategies. Although these coping strategies may be predetermined in the sense that they represent the options available at a particular point in time in relation to a specific event, they are not static but are influenced by knowledge gained through the *adaptive resiliency process*. This process emphasizes adaptive resilience through improvisation and social learning.

The ideas and models summarized place the phenomenon of disaster at the interface between social relations, individual choice and natural forces. The DROP model points to the need for social-structural and ecological manipulations as a part of building adaptive capacity within the broader context of environmental change. While an ecological perspective on disaster is becoming increasingly mainstream, researchers have traditionally viewed disaster primarily as a social disruption that exacerbated preexisting social inequities. Consequently the emphasis was placed on remedy through social change and advances in technology that would lead to better prediction of hazardous events. Researchers generally neglected considerations of how human activity impacts upon the environment and the consequences of human manipulations on the natural world. More recently, conceptual models consider society as a causal force behind disasters and examine disasters and humanitarian response through a socio-political and an ecological lens (Bornstein and Redfield 2010, Hannigan 2012, Webb 2006). This evolution in thinking is reflected in the WorldRiskReport (2012).

THE WORLDRISKINDEX

The concept of the WorldRiskIndex was developed jointly by scientists and development experts to calculate disaster risk at a global level as it relates to natural hazardous events and climate change. The model combines the natural hazard sphere (exposure) with the vulnerability-societal sphere (susceptibility, coping and adaptation) to assess the degree of risk that a society is exposed to by internal and external factors. Susceptibility depends upon infrastructure, nutrition, housing situation and economic framework conditions; coping depends upon governance, early warning and preparation, medical services and social and material coverage; and adaptive capacity refers to the measures and strategies that are used to deal with the negative impacts of natural hazards and climate change at present and into the future. The model's emphasis on adaptive capacity orients disaster risk reduction towards the future and global sustainability goals.

HUMANITY'S RESILIENCE

History suggests that humanity has demonstrated tremendous adaptive resilience to disaster over time; however, the present global reality of increased exposure and vulnerability calls into question the sustainability of many human environmental adaptations and

suggests a global lack of resilience (Furedi 2007). The challenge in the twenty-first century is that inequities in relationships give disaster and risk its disproportionate shape across the globe, and are held in place by historically embedded patterns of dominance and dependency between the North and the South that continue to carry meaning today in the broader context of risk and global processes of change (e.g. population growth, urbanization, consumerism, industrialization, economic pressures, environmental degradation and climate change) (Bankoff 2001). These processes are leading to the increase in the exposure of people and places to natural hazards and are challenging the adaptive capacity of societies over the long term.

Poor nations also experience a disproportionate share of the burden of the negative consequences associated with worldwide environmental degradation and climate change (e.g. vulnerable rural livelihoods, declining ecosystems) (Müller 2008). This is further compounded by poor urban infrastructure and governance and the lack of social protection in the context of broader socio-political and economic processes. Cutter et al (2008) argue that the resilience (and vulnerability) of a community is '… inextricably linked to the condition of the environment and the treatment of its resources' (p. 602), that is, human actions impact on the state of the environment and in turn a degraded environment contributes to natural hazardous events and provides people with less protection and fewer options for adaptation in response to hazardous threats (Adger et al 2005).

PLANETARY RESILIENCE: ENVIRONMENTAL DEGRADATION AND CLIMATE CHANGE

Humanity has been spectacularly successful in modifying the planet to meet the demands of a rapidly growing population (Figure 3-1). Between 1960 and 2000, the human population doubled and economic activity increased sixfold, yet we were able to increase food production by two and a half times (Walker & Salt 2006). The changes made to the environment to meet our growing demands have been so sweeping that cultivated ecosystems now cover more than a quarter of Earth's terrestrial surface and as much as six times more water is held in reserves than flows in natural river channels (Walker & Salt 2006, p. 7). The costs of such gains are mounting rapidly and it is widely apparent that humanity's use of the biosphere is not sustainable (Flannery 2005, Walker & Salt 2006).

Human-induced climate change has emerged as perhaps the most pressing global threat to our health and wellbeing – indeed to our very survival. Almost 20% of dry land ecosystems are degraded and unable to meet the needs of people living in them (Figure 3-2); most marine fisheries are on the verge of over-harvesting or have already collapsed; billions of people face problems of water scarcity and quality; and more than half the world's ecosystem services (such as the benefits ecosystems provide in purifying water, preventing landslides, reducing the magnitude of floods) have been degraded (Flannery 2005, Suzuki & Taylor 2009). We are eroding the resource base upon which our very survival depends and are living beyond our means on a small planet with finite resources. In simple terms, demand is out of balance with supply.

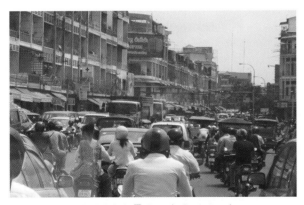

FIGURE 3-1 ■ Population growth.

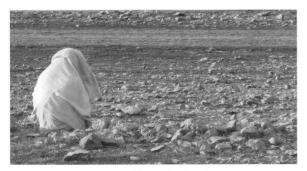

FIGURE 3-2 ■ Famine in Ethiopia.

Furthermore, climate change, through its many aspects, will probably exacerbate the existing inequalities faced by vulnerable groups and threaten to undermine the realization of fundamental rights for many people. Although it is evident that while everyone will ultimately be affected, as we have noted, 'the impacts of climate change will fall disproportionately upon developing countries and the poor persons within all countries, thereby exacerbating inequities in health status and access to adequate food, clean water and other resources' (R K Pachauri, Chairman of the Intergovernmental Panel on Climate Change, DFID 2008).

Depleted natural resources contribute to unsustainable livelihoods and a lower standard of living (including poor health and nutrition) that further compels migratory responses where people relocate to less affected or urban/semiurban areas (IPCC, 2012). These processes are also known to destroy traditional ways of life and can cause the collapse of natural and cultural protections captured in habits and routines (Zebrowski 1997). As conditions deteriorate and access to traditional coping mechanisms and resources shrink, conflict will very likely ensue, further exacerbating social and health inequities and impacts. People with disabilities, children and senior citizens are especially vulnerable and most at risk.

SUSTAINABLE DEVELOPMENT: A WAY FORWARD?

Sustainable development has been promoted as the primary foil to these conditions, together with various disaster mitigation and management strategies and climate change policies.

The central tenets of sustainable development are environmental protection, social equity and economic development, but notions of sustainable development vary according to whose perspective prevails. In 1987, the World Commission on Environment and Development defined it as 'development which meets the needs of the present without compromising the ability of future generations to meet their own needs'. More recently, the Sustainable Development Commission (2011) stated that sustainable development is about '… ensuring a strong, healthy and just society.

This means meeting the diverse needs of all people in existing and future communities, promoting personal wellbeing, social cohesion … and creating equal opportunity'. These are highly laudable aspirations, but in practice they have had limited impact at a global level in addressing the fundamental conditions that are contributing to human-induced climate change which, as noted above, will erode development gains across all sectors.

Development is a human-centred endeavour characterized by socio-economic activity. As conceived from neoliberal economic models, development that directs human activity towards economic growth potentially minimizes the need for regulation that is geared towards protecting the most vulnerable people in our society and ensuring access and opportunities for all. This type of development contributes to environmental degradation, climate change and disaster risk. Economic development can also perpetuate inequitable and unsafe labour arrangements and produce vulnerabilities that affect everyone but the richest in society (Wisner et al 2003). Conversely, 'social' development directs human activity towards addressing poverty and disadvantage and potentially reduces disaster risk by increasing capabilities and freedom and promoting participation, widespread livelihood security and environmental enhancement (Wisner et al 2003).

An interesting paradox with the notion of 'sustainability' is that the term suggests the achievement of *equilibrium* as a final state, when the reality of ecological, and indeed human systems is that they are highly dynamic, complex and adaptive systems. The nature of complex adaptive systems (be they at individual or societal levels) is that they are continually adapting and evolving in response to the interplay between internal and external conditions and pressures. Nothing ever stays the same, which implies that there is always the potential for both loss and opportunity at any given moment in time. This suggests that, along with global crises such as disaster and climate change, there is the potential for transformation and growth, as defined by new patterns of social relations, choices and activities. This dynamic is captured by the conventional Chinese symbol for disaster which combines two characters, one symbolizing 'danger' and the other 'opportunity' (Rodriguez et al 2006).

SOCIO-ECOLOGICAL PERSPECTIVES ON HEALTH, WELLBEING AND JUSTICE

Although social development approaches may promote empowerment, equity and inclusion, the extent to which the underlying conditions that perpetuate ecological deterioration are inherently addressed is widely variable. Climate change is challenging current approaches to sustainable development and is creating a shift towards new models that are framed around concepts of 'adaptation', 'resilience', 'transformation' and 'ecological justice' (Ife 2002, Walker & Salt 2006, Walker et al 2004, Westley et al 2011). The movement towards ecological justice aims to promote the rights, health and wellbeing of ecological habitats – to preserve their integrity for their own sake and not merely as a resource for human use. In contrast to human-centred equity, ecological justice positions people as one species within a broader interdependent ecological biosphere. This potentially changes how people perceive and interact with each other and the environment around them, and experience health and wellbeing.

This movement towards ecological justice emerges from the shadows of neoliberal ideology and Western society's preoccupation with risk, with its emphasis on individualism, competitive relations, freedom of choice and unbridled capitalism (Hay 1996, Wisner et al 2003). Neoliberal ideology and its values associated with individualism, including independence and mastery and control of the environment, potentially conflict with the reality of a finite planet and shared resources. Collectively, as a global society, we need to foster understanding, capabilities and engagement to turn principles and concepts of equity and justice into action within the broader context of achieving sustainable development and safeguarding ecological integrity, while promoting transformative patterns of living and resilience to shocks.

MANAGING COMPLEXITY

It is becoming evident that disaster and development is a particularly dynamic and complex field in which to engage, particularly within the context of managing trauma and transition in a transformative way. Social and ecological dimensions are inextricably bound – disaster begets complexity, not so much due to natural forces that traverse the globe but because it is a social and ecological phenomenon that occurs at the interface where individual choice, social relations and natural dimensions converge. Patterns of social inequity and destructive environmental processes are configuring scenarios of risk that feature greater exposure and escalating effects for people, the planet and all living systems; tipping points abound.

Among a myriad of emerging approaches, concepts such as 'chaos points' and 'chaos windows' are appearing in popular literature and offer alternative ways of empowering people to find innovative solutions to crises facing the contemporary world. These operate in association with disastrous events and tipping points in 'the evolution of a system, in which trends that have brought the system to its present state break down and it can no longer return to its prior states and

modes of behaviour: the system is launched irreversibly on a new trajectory that leads either to breakdown or to breakthrough to a new structure and a new mode of operation' (Laszlo 2006, p. vii).

Disaster and chaos are infused with highly complex social, political, economic and environmental dynamics, generating very significant challenges to the establishment of processes through which positive responses for recovery, adaptation and/or transformation can occur.

At a very practical level, participatory planning, monitoring and evaluation help to ensure planning is locally and culturally relevant, while being coherent with national and global requirements. The project cycle remains a fundamental structure around which to develop both disaster and development initiatives and embed participatory processes (Thomas 2010). Key elements of this cycle are presented in Figure 3-3 and summarized in Box 3-1. It involves a process of assessment (of situations and contexts as well as needs,

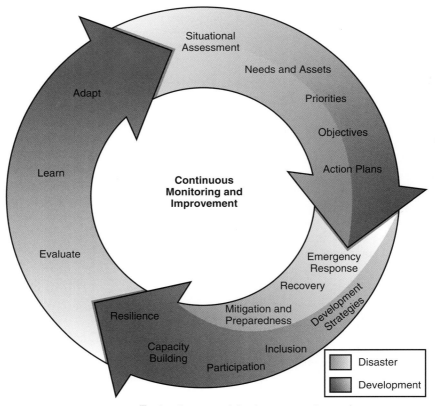

FIGURE 3-3 ■ The disaster and development project cycle.

BOX 3-1
THE DISASTER AND DEVELOPMENT PROJECT CYCLE STEPS

As summarized in Figure 3-3, the key elements are:

- Situational assessment, encompassing problem, need and asset analysis (assets being existing capabilities and resources), as well as risk and vulnerability assessment.
- Agreeing goals and setting objectives, with primary consideration to collaborative development of measurable outcomes for the community, but also implications for agencies and service providers, and other stakeholders.
- Developing action plans, including identifying and agreeing roles and responsibilities, communication and management processes, and key actions across various parameters (e.g. policy and practice; and the three elements of sustainable development – social, economic and ecological), as well as determining and accessing resources, developing a monitoring and evaluation plan, and agreeing who will do what, when and where.
- Implementing and managing actions, maximizing use of participatory strategies that will also inherently build capacity, reduce vulnerability and enhance resilience.
- Evaluating progress and performance at milestone points and at the end of initiatives, again with an emphasis on using participatory, learning and adaptive capacity approaches.
- Monitoring throughout and across the whole process, to directly inform ongoing learning and adaptive capacity.

assets and issues), prioritizing and objective setting, followed by collective planning and action, continual monitoring and periodic evaluation through which learning and change occur (Thomas 2010).

Even in disaster management, planning and participation are critical to achieving appropriate, effective and efficient outcomes. The project cycle applies across the disaster management continuum, usually through iterative processes coinciding with each phase of a disaster, although the timeframes and activities will vary substantially. As indicated in Figure 3-3, disaster management activities and processes are increasingly undertaken within a broader development context, although emergency response and early recovery efforts tend to occur in parallel.

OCCUPATIONAL CONSIDERATIONS

Occupation sits at the nexus between society and the natural world. It is at the heart of human-induced climate change and its consequences based on patterns of human activity and consumption, but it is also the conduit through which we can emerge from disaster and mitigate, adapt, and build resilience.

Occupational therapy practitioners possess knowledge about how individuals, the environment and human occupation (or activity) stimulate participation and health (World Federation of Occupational Therapists 2012). The emergence of the discipline of Occupational Science along with terms such as 'occupational injustice' (Townsend & Wilcock 2004), 'occupational deprivation' (Whiteford 2000, Wilcock 1998) and 'occupational apartheid' (Kronenberg & Pollard 2005) has served to broaden conceptualizations of human occupation and activity along social dimensions and orientate it to human rights. In particular, these changes in perspective have drawn attention to the choices and opportunities people have in life to develop and promote their health and wellbeing (through occupation). This has also provided the impetus for the profession's drive towards occupational justice and social action and change.

More recently, the World Federation of Occupational Therapists (WFOT) has broadened its occupational justice agenda by encouraging occupational therapists to reflect upon practice models and expand clinical reasoning to include sustainable practice (Whitticker & Shann n.d.). The profession's increasing attention to issues of sustainability is represented by the WFOT's position statement on environmental sustainability, perspectives on sustainable development offered by national occupational therapy associations and through research initiatives (e.g. Jenkins 2014), and the emergence of sustainable practice networks such as OT Susnet.

These developments reflect the broader global movement towards sustainable forms of heath care, based on principles of sustainable clinical practice. These include: (1) preventative health care; (2) patient empowerment and supported self-care; (3) continuous quality improvement (i.e. lean methodologies towards efficient health service delivery); (4) lower carbon treatment options (i.e. walking/cycling as treatment). Under this umbrella, clinical practice extends beyond the treatment of individual health conditions to encompass a 'sustainable individual lifestyle approach' that links health with lifestyle choices and indirectly the global issue of climate change and disaster (Pachauri 2009).

For persons in the Southern hemisphere or Western world, disaster risk may appear distant enough to be framed as an individual lifestyle choice – in other words, an effort to decrease one's ecological footprint and improve health and wellbeing. However, in poorer regions of the world where the consequences of human-induced climate change are more direct and disasters more frequent, there is not the luxury of lifestyle choices. On the contrary, climate change and disaster are matters of survival.

If the profession is to adopt a broader occupational justice agenda related to disaster risk, resilience and sustainability, interventions will need to extend beyond individual health and wellness to address these social inequalities and their impact upon people's choices and the options available for recovery and resilience.

As occupational therapists engaged in disaster response and recovery efforts have reported, 'people's lives have been turned upside down … devastated … changed forever' and the dislocation and suffering caused by extreme events can linger for years, long into 'recovery'. We are gaining ability to support interventions and action that understand these effects in accord with human capabilities and socio-cultural contexts and that promote sustainable development; critically, we must now evolve ways to facilitate transformative shifts in patterns of recovery and living that actively nurture ecological sustainability, adaptability and resilience. And we need to do this at individual and societal levels.

SUMMARY

Disaster represents the complex and emergent relationships between people and nature. Throughout time and civilization it has inspired humanitarian efforts to alleviate suffering that have become increasingly sophisticated in response to social challenges and global processes of change. In particular, in the twenty-first century, social inequality and global forces are reconfiguring scenarios of risk, as defined by greater exposure to natural hazards, coupled with the inability of the

most vulnerable groups to cope with disaster. Furthermore, it is evident that unsustainable environmental practices are increasing societal vulnerability in the manner that they cause ecological damage and reduce the opportunities for people (and largely those living in poverty) to avoid or mitigate disaster. Research in the field has increasingly focused on the interactive nature of natural and human systems and has sought to delineate the relationships between hazards and vulnerability in order to mitigate disaster with increased attention to resilience and adaptive capacity in the broader context of planetary viability. Widespread social and ecological change and transformation is required.

The occupational therapy profession's increasing attention to global issues and a 'sustainable individual lifestyle approach' to health is a promising development that potentially aligns occupational therapy practice with approaches to disaster and development. In particular, the discipline of occupational therapy may be well positioned to contribute to vulnerability and risk reduction from the perspective of transforming everyday patterns of activities (occupations) to reflect more equitable and sustainable social relations and choices. However, the transformative potential of occupation should not be limited to the individual sphere of occupation and activity. Rather, occupational therapists may be well positioned to adopt a broader occupational justice agenda. The chapters that follow offer perspectives on occupation in contexts of disaster and insights into its transformative potential. This lays the foundation for an occupational perspective on disaster and development to emerge and deepen the profession's involvement in the field.

REFERENCES

Adger, W.N., Arnell, N.W., Tompkins, E.L., 2005. Successful adaptation to climate change across scales. Global Environ. Chang. 15 (2), 77–86.

Alexander, D., 1991. Natural disasters. A framework for research and teaching. Disasters 15 (3), 209–226.

Alexander, D., 1997. The study of natural disasters, 1977–1997: some reflections on a changing field of knowledge. Disasters 21 (4), 284–304.

Alexander, D., 2008. Disaster planning and management. Managing hazards and disasters: new theories, new imperatives. Retrieved January 16, 2014, from: <http://emergency-planning.blogspot.ca/2008_02_01_archive.html>.

Ansbacher, H.L., Ansbacher, R.R. (Eds.), 1964. The Individual Psychology of Alfred Adler. Harper Torchbooks, New York, NY.

Ansbacher, H.L., Ansbacher, R.R. (Eds.), 1979. Superiority and Social Interest: A Collection of Later Writings. W.W. Norton, New York, NY.

Bankoff, G., 2001. Rendering the world unsafe. Vulnerability as western discourse. Disasters 25 (1), 19–35.

Beaudoin, C.E., 2007. News, social capital and health in the context of Katrina. J. Health Care Poor Underserved 18, 418–430.

Beck, U., 1999. World Risk Society. Polity Press, Cambridge, UK.

Bernstein, P.L., 1996. Against the Gods – The Remarkable Story of Risk. John Wiley and Sons, Inc., New York, NY.

Blaikie, P., Cannon, T., Davis, I., Wisner, B., 1994. At Risk: Natural Hazards, People's Vulnerability, and Disasters. Routledge, London, UK.

Bornstein, E., Redfield, P., 2010. Forces of Compassion. Humanitarianism Between Ethics and Politics. School for Advanced Research Press, Santa Fe, CA.

Bourdieu, P., 1986. The forms of capital. In: Richardson, J.G. (Ed.), Handbook of Theory and Research for the Sociology of Capital. Greenwood Press, New York, NY.

Cannon, T., 2000. Vulnerability analysis and disasters. In: Parker, D.J. (Ed.), Floods. Routledge, Oxford, UK.

Cohen, S., Wills, T.A., 1985. Stress, social support, and the buffering hypothesis. Psychol. Bull. 98, 310–357.

Commission on Climate Change and Development, 2008. Closing the gaps. Disaster risk reduction and adaptation to climate change in developing countries. Retrieved from: <http://reliefweb.int/report/world/closing-gaps-disaster-risk-reduction-and-adaptation-climate-change-developing-countries>.

Cutter, S.L., 1996. Vulnerability to environmental hazards. Prog. in Hum. Geog. 20 (4), 529–539.

Cutter, S.L., Barnes, L., Berry, M., Burton, C., Evans, E., Tate, E., et al., 2008. A place-based model for understanding community resilience to disasters. Glob. Environ. Change 18, 598–606.

Cutter, S.L., Boruff, J., Shirley, W.L., 2003. Social vulnerability to environmental hazards. Soc. Sci. Q. 84 (2), 242–261.

Enarson, E., 2000. InFocus programme on crisis response and reconstruction. Gender and natural disasters (Working Paper 1. ISBN No. 92-2-112260-3). Retrieved November 18, 2013, from ILO Recovery and Reconstruction Department website: <http://www.ilo.int/wcmsp5/groups/public/---ed_emp/---emp_ent/---ifp_crisis/documents/publication/wcms_116391.pdf>.

Fine, S.B., 1991. Resilience and human adaptability: who rises above adversity? 1990 Eleanor Clarke Slagle Lecture. Am. J. Occup. Ther. 45 (6), 493–503.

Flannery, T., 2005. The Weather Makers. The History and Future Impact of Climate Change. The Text Publishing Company, Melbourne.

Freud, A., 1966. The Ego and the Mechanisms of Defence, revised ed. Hogarth Press and Institute of Psycho-Analysis, London, UK.

Furedi, F., 2007. The changing meaning of disaster. Royal Geographical Society 39 (4), 482–489.

Gaillard, J.C., 2007. Resilience of traditional societies in facing natural hazards. Disaster Prev. Manag. 6 (4), 522–544.

Gall, M., 2007. Indices of social vulnerability to natural hazards: a comparative evaluation. Doctoral dissertation. Department of Geography, University of South Carolina. Available from ProQuest Dissertations and theses database. (UMI Microform 3272445).

Giddens, A., 1990. The Consequences of Modernity. Stanford University Press, Stanford, CA.

Hall, D.R., 2002. Risk society and the second demographic transition. Can. Stud. Popul. 29 (2), 173–194.

Hannigan, J., 2012. Disasters Without Borders. The International Politics of Natural Disasters. Polity Press, Cambridge, UK.

Hay, I., 1996. Neoliberalism and criticisms of earthquake insurance arrangements in New Zealand. Disasters 20, 34–48.

Holzmann, R., Jørgensen, S., 2001. Social risk management: a new conceptual framework for social protection, and beyond. Int. Tax Public Finan. 8 (4), 529–556.

Hutton, D., 2001. Psychosocial aspects of disaster recovery: integrating communities into disaster planning and policy making (ICLR Research Paper Series No. 4). Retrieved from Institute for Catastrophic Loss Reduction website: <http://www.iclr.org/healthimpactspsychologic.html>.

Ife, J., 2002. Community Development. Community-Based Alternatives in an Age of Globalisation, second ed. Longman, Frenchs Forest, NSW.

IPCC, 2012. Managing the risks of extreme events and disasters to advance climate change adaptation. Special report of working groups I and II of the intergovernmental panel on climate change. Field, C.B., Barros V., Stocker T.F., et al. (Eds.) Retrieved from: <https://www.ipcc.ch/pdf/special-reports/srex/SREX_Full_Report.pdf>.

Jenkins, K., 2014. WFOT policy and sustainable development. Occupational Therapy (Honours) research proposal, University of South Australia.

Kaniasty, K., Norris, F.H., 2004. Social support in the aftermath of disasters, catastrophes, and acts of terrorism: altruistic, overwhelmed, uncertain, antagonistic and patriotic communities. In: Ursano, R.J., Norwood, A.E., Fullerton, C.S. (Eds.), Bioterrorism: Psychological and Public Health Interventions. Cambridge University Press, Cambridge, UK.

Kronenberg, F., Pollard, N., 2005. Overcoming occupational apartheid: a preliminary exploration of the political nature of occupational therapy. In: Kronenberg, F., Simó Algado, S., Pollard, N. (Eds.), Occupational Therapy without Borders: Learning from the Spirit of Survivors. Elsevier–Churchill Livingstone, Oxford, UK, pp. 58–86.

Laszlo, E., 2006. Chaos Point 2012 and Beyond. Our Choices between Global Disaster and a Sustainable Planet. Hampton Roads Publishing Company, Charlottesville, VA.

Lin, N., 2000. Inequity in social capital. Contemp. Sociol. 29 (6), 785–795.

Manyena, S.B., 2006. The concept of resilience revisited. Disasters 30 (4), 433–450.

Müller, B., 2008. Equity in climate change. The great divide. Glob. Environ. Change 18 (4), 598–606. Oxford Institute for Energy Studies. Retrieved from the Oxford Climate Policy website: <http://www.oxfordclimatepolicy.org/publications/documents/The_Great_Divide-Executive_Summary.pdf>.

Norris, F.H., Perilla, J.L., Riad, J.K., Kaniasty, K., Lavizzo, E.A., 1999. Stability and change in stress, resources, and psychological distress following natural disaster: findings from hurricane Andrew. Anxiety Stress Copin. 12 (4), 363–396.

Pachauri, R.K., 2008. Chairman Intergovernmental Panel on Climate Change. DFID.

Pachauri, R.K., 2009. Foreword. In: The Health Practitioner's Guide to Climate Change. Diagnosis and Cure. Earthscan, London.

Perry, R.W., 2006. What is disaster? In: Rodriguez, H., Quarantelli, E.L., Dynes, R.R. (Eds.), The Handbook of Disaster Research. Springer, New York, NY, pp. 1–15.

Perry, R.W., Quarantelli, E.L., 2005. What is a Disaster? New Answers to Old Questions. Xlibris, Philadelphia, PA.

Reisberg, D. (Ed.), 2013. The Oxford Handbook of Cognitive Psychology. Oxford University Press, Oxford, UK.

Rodriguez, H., Quarantelli, E.L., Dynes, R.R., 2006. The Handbook of Disaster Research. Springer, New York, NY.

Schuurman, F.J., 2003. Social capital: the politico-emancipatory potential of a disputed concept. Third World Q. 24 (6), 991–1010.

Sustainable Development Commission, 2011. What is sustainable development?, Retrieved from: <http://www.sd-commission.org.uk/pages/what-is-sustainable-development.html>.

Suzuki, D., Taylor, D.R., 2009. The Big Picture: Reflections on Science, Humanity, and a Quickly Changing Planet. Indigo, Canada.

Tarn, J.M., Wen, H.J., Shih, S.C., 2008. A theoretical perspective of man-made system disasters: social-technical analysis and design. Disaster Prev. Manag. 17 (2), 256–280.

Thomas, K., 2010. Planning for Change and MERI (Monitoring, Evaluation, Reporting and Improvement): Training Materials. interPART, Macclesfield, South Australia.

Townsend, E., Wilcock, A.A., 2004. Occupational justice and client-centred practice: a dialogue in progress. Can. J. Occup. Ther. 71 (2), 75–87.

USAID, 2012. Building resilience to recurrent crisis. USAID Policy and Program Guidance. Retrieved from: <http://www.usaid.gov/sites/default/files/documents/1870/USAIDResiliencePolicyGuidanceDocument.pdf>.

Van den Eynde, J.A., Veno, A., 1999. Coping with disastrous events: an empowerment model of community healing. In: Gist, R., Lubin, B. (Eds.), Response to Disaster: Psychosocial, Community and Ecological Approaches. Brunner/Mazel, USA, pp. 167–192.

Walker, B., Holling, C.S., Carpenter, S.R., Kinzig, A., 2004. Resilience, adaptability and transformability in social–ecological systems. Ecol. Soc. 9 (2), 5.

Walker, B., Salt, D., 2006. Resilience Thinking. Sustaining Ecosystems and People in a Changing World. Island Press, Washington DC.

Webb, G.R., 2006. The popular culture of disaster: exploring a new dimension of disaster research. In: Rodriguez, H., Quarantelli, E.L., Dynes, R.R. (Eds.), The Handbook of Disaster Research. Springer, New York, NY, pp. 430–440.

Westley, F., Olsson, P., Folke, C., Homer-Dixon, T., Vredenburg, H., Loorbach, D., et al., 2011. Tipping toward sustainability: emerging pathways of transformation. AMBIO 40 (7), 762–780.

Whiteford, G., 2000. Occupational deprivation: global challenge in the new millennium. Br. J. Occup. Ther. 63 (5), 200–204.

Wilcock, A.A., 1998. An Occupational Perspective of Health. Slack Inc., Thorofare, NJ.

Wisner, B., Blaikie, P., Cannon, T., Davis, I., 2003. At Risk: Natural Hazards, People's Vulnerability and Disasters, second ed. Retrieved from: <http://www.preventionweb.net/files/670_72351.pdf>.

World Federation of Occupational Therapists, 2012. Definition of occupational therapy, Retrieved from: <http://www.wfot.org/AboutUs/AboutOccupationalTherapy/DefinitionofOccupationalTherapy.aspx>.

WorldRiskReport, 2012. Focus: environmental degradation and disasters. Alliance Development Works. Retrieved from: <http://www.ehs.unu.edu/article/read/worldriskreport-2012>.

Zebrowski, E., 1997. Perils of a Restless Planet: Scientific Perspectives on Natural Disasters. Cambridge University Press, Cambridge, UK.

4

DISASTER, DAILY LIFE AND MEANING

DIKAIOS SAKELLARIOU ▪ SUSANN BAEZ ULLBERG

INTRODUCTION

Disasters are extraordinary totalizing events 'sweeping across every aspect of human life' (Oliver-Smith 2004, p. 10). They put community integration at risk and can lead to impoverishment, high prevalence of disease and increased morbidity in both resource poor and resource rich contexts (Norris et al 2002, 2005, PAHO 2000) – issues that in and of themselves are determinants of access to occupation (Wilcock 2006). In disaster contexts, a combination of factors associated with disruption of everyday life patterns is often present, making it difficult to distinguish one factor from the other in accounts of individual experience. Populations in disaster affected areas are likely to experience loss of livelihood, shortage of food, disruption of access to health services, forced evacuation or trauma (Noji 1997). Increased incidence of post-traumatic stress disorder (Crighton et al 2003) and intrafamilial violence (Curtis et al 2000) has been observed after disasters, and increased morbidity and incidence of illness or epidemics are common (Norris et al 2002). The Hyogo Framework for Action 2005–2015 (United Nations 2005) states that disasters severely compromise community development efforts and can lead to a downward spiral of poverty. Disasters are affecting large numbers of people around the world. As such it is important to achieve an understanding of their social impact, while equally crucial to understand how they are experienced by affected individuals. The Hyogo declaration and the subsequent policy work at global, regional and national levels hitherto specifically states that active involvement of affected communities is essential in disaster preparedness and vulnerability reduction efforts. This cannot be achieved without exploring how communities and individuals themselves experience disaster and its impact on their everyday occupations and lives.

Giving voice to individual and community experiences of disaster and occupation also means gaining an insight on the historical construction of disasters. Models that view disasters as one-off events inevitably neglect the underlying factors that shape disaster vulnerability and risk. Moreover, disaster prevention strategies do not always address the underlying causes of disasters. Disasters can thus be said to have a 'double nature'. While they are perceived as disruptive events from a relative 'normal' everyday life, they are at the same time social processes that are not only historically embedded in economic, political and cultural structures but also subject to contestations and negotiations on their meaning.

The aim of this chapter is to discuss the experience of disaster as it unfolds in everyday individual and social life, by forwarding some key theoretical concepts in this context such as public bad, communality and heteroglossia. To illustrate the discussion, we draw on examples from different empirical studies on how disaster affects individuals and communities, and in particular on the case of the 2003 flood in the city of Santa Fe in the north-east of Argentina.

NATURAL DISASTER AS CULTURAL MYTH AND PUBLIC BADS

The use of the word 'natural' in relation with disasters has a dual meaning. It refers on the one hand to disasters caused by natural hazards (floods, earthquakes, drought, etc.) but it also implies a notion of naturalness and inevitability. 'Natural disasters' are often considered random events that can affect anyone, anywhere and at any time. This has been called the cultural myth of natural disasters (Wisner et al 2004) in light of research that shows that the impact of disasters is unequally spread across the population along lines of class, gender and ethnicity. The only natural thing about such disasters is the hazardous force emerging from nature but, even so, it can be held that many phenomena involving nature are in fact produced by humans. Climate change is currently the most emblematic example of this. Oliver-Smith (1999) argues that disasters are socially embedded events, symptomatic of societies' failure to adapt to changing circumstances. 'Natural disasters' can in this vein be conceptualized as the outcomes of a dynamic interaction between geophysical hazards and the vulnerable conditions of a population (Blaikie et al 1994, McEntire 2001, Weichselgartner 2001, Wisner et al 2004, 2012). Boyce (2000, p. 256) has described vulnerability as 'public bads', which, just like public goods, are not distributed equitably across the population. Empirical examples abound in the disaster literature, but just to mention a few we refer to Chou et al's (2004) study on the aftermath of the 1999 earthquake in Taiwan, which showed that risk of death is positively correlated with low socioeconomic status and disability, and there is extensive evidence from other settings on the relationship between socioeconomic status and increased disaster impact (see, for example, Ahern & Galea 2006, Chen et al 2007). Another example can be taken from the dry zone of Nicaragua. Here drought is a recurrent problem in general for poor people in rural areas, yet men and women employ different coping practices, which in the long run in fact make women more vulnerable to droughts than men (Segnestam 2009).

Disasters, in this sense, do not strike randomly, and their impact is, to an extent, preventable (Bauman 2006) or at least predictable. This is particularly true when it comes to 'natural' disasters. Communities living in naturally hazardous environments are generally well aware of the risks they live with and develop practices in order to mitigate such risks. In the city of Santa Fe, in the north-west of Argentina, people know that extraordinary floods will occur every now and then from the Paraná and the Salado rivers. Historically people have settled on higher ground as a common strategy to mitigate the effects of the floods. Yet urban sprawl and growing social inequalities in the twentieth century increasingly forced poor people to settle in lowland flood-prone areas, where evacuation and reliance on governmental disaster relief have become their only means to cope with the recurrent floods (Ullberg 2013). Yet, as the concept of 'public bad' indicates, such practices are not equally accessible to every member in a community and are furthermore subject to differentiation along lines of gender, age, ethnicity and class, as well as to changes over time. These categories are not to be taken deterministically, however. As Fjord & Manderson warn, such categories 'often replicate the explanation that people's characteristics are responsible for tragic outcomes rather than the social inequalities that ensure they will be harmed. That they are poor, they are children, or they use a wheelchair becomes an easy rationale for their suffering' (2009, p. 65). Focusing on vulnerability as a public bad thus implies the need to address issues of social inequality between social categories rather than any inherent vulnerability of the categories per se.

THE VULNERABILITY APPROACH

Disability as one such category is increasingly being paid attention to in disaster contexts, ranging from the UN Convention on the Rights of Persons with Disabilities to more scholarly work (cf. Kett & Twigg 2007, Fjord & Manderson 2009). Aspects such as the conveying of vital information through live text feed on television that are inaccessible to people with visual impairments due to the lack of audio description (Gerber 2009), or denial of shelter access to people with obvious impairments, as has been reported was the practice by the American Red Cross in the aftermath of Hurricane Katrina (National Council on Disability 2006), are practices that reinforce lines between people. Social inequalities do not vanish in the context of disasters; on the contrary, they are often exacerbated. Individuals experience disaster in different ways, depending on their specific vantage point and the resources to which they have access within a larger social and cultural context. It is important that disaster preparedness and prevention models take into account social inequalities and how these impact on individuals in the context of disasters, as quite simply these are often the deciding factors between surviving and perishing.

The vulnerability approach has been criticized for its objectivism and for not taking account of either resilience as a means of coping with disaster or the point of view of those that have to cope with them (Birkmann 2006, Hewitt 1997, Hogan & Marandola 2005, Oliver-Smith 2004). The meanings people make of a disastrous event are culturally contingent as well as shaped by individual experience. Thus, while vulnerability as an approach is fruitful and crucial in the analysis of causality because it encompasses the multiple dimensions of disaster impacts, that is, its political, economic and cultural nature, its materiality and temporality as well as its individual and collective dimensions, it also needs to be unpacked (Oliver-Smith 2002, p. 29). This is necessary in order to forward our understanding, not only of how disasters are socially produced but also how they are culturally and individually experienced in and through everyday life.

COMMUNITY AND COMMUNALITY

The notion of 'community' is important in exploring everyday life after a disaster, as is the significance of the immediate social group (family, neighbourhood, greater community) that often offers support to disaster victims. Survivors of disasters have reported receiving more support from their social networks than from institutions meant to provide relief (Ibanez et al 2003). Social networks, trust and support in a community are generally thought to promote more effective disaster recovery and preparedness (Nakagawa & Shaw 2004). Many scholars use the concept 'social capital' to analyse such processes. Social capital is a concept with multiple definitions and applications (Bourdieu 1986, Coleman 1990, Jacobs 1961, Putnam 1993, 2000) that is widely used also in disaster research, predominantly drawing on Putnam's definition. However, in line with the critique that states that social capital represents an economic reductionist view of social relations (Navarro 2002) and is an analytical concept with ideological connotations (Smith & Kulynych 2002) that disregards power and politics as

constitutive to social relations, we prefer Erikson's concept 'communality' (1976a) to describe such social relations.

Informal social networks and the support they provide can contribute to the rebuilding of civil society after a disaster, as the example of the social mobilization after the Kobe earthquake illustrates. Here, listening to the survivors' voices was an important stage in the community rebuilding efforts that were initiated by the affected community and resulted in the development of the Kobe Action Plan (Shaw & Goda 2004). Yet it is necessary to look into the quality of those networks and not assume that because they exist they are inherently good. Erikson's early study (1976a, 1976b) on the Buffalo Creek flooding in the USA in 1976 shows that the disaster worked as a catalyst in further weakening the already strained preexisting social relations within the small community shaped by increasing unemployment and poverty in the Appalachians. An analogy can be made with the situation of the Ik in Uganda in the 1970s where large-scale social and political processes of disastrous scope had, through the previous decades, generated a starving people largely mistrustful of each other and internally divided (Turnbull 1972). In the Argentinean city of Santa Fe, despite efforts to mitigate recurrent flooding by technological means (embankments, water pumps, etc.), social vulnerability has been a constant among the poorest sectors of the community through the reproduction of historical class relations and the social category of the *inundado*, the flooded subject. This has contributed to the normalization of this natural disaster in Santa Fe. Every flood would operate to reinforce existing class differences, hence perpetuating them (Ullberg 2013). Thus, we suggest that the notion of communality and the importance of preexisting bonds for disaster coping must be empirically explored, because it is also a well documented phenomenon that solidarity in a community struck by disaster emerges regardless of preexisting communality. This has been conceptualized as 'city of comrades' (Prince 1920), 'therapeutic community' (Fritz 1961), 'altruistic community' (Barton 1969), 'community of suffering' (Oliver-Smith 1986) and 'brotherhood of pain' (Oliver-Smith 1999). Disasters tend to work as a bonding experience among people, creating 'communitas' (Turner 1974, Turner 2012). The emergence of what Malkki calls 'accidental communities of memory' (1995, p. 186) suggests that collective trauma can operate as a 'spiritual kinship' among people who have experienced the same event, thus bringing a community together even where people did not know each other before the catastrophe.

In all cases there seem to be reasons to follow this process of communality over time, as social relations are dynamic processes. Some social relations, such as kinship, are generally thought of as more resilient, while other social networks can fade and disappear. The trust in this social network produced through the shared experience of being victims of a disaster thus diminished or disappeared with time, which affected negatively the sense of support for individuals. The role and quality of communality must thus not be taken for granted but rather strived for to be inclusive and to bridge preexisting as well as emerging differences within a community.

For social networks to be efficient in coping with disaster, there must be an understanding of needs, desires and experiences between disaster survivors and people working in the reconstruction phase after a disaster. However, as illustrated above, often all these actors express different realities and different representations of everyday life after a disaster. The way people talk is a means through which they represent the world around them; talk expresses people's realities, their meaning-worlds. Cordasco et al (2007) illustrate how different agendas between disaster survivors and officials can lead to distrust towards authorities. This can prove a challenging issue to deal with when designing disaster preparedness and mitigation strategies, not least when it comes to contexts where hazards are recurrent, such as climatic and geophysical ones. The institutional loss of credibility, as an expression of lack of trust, is a serious matter when the worst happens (Box 4-1).

STORIES OF DISASTER AND EVERYDAY LIFE

A disaster, defined as an event/process that disrupts the social order (Oliver-Smith & Hoffman 2002), creates a volatile environment where infrastructure, social networks and institutions are greatly affected. What people did before and do after the disaster can be very

---

BOX 4-1
LA INUNDACIÓN

On April 29, 2003, the lives of many people in the city of Santa Fe, Argentina, would change forever. That was the day of La Inundación, the disastrous flood that killed at least 23 people and forced 130 000 to evacuate for weeks and months. While local, provincial and national government provided scarce emergency relief, people from the whole of Argentina became engaged and all kinds of donations were received. Yet there was no organization in place to take care of this virtual flood of goods. Flood victims had to put up with bureaucratic odysseys to get registered as 'inundados' (flood victims) in order to receive assistance during the evacuation. The presence of navy military forces for the evacuation and the distribution of food and clothing was also traumatic to many – the last military dictatorship cast long shadows even in this context. There was a prevailing sense of chaos and abandonment long after the waters had receded. Many suffered from what they felt was arrogance and disrespect from authorities due to their condition of being an 'inundado' – a sense of indignity. 'They treated us like livestock in the evacuation centres as well as in the lines for food and clothes', a young woman complained. It was equally traumatic to finally return home just to find it ruined, completely covered in foul-smelling mud and all belongings damaged or destroyed. People had to throw away ruined furniture, electronic devices and personal belongings. In fact, local authorities recommended they did so for health and sanitary reasons. Mirta, a middle-aged woman from the middle-class district of Cavas, spoke about her ruined family albums: 'It was as if my whole life had vanished ... [the pictures] were filled with clay and shit from the dirty flood water ... having to take them out of the house and just throw them away ... there's no way I can explain the pain that I felt ... a mix of pain, sadness, hate and anger'.

---

different. Changes in the physical, political and social environment create new demands and impose additional restrictions on what individuals and groups can do in their communities. The way people perceive and talk about everyday life can be viewed as a meaning-making mechanism.

The importance of stories according to Frank (2002) is that by giving lives a sense of continuity and meaning they make them legible, and thus they enable people to communicate towards a negotiated common understanding. Storytelling is thus essentially a social practice. Molineux & Rickard (2003, p. 54) argue that storied approaches to exploring occupation are a powerful tool as they 'provide insight into … human action which is socially and culturally situated'. Now, the stories that people tell, what they communicate and how, depend on whom they interact with (Moen 2006). Stories then are not, and cannot be, about everlasting truths. The way people construct their reality and make sense of their world is dynamic, subjective and contingent not only upon who tells the story and to whom but also upon the context in which the story is told. Individual and social actors alike are driven by different motives and logics in their storytelling. Taken together, these different voices constitute what Bakhtin (1995a) has called a heteroglossic discourse.

HETEROGLOSSIA

Heteroglossia refers to the presence of 'another's speech in another's language', for example the presence of multiple perspectives within a novel, those of the author and those of the protagonists. In an analogy with the textual construction of a novel, where heroes are situated in interactions initiated by the author and act within preset boundaries, social actors operate within an inescapable dominant cultural discourse. These multiple 'languages', the diverse perspectives of the various actors together with the scripts, beliefs and attitudes present in society, comprise the social whole that is the setting of human action. The various vantage points from which people view the world, their different perspectives and the different 'languages' they speak are intertwined in relationships of power. In exploring individual stories from different vantage points it is therefore necessary to acknowledge the presence and validity of a multitude of voices.

Experiences of everyday life in the context of disaster are rarely heard, leading to a devaluation of community and individual perspectives. As Button (2002) stresses, the origin of the interpretations heard in the aftermath of a disaster, who can and who cannot talk about it, is of crucial importance in guiding reconstruction efforts, developing future policies and influencing the public discourse. Disabled people in particular often find that their voices, including vital knowledge on disaster prevention, response and mitigation for all, are silenced and their needs are not heard. Yet the flood victims in Santa Fe contradict this view. As an 'accidental community of memory' they

enact public street manifestations on a regular basis (Box 4-2) and often take spectacular actions that call the attention of local and even national media (Ullberg 2010). They have also published and produced a vast number of books and films (mainly in the documentary genre) that 'tell their story'. These stories are founded in the Latin American literary genre of *testimonio* which addresses 'wounds that have yet to heal because they have never fully been acknowledged' (Argenti 2007, p. 25).

Reality is shaped subjectively in heterogeneous contexts, thus meanings of events are likely to be subject to contestation. In the context of disaster, such struggles occur both in the acute phase and in the post-disaster phase when different people frame the events in varying ways (Goffman 1959) and thus enact different responses to it. In the Boliden mine spill in southern Spain in 1998, three different meanings were ascribed to the disaster: that of the company, which saw it as a loss of production and image; that of the local government and national public opinion, which framed it as an environmental catastrophe due to its vast ecological effects, not least in the adjacent Doñana National Park; and that of the local farmers and inhabitants, who experienced it as a blow to the local economy and their farming livelihood (Ullberg 2001).

STORIES OF DISASTER IN A HETEROGLOSSIC CONTEXT

As Bakhtin (1995a, 1995b) reminds us, language can never be neutral, but it is always rich with meaning, constituting an operational means for social discourse. Disasters are revelatory because '… the fundamental features of society and culture are laid bare in stark relief by the reduction of priorities to basic social, cultural, and material necessities' (Sahlins 1972, cited in Oliver-Smith 1996, p. 304). This is a heterogeneous context in which several discourses coexist: official and vernacular, personal and political, explicit and implicit, scientific and narrative. The words used in each case are embedded within unique conceptual systems, each of them trying to enter into dialogue with the other systems. Survivors, for example, will need to get their voices heard and their needs known; they will want to be part of the reconstruction of their own lives.

BOX 4-2
THE BLACK TENT OF MEMORY AND DIGNITY

In May 2003, one month after the flood, it had become publicly known in Santa Fe that 200 metres of the levee that was intended to protect the city from the Salado river floods had in fact never been built and that through this 'entrance' the flood had entered the city. The governor of the time had in a press conference declared that 'nobody had informed him' either about the infrastructural problems, or about the severity of the flood, accounting for the negligence of the local authorities in terms of disaster preparedness. This outraged those Santafesinos who had lost everything. The inundados chose the main plaza to stage a manifestation. The protest was set up by raising a tent in the middle of the plaza, the Black Tent of Memory and Dignity' (Figure 4-1), which would be the beginning of a new political horizon in Santa Fe.

On April 29th our lives were transformed in all senses. We lost our lives, the everyday life; that which we have now discovered – now that we don't have it – gives us an order that each and every one of us constructs at home, with our flowers, our animals, in every corner, in the backyard, on the street, with our neighbours. Everyday life changed into the extraordinary ... we realised that living from now on would be a difficult task. So, we met in the street corners, we improvised meetings, we talked everybody at the same time because it was all mixed up; the need, the pain, the anger, the powerlessness. We suddenly realised that we were on our own ... the census, the lining up, the distribution [of relief assistance], everything turned into a torture! We hit the roof, but nobody would listen. Every 29th we would meet in the street, increasingly worried and rebelling against the certainty that we were being forgotten ... So ... with the support of the people today in this square the Tent of the 'Inundados' is raised to resist. No water or mud this time, but with the same pain and sense of abandonment. We raise this tent for dignity, for justice, for recovery, for our dead and sick. No to impunity! We have learned from this disaster that we live in an insecure city and that we have rulers that ignore a large part of the population which only claims to be treated as citizens.

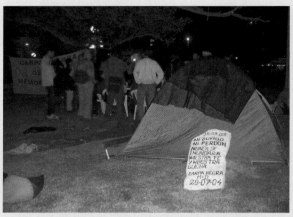

FIGURE 4-1 ■ The Black Tent of Memory and Dignity, Santa Fe, 2004.

Yet the various vantage points from which people view the world and construct their reality in stories are intertwined in relationships of power. In a study on representations of experience after a natural disaster, Cox et al (2008) argued that the voice heard was male, authoritative and institutionalized, perpetuating public discourse of disaster survivors as helpless, needy and in need of 'expert knowledge'. Analysing newspaper articles in the aftermath of the disaster they found that voices of survivors were not heard and did not inform the public discourse on recovery; the voices of survivors were discredited. The victims of the 2003 flood in Santa Fe have made efforts to contest such discrediting discourse, not only through numerous and consistent street protests, but also by publishing testimonies of the disaster. Numerous books, films, monuments, street graffiti and internet interfaces have been produced in the wake of this flood, constituting a counter discourse to that of the local government (Ullberg 2013).

Different perspectives and voices need to be heard and taken into account so that a common ground for negotiated understanding can be established. Through the exploration of personal testimony and the promotion of exchange of such testimonies, a shared understanding of everyday life after natural disasters can be established (Garro 2000, Mattingly & Garro 2000) through which reconstruction after the catastrophe can be facilitated. Each individual's narrative depicts a cycle of events, causes and motivations which may ultimately be interrelated, directly or less directly (Ricoeur 1990). The development of heteroglossic awareness would inform disaster preparedness and prevention efforts and community development strategies. It would enable people professionally involved in these to effectively 'translate' and make sense of the various ways everyday life is affected after a disaster.

CONCLUSION

Throughout this chapter our aim has been to introduce an occupational perspective that takes account of people's experiences from disasters. Affected communities need to be actively involved in the disaster preparedness and response process. This would enhance our understanding of how people make meaning of such disruptive events in everyday life and how they act upon them. It can get us closer to people's experiences when the worst happens. Such an understanding can enhance disaster preparedness and improve mitigative as well as reconstruction efforts. In order to establish a notion of collaboration and negotiated understanding it is important to explore the experience of everyday life after a disaster, taking account of social inequalities and the multiplicity of voices that shape experience.

REFERENCES

Ahern, J., Galea, S., 2006. Social context and depression after a disaster: the role of income inequality. J. Epidemiol. Community Health 60, 766–770.

Argenti, N., 2007. The Intestines of the State: Youth, Violence and Belated Histories in the Cameroon Grassfields. University of Chicago Press, Chicago, p. 25.

Bakhtin, M., 1995a. Heteroglossia in the novel. In: Dentith, S. (Ed.), Bakhtinian Thought: An Introductory Reader. Routledge, London, pp. 195–224.

Bakhtin, M., 1995b. The heteroglot novel. In: Morris, S. (Ed.), The Bakhtin Reader; Selected Writings of Bakhtin, Medvedev, Voloshinov. Arnold, London, pp. 112–122.

Barton, A.H., 1969. Communities in Disaster. Doubleday, New York.

Bauman, Z., 2006. Liquid Fear. Polity, Cambridge.

Birkmann, J., 2006. Measuring vulnerability to promote disaster-resilient societies: conceptual frameworks and definitions. In: Birkmann, J. (Ed.), Measuring Vulnerability to Natural Disasters: Towards Resilient Societies. United Nations University, Tokyo, pp. 9–54.

Blaikie, P., Cannon, T., Davis, I., Wisner, B., 1994. At Risk; Natural Hazards, People's Vulnerability and Disasters. Routledge, London.

Bourdieu, P., 1986. The Forms of Capital. In: Richardson, J.G. (Ed.), Handbook of Theory and Research for the Sociology of Education. Greenwood, Westport, CT.

Boyce, J., 2000. Let them eat risk? Wealth, rights and disaster vulnerability. Disasters 24 (3), 254–261.

Button, G., 2002. Popular media reframing of man-made disasters: a cautionary tale. In: Hoffman, S., Oliver-Smith, A. (Eds.), Catastrophe and Culture: The Anthropology of Disaster. School of American Research Press, Santa Fe, pp. 143–158.

Chen, A., Keith, V., Airriess, C., Li, W., Leong, K., 2007. Economic vulnerability, discrimination, and hurricane Katrina: health among Black Katrina survivors in Eastern New Orleans. J. Am. Psychiatr. Nurses Assoc. 13, 257–266.

Chou, Y., Huang, N., Lee, C., Tsai, S., Chen, L., Chang, H., 2004. Who is at risk of death in an earthquake? Am. J. Epidemiol. 160 (7), 688–695.

Coleman, J.S., 1990. Foundations of Social Theory. Harvard University Press, Cambridge, MA.

Cordasco, K., Eisenman, D., Glik, D., Golden, J., Asch, S., 2007. 'They blew the levee': distrust of authorities among hurricane Katrina evacuees. J. Health Care Poor Underserved 18, 277–282.

Cox, R., Long, B., Jones, M., Handler, R., 2008. Critical discourse analysis of natural disaster media coverage. J. Health Psychol. 13 (4), 469–480.

Crighton, E., Elliott, S., van der Meer, J., Small, I., Upsur, R., 2003. Impacts of an environmental disaster on psychosocial health and wellbeing in Karakalpakstan. Soc. Sci. Med. 56, 551–567.

Curtis, T., Miller, B., Berry, E., 2000. Changes in reports and incidence of child abuse following natural disasters. Child Abuse Negl. 24 (9), 1151–1162.

Erikson, K.T., 1976a. Everything in Its Path: Destruction of Community in the Buffalo Creek Flood. Simon and Schuster, New York.

Erikson, K.T., 1976b. Disaster at Buffalo Creek. Loss of communality at Buffalo Creek. Am. J. Psychiatry 133, 302–305.

Fjord, L., Manderson, L., 2009. Anthropological perspectives on disasters and disability: an introduction. Hum. Organ. 68 (1), 64–72.

Frank, A., 2002. Why study people's stories? The dialogical ethics of narrative analysis. Int. J. Qual. Meth. 1 (1), Article 6. Online. Available from: <http://ejournals.library.ualberta.ca/index.php/IJQM/index>.

Fritz, C., 1961. Disasters. In: Merton, R., Nisbet, R. (Eds.), Contemporary Social Problems. Harcourt, New York, pp. 651–694.

Garro, L.C., 2000. Cultural knowledge as resource in illness narratives. In: Mattingly, C., Garro, L.C. (Eds.), Narrative and the Cultural Construction of Illness and Healing. Berkley, California, pp. 70–87.

Gerber, E., 2009. Describing tragedy: the information access needs of blind people in emergency-related circumstances. Hum. Organ. 68 (1), 73–81.

Goffman, E., 1959. The Presentation of Self in Everyday Life. Doubleday Anchor, New York.

Hewitt, K., 1997. Regions of Risk: A Geographical Introduction to Disasters. Addison Wesley Longman, Essex.

Hogan, D., Marandola, E., 2005. Towards an interdisciplinary conceptualisation of vulnerability. Popul. Space Place 11, 455–471.

Ibanez, G., Katchikian, N., Buck, C., Weishaar, D., Abush-Kirsh, T., Lavizzo, E., et al., 2003. Qualitative analysis of social support and conflict among Mexican and Mexican-American disaster survivors. J. Community Psychol. 31 (1), 1–23.

Jacobs, J., 1961. The Death and Life of the Great American Cities. Vintage, New York.

Kett, M., Twigg, J., 2007. Disability and disasters: towards an inclusive approach. In: World Disaster Report 2007. International Federation of the Red Cross and the Red Crescent, Geneva.

Malkki, L., 1995. Purity and Exile: Violence, Memory, and National Cosmology Among Hutu Refugees in Tanzania. Chicago University Press, Chicago.

Mattingly, C., Garro, L.C., 2000. Narrative as construct and construction. In: Mattingly, C., Garro, L.C. (Eds.), Narrative and the Cultural Construction of Illness and Healing. Berkley, California, pp. 1–49.

McEntire, D., 2001. Triggering agents, vulnerabilities and disaster reduction: towards a holistic paradigm. Disaster Prev. Manag. 10 (3), 189–196.

Moen, T., 2006. Reflection on the narrative research approach. Int. J. Qual. Meth. 5 (4), Article 5. Online. Available from: <http://ejournals.library.ualberta.ca/index.php/IJQM/index>.

Molineux, M., Rickard, W., 2003. Storied approaches to understanding occupation. J. Occup. Sci. 10 (1), 52–60.

Nakagawa, Y., Shaw, R., 2004. Social capital: a missing link to disaster recovery. Int. J. Mass Emerg. Disasters 22 (1), 5–34.

National Council on Disability. The Impact of Hurricanes Katrina and Rita on People with Disabilities: A Look Back and Remaining Challenges. Washington, DC: 2006. Online. Available from: <http://www.ncd.gov/publications/2006/Aug072006>.

Navarro, V.A., 2002. Critique of social capital. Int. J. Health Serv. 32 (3), 423–432.

Noji, E., 1997. The nature of disaster: general characteristics and public health effects. In: Noji, E. (Ed.), The Public Health Consequences of Disasters. Oxford University Press, New York, pp. 3–20.

Norris, F., Friedman, M., Watson, P., Byrne, C., Diaz, E., Kaniasty, K., 2002. 60,000 disaster victims speak, part I: an empirical review of the empirical literature, 1981–2000. Psychiatry 65 (2), 207–239.

Norris, F., Baker, C., Murphy, A., Kaniasty, K., 2005. Social support mobilization and deterioration after Mexico's 1999 flood: effects of context, gender and time. Am. J. Community Psychol. 36 (Nos 1/2), 15–28.

Oliver-Smith, A., 1996. Anthropological research on hazards and disasters. Annu. Rev. Anthropol. 25, 303–328.

Oliver-Smith, A., 1999. What is a disaster? Anthropological perspectives on a persistent question. In: Oliver-Smith, A., Hoffman, S. (Eds.), The Angry Earth: Disaster in Anthropological Perspective. Routledge, New York, pp. 18–34.

Oliver-Smith, A., 2002. Theorizing disasters: nature, power, and culture. In: Hoffman, S., Oliver-Smith, A. (Eds.), Catastrophe and Culture; The Anthropology of Disaster. School of American Research Press, Santa Fe, pp. 23–47.

Oliver-Smith, A., Hoffman, S., 2002. Introduction: why anthropologists should study disasters. In: Hoffman, S., Oliver-Smith, A. (Eds.), Catastrophe and Culture; The Anthropology of Disaster. School of American Research Press, Santa Fe, pp. 3–22.

Oliver-Smith, O., 2004. Theorizing vulnerability in a globalized world: a political ecology perspective. In: Bankoff, G., Frerks, G.,

Hilhorst, D. (Eds.), Mapping Vulnerability: Disasters, Development and People. Earthscan, London, pp. 10–24.

PAHO (Pan American Health Organization), 2000. Natural Disasters: Protecting the Public's Health. Pan American Health Organization, Washington, DC.

Prince, S., 1920. Catastrophe and Social Change. Columbia Studies in the Social Sciences, 94(1). Columbia University, New York.

Putnam, R., 1993. Making Democracy Work: Civic Traditions in Modern Italy. Princeton University Press, Princeton, N.J., pp. 28–29.

Putnam, R., 2000. Bowling Alone: The Collapse and Revival of American Community. Simon and Schuster, New York.

Ricoeur, P., 1990. Time and Narrative, vol. 1. Translated by Kathleen McLaughlin and David Pellauer. University of Chicago Press, Chicago.

Segnestam, L., 2009. Division of capitals – what role does it play for gender-differentiated vulnerability to drought in Nicaragua? Community Dev. 40 (2), 154–176.

Shaw, R., Goda, K., 2004. From disaster to sustainable civic society: the Kobe experience. Disasters 28 (1), 16–40.

Smith, S.S., Kulynych, J., 2002. It may be social, but why is it capital? The social construction of social capital and the politics of language. Polit. Soc. 30 (Nr.1), 149–186.

Turnbull, C., 1972. The Mountain People. Simon & Schuster, New York.

Turner, E., 2012. Communitas: The Anthropology of Collective Joy. Palgrave Macmillan, New York.

Turner, V., 1974. Dramas, Fields, and Metaphors: Symbolic Action in Human Society. Cornell University Press, pp. 273–274.

Ullberg, S., 2001. Environmental Crisis in Spain: The Boliden Dam Rupture. Crisis Management Europe Research Program, vol. 14. ÖCB/The Swedish Agency for Emergency Planning, Stockholm.

Ullberg, S., 2010. De inundados a Inundados: posdesastre y movilización social en Santa Fe, Argentina. In: Visacovsky, S. (Ed.), Estados Críticos. Estudios Sobre La Experiencia Social De La Calamidad. Editorial Antropofagia, Buenos Aires.

Ullberg, S., 2013. Watermarks: Urban Flooding and Memoryscape in Argentina. (Doctoral Dissertation). Acta Universitatis Stockholmiensis, Stockholm.

United Nations, 2005. Report of the World Conference on Disaster Reduction, Kobe. Online. Available from: <http://www.unisdr.org/2005/wcdr/thematic-sessions/WCDR-proceedings-of-the-Conference.pdf>.

Weichselgartner, J., 2001. Disaster mitigation: the concept of vulnerability revisited. Disaster Prev. Manag. 10 (2), 85–94.

Wilcock, A., 2006. An Occupational Perspective of Health, second ed. Slack Inc, Thorofare, NJ.

Wisner, B., Blaikie, P., Cannon, T., Davis, I., 2004. At Risk; Natural Hazards, People's Vulnerability and Disasters. Routledge, London.

Wisner, B., Gaillard, J.C., Kelman, I. (Eds.), 2012. Handbook of Hazards and Disaster Risk Reduction. Routledge Handbooks, London.

5

LOST IN THE MIX: A CASE FOR INCLUSIVE AND PARTICIPATORY APPROACHES TO DISASTER AND DEVELOPMENT

NANCY RUSHFORD

INTRODUCTION

This chapter looks at the issue of social inequality in disaster through the lens of disability. People with disabilities are among the most socially disadvantaged in society. They are especially at risk in situations of disaster and face significant barriers to accessing critical supports for recovery. The occupational therapy profession espouses a social vision of a healthy, just and inclusive society, within which experiences of disability have been of longstanding interest to the profession. This chapter aligns occupational therapy practice with inclusive and participatory approaches to disaster and development as it involves persons with disabilities. Disability serves as a foundation to develop ideas around the integration of occupation with disaster and development.

A STORY OF SURVIVAL AND RESILIENCE

The Letter ...

His letter arrived three years after the 2004 Indian Ocean tsunami. It rested on my doorstep remarkably intact, having forged a rather uncertain path from its place of origin, a small, once devastated village on the northeast coast of Aceh, Indonesia, to its final destination – my home on the east coast of Australia. The impressive fact about this letter was that it arrived, against all odds, with little and at times no formal infrastructure to carry it along its way. The small community in which it originated was rendered largely

inaccessible by the disaster, so the letter travelled via an informal network of people who carried it by foot, motorcycle, vehicle and plane. It rested in satchels and suitcases along the way and somewhere in safe-keeping was translated then set back on its path. When I finally held it in my hand it represented more to me than a message relayed between two people from different parts of the world. Rather, it illuminated the transformative potential of human occupation and revealed how that simple connection between two people can spark an entire network of support capable of traversing great distance.

Social Change and Personal Transformation

The letter itself told a story about personal transformation and collaborative engagement. I opened it carefully, gently tugging on the edge of thin paper until both it and a photograph broke free from the envelope. A young man's face grinned at me. He was seated in a wheelchair in front of a village shop, surrounded by hanging baskets of food, candies and everyday conveniences to sell. He looked proud. I barely recognized him.

His name was Bima[1] and I had met him while working with a local outreach team in the rehabilitation and recovery efforts following the tsunami. Bima was paralysed, having sustained a spinal cord injury prior to the tsunami. When disaster struck he had managed to get to safety with the help of his father and a nurse who hoisted him to the roof of the hospital. Although Bima was dependent on others for survival

---

[1]Name changed to protect identity.

41

during the emergency, he was far from helpless; his potential, however, was eclipsed by the actions and attitudes of others who believed the contrary.

Rehabilitation and Recovery

When we met Bima he was bedridden, physically weak and mentally exhausted. His body showed signs of muscle wasting and skin breakdown; his mind was plagued by anxiety and nightmares. Bima spent most of his day unoccupied and alone while others worked to rebuild their lives. He was so isolated in his experience that there appeared no alternative beyond the confines of his bed. Bima was caught in a cycle of dependency; his family did everything they could for him. But the more they did, the weaker he became in body, mind and spirit. Ironically, the weaker he became, the less chance he had of receiving the support he needed to live – to create and sustain a livelihood. As a person with a disability, Bima was either invisible to the aid and development agencies offering assistance in the area or was denied support on the basis that he 'did not qualify'.

We instinctively responded to Bima's discouragement on a human level by sharing with him stories of others as a way of offering hope. These stories were about the experiences of other people with disabilities, also affected by disaster, who had carved out a livelihood from the loss and injustice that had pervaded their lives. They offered alternatives to Bima's situation and illuminated possibility within his experience of darkness. The stories struck a chord within him. This was revealed through one spontaneous yet symbolic gesture…

A Symbolic Gesture

He took hold of a rope.

Not a lifeline thrown to him but one thrown by him.

The rope served a practical purpose; tied to the ceiling above his bed, it enabled him to sit up and in time transfer out of bed independently. But on a symbolic level, Bima's reality transformed the moment his family helped him attach the rope.

The life-changing effect of this action within the environment around him was remarkable. Once he took hold of the rope he became visible and his goals crystallized. He told us he wanted to run a local shop.

Astonishingly, people mobilized around him, including ourselves, to help him reach his goal.

Information was passed through community networks; resources were secured and made available by agencies that had previously denied him. In time, but not without setbacks, Bima regained a livelihood and a life. A shop was constructed, it was made accessible and he proudly became a vendor within his community.

The Power of Human Connection

Bima's letter and story illuminated to me the power of human connection and collective action. As a mobilizing force it has the potential to transform – to spark networks that connect people and strengthen communities. Relating to the experiences of others through stories that offered hope gave Bima the strength to grab the rope. It mobilized a community around his goals and broke the cycle of dependency that defined his daily life.

Standing there on my doorstep with that letter in hand, I stared intently at its author – a protagonist within his own story; once isolated and 'helpless', he had emerged … reconnected and resilient.

Two Years On …

Two years later, and with further advancements in social media and technology, I received a message from Bima's brother via Facebook. He told me that Bima was well and had become a respected shaman in his village. Once again he had reinvented himself.

At the heart of Bima's recovery was his ability to adapt: to explore alternatives and modify his actions and occupations in response to changing circumstances in life. Bima did not do this on his capabilities alone. It necessitated a supportive and enabling environment with the requisite community skills, ability and resources to support his recovery. With the 'right' kind of support, assistance and opportunity, Bima's daily life and experience changed. His story took a different course.

DISABILITY AND DISASTER

People with disabilities are not only the most deprived of human beings in the developing world, they are also the most neglected. It is important to acknowledge that more than 600 million people in the world live with some form of disability. More than 400 million of them live in developing countries often amid poverty, isolation and despair (Sen & Wolfensohn 2004).

To this point within the book, we have illuminated the social and ecological dimensions of disaster and its inherent complexities as they play out in the field. Further to this, we have emphasized the importance of listening to the voices of survivors relating their individual and community experience and the occupations of everyday life. Disaster tells a story about people and their relationships with each other and the environment that is largely characterized by social inequality and exclusion. Within that story, people with disabilities represent a particularly vulnerable group in that they are frequently trapped in cycles of poverty and disadvantage (WHO 2011). People with disabilities are more likely to live in hazard-prone areas and lack the power and resources to cope with disaster or avoid hazardous threats (UNISDR 2013). As such, disability is more than an individual issue; it is a social issue. It is not only a health issue, but is one that cuts across disaster and development. In other words, disability is about people and their social relationships; it reflects interaction with the community and the environment (Parnes 2008).

The profession of occupational therapy ultimately aims to support health and participation by promoting engagement in occupation based on the belief that 'all people need to be able or enabled to engage in the occupations of their need and choice and to grow through what they do ...' (Wilcock & Townsend 2008, p.198). This vision resonates with a social development perspective and its emphasis on expanding people's choices and opportunities within a sustainable development context. Enabling equal opportunity for all persons to access and participate in a range of meaningful occupations is of fundamental importance to occupational therapists who carry with them into the field of disaster and development the profession's commitment to occupational justice and self-determination (Figure 5-1).

PERSPECTIVES ON DISABILITY AND DISASTER

Similar to changes in society's perception of disaster over time, perspectives on disability have evolved from

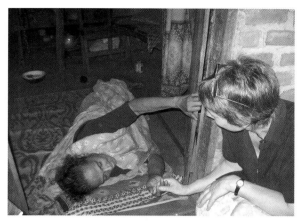

FIGURE 5-1 ■ An older woman immobilized following a disaster-related injury. Older, female people with disabilities are among the most vulnerable and marginalized in disaster contexts. A visiting occupational therapist worked with local disability and aged care volunteers to facilitate mobilization, functional capacity and social interaction with other older people and those experiencing disabilities before and after the disaster, as well as supported access to mainstream health and community-based rehabilitation services.

a medical to a social model of disability, and from a charity to a human rights based approach. The social model of disability defines disability as the consequence of discrimination at the social and institutional level (Oliver 1996). This model contrasts with a medical model that historically has viewed disability as the consequence of individual deficits or impairments. The social model shifts the focus of intervention from the individual towards the environment and improving the socio-economic conditions in which people with disabilities find themselves, ultimately towards an inclusive, barrier-free and rights-based society. The International Classification of Functioning, Disability and Health (ICF) (WHO 2002) integrates individual and societal perspectives through the notion of the 'context' and its role in health, functioning and disability. The ICF describes the relationship between health conditions, activity and participation in daily life in what has been referred to as a 'biopsychosocial framework'.

Comprehensive approaches to managing disaster and reducing risk seek to address the root causes of vulnerability through participatory and community-based processes that aim to engage all persons and households affected by disaster (CBM n.d, UNISDR 2006). These approaches drive a process of social development and change that ultimately reconfigures patterns of vulnerability and risk. Addressing the routines of everyday life as socially and culturally embedded is a key aspect of identifying and mitigating vulnerabilities and risks. People with disabilities tend to be excluded from these processes, and thus their specific needs and interests remain largely unmet and their equal rights unfulfilled in disaster and development contexts (UN enable n.d.a, WHO 2011).

Historically researchers assumed that disaster would inevitably lead to major changes in organizations and people without the need for targeted interventions that identify particularly vulnerable groups and, further, that altruistic behaviour would prevail in situations of disaster. On the contrary, disaster research has shown that an initial period of altruism gives way to disillusionment as limited resources fail to meet the overwhelming needs of populations. Under these circumstances, preexisting patterns of social inequality resurface. Hewitt (1983) asserts that the normal order of things in pre-disaster situations is marked by social conditions such as inequality and subordination (Hewitt 1983). People hold these preexisting patterns and relationships in place as they try to reestablish a sense of normality following disaster, even if those patterns are maladaptive and place some people at even greater risk (Gall 2007, Henry 2011, Stallings 1998). The neglect of people with disabilities in situations of disaster is a testament to the persistence of inequitable social relations and structures of domination.

SOCIAL EXCLUSION

The World Report on Disability documents widespread evidence of barriers that contribute to the degree of risk and disadvantage experienced by people with disabilities, including inadequate policies and standards, negative attitudes, lack of provision of services, problems with service delivery, inadequate funding, lack of accessibility, lack of consultation and involvement, and lack of data and evidence (WHO 2011). In emergency situations, people with disabilities may not receive critical information, may be less able to escape, may lose assistive devices or essential medication and may be left behind, abandoned or displaced. People with disabilities who live in displaced persons camps are often invisible to emergency registration systems and are unable to access the general distribution of relief (WHO 2005). Attitudes and environmental barriers within the camps also prevent their access to basic entitlements such as food, water, shelter, latrines and health care services (WHO 2013). Women and children with disabilities are especially vulnerable and face additional risks in terms of their safety and security in these camps. Furthermore, displacement and the breakdown of social supports and traditional caring mechanisms erode the independence and dignity of persons with disabilities. Emergencies may also reduce the capacity of caregivers to support people with disabilities. Researchers now largely agree that the potential for change in these circumstances is a matter of power and resources and, further, that recovery depends upon profound changes in social relations and structures (Blaikie et al 1994, Wisner et al 2004).

A VISION OF INCLUSION

The global perspective on disability espouses a vision of an inclusive world in which all people have freedom to choose, and are able to live a life of health, comfort and dignity (Universal Declaration of Human Rights, http://www.un.org/en/documents/udhr/resources .shtml); furthermore, each person affected by conflict or disaster is able to access assistance and protection to support a life with dignity (Sphere 2011, UN 2006).

An inclusive social vision has emerged over time through effective lobbying efforts of people with disabilities and disabled people's organizations (DPOs) and the development and evolution of international human rights instruments such as the Standard Rules on the Equalization of Opportunities for Persons with Disabilities (UN enable, n.d.b) and the Convention on the Rights of Persons with Disabilities (CRPD). Landmark texts such as Michael Oliver's *Understanding Disability* (1996), the World Report on Disability and initiatives such as the International Disability and Development Consortium (IDDC) have also helped to position disability as a cross-cutting issue in development and raise the profile of disability in disaster. Inclusive approaches to disaster and development are based upon the equitable distribution of humanitarian aid and development assistance and the active participation and representation of particularly vulnerable groups, such as people with disabilities, in response, recovery and risk reduction activities. Guidelines and frameworks have been developed to fulfil the values and goals of equity and participation, some of which include a disability perspective. The Sphere guidelines emphasize human rights and specify a disability component to better ensure that practitioners are sensitized to the specific needs and issues of people with disabilities. Moreover, the Draft Guidance Note on Disability and Emergency Risk Management for Health (WHO, 2013) represents a global initiative to elaborate and provide support in addressing disability-specific considerations in disaster response. However, on a higher policy level, the Hyogo Framework for Action is arguably not disability inclusive. Nevertheless, the emphasis on human rights and the development of international human rights instruments has drawn attention to disability in the field and has translated into national and global commitments to disability-inclusive approaches to disaster and development.

INTERNATIONAL INSTRUMENTS

International attention to the issue of disability was marked by the UN's proclamation that 1982–1992 was the 'decade of disabled persons'. This dedication influenced a change in practice from a curative or care approach to disability towards a human rights approach that emphasizes the equal rights of people with disabilities to participate in societal processes. The human rights approach focuses not only on enabling access to specific prevention and rehabilitation services but on participation in all aspects of society, where people with disabilities, their families and disabled people's organizations are active partners in procuring their rights.

The Decade of Disabled Persons led the UN General Assembly to adopt the Standard Rules on the Equalization of Opportunities for Persons with Disabilities. These rules provided a universal framework to integrate the rights of people with disabilities into national legislation. Consequently many governments developed disability legislation and began to incorporate disability in their development policies and agenda. Governments in Asia and the Pacific formed the Biwako Millennium Framework for Action (2003–2012), a regional framework for an inclusive, barrier-free and rights-based society for persons with disabilities. Despite these achievements, the Standard Rules were a political guideline and not binding, thus the needs and interests of people with disabilities were not adequately reflected in national and international development policies and strategies. This challenge prompted the development of the CRPD.

THE CONVENTION ON THE RIGHTS OF PERSONS WITH DISABILITIES (CRPD)

The CRPD defines persons with disabilities as those who have long-term physical, mental, intellectual or sensory impairments which, in interaction with various barriers, may hinder their full and effective participation in society on an equal basis with others (UN 2006). The Convention promotes awareness of disability among policy makers and practitioners in the field and puts pressure on agencies to integrate disability policies into development assistance. The CRPD's explicit social development dimension compels integrated and inclusive policy and practice. However, it is important to note that some people in the disability movement claim the emphasis on human rights neglects the radical societal changes needed to address the barriers to disability equality, including those that are largely driven by a competitive market social system (Yeo 2005).

FROM RHETORIC TO REALITY: THE TWIN-TRACK APPROACH

Inclusion is about changing society to accommodate difference, and combating discrimination. Through an inclusive lens, society is the problem, not the person or the impairment. To achieve inclusion, a twin-track approach is needed (Figure 5-2): focus on the society to remove the barriers that exclude (mainstreaming), and focus on the group of persons who are excluded, to build their capacity and support them to lobby for their inclusion (Stubbs 2008). There are four fundamental principles that inform the way in which

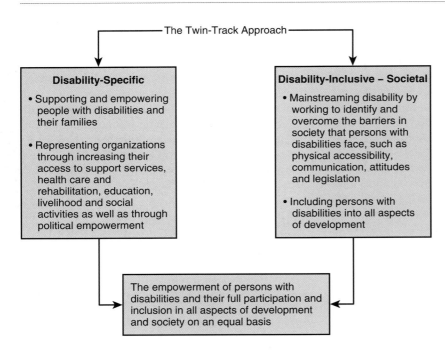

FIGURE 5-2 ▪ The twin-track approach. Sources: http://www.cbm.org/The-Twin-Track-approach-250816.php; http://www.cbm.org/article/downloads/54741/Twin-Track_Paper_final_version_October2008.pdf; http://www.inclusive-development.org/cbmtools/part1/twin.htm

disability is included in disaster preparedness, response and recovery.

Core Principles

- Human rights and equity – disaster preparedness and management must be firmly set within a human rights framework, demonstrating commitment to equitable and inclusive practice (IFRC 2007, Plan-CBM-Nossal 2011, Sphere 2011, UN-CRC 1989, UN 2006, UN-DHR 1948, WHO 2011); this includes promoting non-discrimination and facilitating equity in access to disaster planning and programmes.
- Participation – representation and inclusion of persons with disabilities and their families is not only a right but is essential to effective disaster management; participation of persons with disabilities in decision-making across the disaster management continuum and throughout the project cycle helps ensure that programmes are equitable and effective (Atlas Alliance and CBM 2011, Bonn Declaration 2007, IFRC 2007, Plan-CBM-Nossal 2011, Shafallah Forum 2012, UN 2006, WHO 2011).

- Capacity building – utilize and build on available disability-related resources and capacity, and promote self-help, while also building disability awareness, understanding, skills and confidence among non-disabled actors (Bonn Declaration 2007, Plan-CBM-Nossal 2011, Shafallah Forum 2012, Thomas 2008, UN 2006, WHO 2011).
- Disability prevention – prevent impairment and disability, and promote functional ability; the immediate cost of preventive actions is significantly less than the long-term cost of disability to individuals, families, communities and economies (Oosters 2005, WHO 2005, 2011). It requires attention to both person and environment factors (WHO 2011).

The twin-track approach is the vehicle through which these principles translate into action. The application of the twin-track approach to disaster promotes the fulfilment of disabled people's basic and specific needs and human rights across the disaster cycle and potentially reduces their vulnerability through poverty reduction and other risk reduction strategies.

The twin-track approach is rooted in the development sector and efforts to ensure that the considerations of particularly vulnerable groups are integrated into development cooperation. It encompasses a wide spectrum of micro- and macro-interventions incorporated within a range of strategies, such as community-based rehabilitation (CBR), social capital building, and advocacy and policy reform, based on a rights perspective (Kett et al 2004). The approach is well supported on an international level through the activities of multilateral organizations such as the WHO, UNICEF and World Bank, and government aid/development agencies, international nongovernmental organizations, and disability-focused organizations (e.g. Christian Blind Mission and Handicap International). Many of the humanitarian aid and development organizations that have adopted the twin-track approach as a core element of policy on disability and development are incorporating the approach into their disaster-related work. Furthermore, organizations that have adopted CBR as an inclusive development strategy are guided in its application to crisis situations through a set of guidelines developed by the UN and civil society organizations including disabled people's organizations (WHO 2010).

MERGING OCCUPATION AND OCCUPATIONAL THERAPY PRACTICE

Ultimately the outcomes of the twin-track approach hinge upon its potential to influence the various perspectives and positions of multiple stakeholders involved and foster new and inclusive patterns of engagement. On this subject, Yeo (2005) contends that changes in language and documentation about disability may be the first step to more practical progress, or a smokescreen that pacifies the movement without changing anything in practice (Yeo 2005, p. 4). *Real change is evidenced by new patterns of engagement.*

These patterns are represented by the activities of everyday life as they are embedded in social structures, relationships and routines. Townsend & Polatajko (2007) describe these occupational patterns as 'windows on the lifestyles of individuals, cultures, and eras and – over time – are evidence of social change' (p. 7). The implication is that occupation is an important medium in disaster and development and could be used as a tool to support and potentially strengthen the twin-track approach.

There is a need to explore how occupation can be applied to both disability-specific and disability-inclusive (mainstreaming) tracks of the approach, and across micro- and macro-interventions, to fully realize this potential. Traditional occupational therapy practice readily translates into disability-specific activities as they involve rehabilitation and supporting and empowering people with disabilities and their families within the individual or household realm of occupation and activity. However, less is understood about how occupation and occupational therapy practice could support disability equality through community building in contexts of disaster. Community development in occupational therapy is not a new concept, and there is growing interest in articulating the contribution of occupational therapy to the field (CAOT 2008), particularly as it involves CBR (CAOT 2008, McColl 1998, Pollard et al 2005, Pollard & Sakellariou 2012, Twible & Henley n.d., WFOT 2004). To further this aim, the profession has defined community development in terms of relationship building in the broader context of a multilayered, community-driven process (Wilcock 1998). More could be learned about how occupation could be used as medium to assess, better understand and ultimately build relationships as aligned with a human rights-based and inclusive vision of health, wellbeing and participation.

SUMMARY

Disaster tells a story about people and their relationships with each other and the environment that is largely characterized by social inequity and exclusion in the broader context of global risk drivers and processes of change. Within that story, people with disabilities represent a particularly vulnerable group. They are more likely to be poor and to live in hazard-prone areas, and they lack the power and resources to cope with disaster or avoid hazardous threats. As such, disability extends beyond an individual health issue to represent a pressing social issue – one that cross-cuts disaster and development. The twin-track approach to disability equality in disaster and development focuses on removing societal barriers and building the capacity of people with disabilities through the combination of micro- and macro-level interventions, based on a core set of principles. Traditional occupational therapy practice is well aligned with capacity development at individual and household levels; however, much more could be learned about the role of occupation in relationship building, as it represents the cornerstone of community development and capacity building processes.

REFERENCES

Atlas Alliance and CBM, 2011. *Disability in conflicts and emergencies fact sheet.* <www.atlas-alliansen.no/English>.

Biwako Millennium Framework for Action, 2003–2012. Retrieved from: <http://www.mukesh.myehome.in/circulars/NHRC%20Disability%20Manual/Annexure7.html>.

Blaikie, P., Cannon, T., Davis, I., Wisner, B., 1994. At Risk: Natural Hazards, People's Vulnerability, and Disasters. Routledge, London, UK.

Bonn Declaration, 2007. Composed and published from the international conference 'Disasters are always inclusive. Persons with Disabilities in Humanitarian Emergency Situations', 7–8 November 2007. Disability and Development Cooperation (bezev), Kindernothilfe, CMB, Caritas Germany, Handicap International, and Der Paritatische Gesamtverband, Bonn, Germany.

CAOT (Canadian Association of Occupational Therapists), 2008. Hot Topic. Occupational Community Development. Retrieved from: <http://www.caot.ca/pdfs/Community%20Dev.pdf>.

CBM, n.d.. Disability Inclusive Disaster Risk Management. Voices from the field and good practices. Retrieved from: <http://www.iddcconsortium.net/sites/default/files/resources-tools/files/disability_inclusive_disaster_risk_management_cbm.pdf>.

Gall, M., 2007. Indices of social vulnerability to natural hazards: a comparative evaluation. Doctoral dissertation, Department of Geography, University of South Carolina. Available from ProQuest Dissertations and theses database. (UMI Microform 3272445).

Henry, J., 2011. Continuity, social change and Katrina. Disasters 35 (1), 220–242.

Hewitt, K. (Ed.), 1983. Interpretations of Calamity. Allen and Unwin, Boston, MA.

IFRC, 2007. World Disasters Report. International Federation of Red Cross and Red Crescent Societies, Geneva.

Kett, M., Lang, R., Trani, J.F., 2004. Disability, development and a dawning of a new convention. A cause for optimism? J. Int. Dev. 21 (5), 649–661.

McColl, M.A., 1998. What do we need to know to practice occupational therapy in the community? Am. J. Occup. Ther. 52 (1), 11–18.

Oliver, M., 1996. Understanding Disability, from Theory to Practice. Macmillan, London, UK.

Oosters, B., 2005. Looking with a disability lens at the disaster caused by the Tsunami in South-East Asia, CBM International. Informed the Disability-Tsunami Emergency Response Summary for the Australian Council for International Development. <http://hpod.org/pdf/looking-with-disability-lens.pdf>.

Parnes, P., 2008. Research on Disability and Development. Report submitted to CIDA. (Project number 7048320). International Centre for Disability and Rehab. University of Toronto. Retrieved from the ADDC website: <http://www.addc.org.au/documents/resources/20080430-research-on-disability-and-development_544.pdf>.

Plan-CBM-Nossal, 2011. Guidance Note in Disability Inclusion in Humanitarian Action. Plan-CMB-Nossal Institute, 13th June 2011. Australia.

Pollard, N., Sakellariou, D., 2012. Politics of Occupation-Centred Practice. Reflections on Occupational Engagement Across Cultures. Wiley-Blackwell, Oxford, UK.

Pollard, N., Alsop, A., Kronenberg, F., 2005. Reconceptualising occupational therapy. Br. J. Occup. Ther. 68 (11), 524–526.

Sen, A., Wolfensohn, J.D., 2004. Helping Disabled People Out of the Shadows. Originally titled '[Nobel Laureates] Helping Disabled People Out of the Shadows' from The Korea Times, 12/21/2004. Retrieved from: <http://disabilityworld.org/12-02_05/news/outof shadows.shtml>.

Shafallah Forum, 2012. Shafallah Declaration on Crisis, Conflict and Disability, 24th January 2012. Doha, Qatar.

Sphere project, 2011. 2011 Edition of the Sphere Handbook: What is New? Retrieved August 6, 2013 from: <http://www.sphereproject.org/silo/files/what-is-new-in-the-sphere-handbook-2011-edition-v2.pdf>.

Stallings, R.A., 1998. Disaster and the theory of social order. In: Quarantelli, E.L. (Ed.), What is a Disaster? Perspectives on the Question. Routledge, London, pp. 127–145.

Stubbs, S., 2008. What is inclusive development? Jan 8, 2008. IDDC website. Retrieved from: <http://www.make-development-inclusive.org/inclusivedevelopment.php?spk=en>.

Thomas, K., 2008. Fostering Pioneers. An Evaluation of the Sri Lanka Tsunami Extended Response Program. HelpAge Sri Lanka and HelpAge International.

Townsend, E.A., Polatajko, H.J., 2007. Enabling Occupation II: Advancing an Occupational Therapy Vision for Health, Wellbeing and Justice through Occupation. CAOT publications ACE, Ottawa, ON.

Twible, R.L., Henley, E.C., n.d.. Preparing occupational therapists and physiotherapists for community based rehabilitation. Retrieved from: <http://english.aifo.it/disability/apdrj/selread100/ot_pt_for_cbr_twible_henley.pdf>.

UN, 2006. Convention on the Rights of Persons with Disabilities, United Nations, Geneva. Retrieved from: <http://www.un.org/disabilities/convention/conventionfull.shtml>.

UN-CRC, 1989. Convention on the Rights of the Child, United Nations, Geneva.

UN-DHR, 1948. The Universal Declaration of Human Rights, United Nations, Geneva.

UN enable, n.d.a. Development and Human Rights for All. Disability, Natural Disasters and Emergency Situations. Retrieved from: <http://www.un.org/disabilities/default.asp?id=1546>.

UN enable, n.d.b. The standard rules on the equalization of opportunities for persons with disabilities. Retrieved from: <http://www.un.org/esa/socdev/enable/dissre00.htm>.

UNISDR, 2006. A guide to community-based disaster risk reduction in Central Asia. Retrieved from: <http://www.unisdr.org/files/2299_ACommunityGuideeng.pdf>.

UNISDR, 2013. UN global survey explains why so many people living with disabilities die in disasters. Retrieved from: <http://www.unisdr.org/archive/35032>.

WFOT, 2004. Position Paper on Community Based Rehabilitation (CBR). Retrieved from: <http://www.ruralrehab.co.za/uploads/3/0/9/0/3090989/wfot_position_paper_cbr_2004.pdf>.

WHO, 2002. Towards a common language for functioning, disability and health. ICF. The international classification of functioning, disability and health. Retrieved from: <http://www.who.int/classifications/icf/training/icfbeginnersguide.pdf>.

WHO, 2005. Disasters, disability and rehabilitation, Department of Injuries and Violence Prevention, World Health Organization, Geneva. Retrieved from: <http://www.who.int/violence_injury_prevention/other_injury/en/disaster_disability.pdf>.

WHO, 2010. Community based rehabilitation. CBR Guidelines. Supplementary Booklet. Retrieved from: <http://whqlibdoc.who.int/publications/2010/9789241548052_supplement_eng.pdf>.

WHO, 2011. World Report on Disability. Retrieved from: <http://whqlibdoc.who.int/publications/2011/9789240685215_eng.pdf>.

WHO, 2013. Guidance note on disability and emergency risk management for health. Retrieved from: <http://apps.who.int/iris/bitstream/10665/90369/1/9789241506243_eng.pdf>.

Wilcock, A.A., 1998. An Occupational Perspective of Health. Slack Incorporated, Thorofare, NJ.

Wilcock, A.A., Townsend, E.A., 2008. Occupational Justice. In: Crepeau, E.B., Cohn, E.S., Schell, B.B. (Eds.), Willard and Spackman's Occupational Therapy, eleventh ed. Lippincott Williams and Wilkins, Baltimore, pp. 192–199.

Wisner, B., Blaikie, P., Cannon, T., Davis, I., 2004. At Risk: Natural Hazards, People's Vulnerability and Disasters, second ed. Routledge, New York, NY.

Yeo, R., 2005. Disability, Knowledge and Research. Disability, poverty and the new development agenda. Retrieved from: <http://hpod.org/pdf/Developmentagenda.pdf>.

PART II   Case Series – Stories from Experience

P art II presents a collection of stories about disaster from different perspectives and cultures. These stories are loosely organized according to phases of the disaster cycle and perspectives on entering the field. The voices of survivors and practitioners come to life through these stories and communicate the realities of surviving disaster and working in the field. Many but not all of these practitioners have been trained as occupational therapists. Some are both survivors and practitioners. Challenges, tragedy and injustices are portrayed but also triumphs and transformations of a personal and social nature. The contributors offer hope, guidance and concrete strategies to help practitioners connect to the experiences of survivors and negotiate the complex terrain of disaster and development.

6

LISTENING TO THE VOICES OF SURVIVORS: THE FLOODS OF 2003 IN SANTA FE, ARGENTINA

MARÍA DE LOS MILAGROS DEMIRYI ■ CARLA BOGGIO ■ MARIANA BOFFELLI ■ DANIELA CHIAPESSONI ■ MAURO DEMICHELIS ■ MARÍA DEL CARMEN HEIT

This chapter documents the story of a group of Argentinian occupational therapy practitioners, some of whom were affected by the 2003 floods in Santa Fe, Argentina, and felt compelled to try to understand the experience of disaster from the perspective of occupation and occupational therapy. The stories of survivors caused them to reexamine the theories and practical knowledge that guide their practice and illuminated occupational dimensions of disaster, resilience and recovery.

The floods of 2003 marked our lives forever. The event was so unexpected, so cruel and sudden that there was no way of anticipating it … We did what we could with it and within it … We are sure of one thing … We are no longer the same.

INTRODUCTION

In a few seconds the violent and sudden burst of water transformed reality at every level of life.

I got up because I could hear a lot of noise coming from the house. I started to look around and saw that water was coming in; I desperately tried to mop up the water – tried to dry up what was coming in fast through the grates but I soon realized that it was useless.

Uncertain, I stayed until it got to the point that I told myself that I either had to go or I would die … GO or DIE … and then I managed to go forward, one step at a time, against the water that had already risen up to my waist.

Every person affected by the floods that day responded to the situation in the best way they could under the most challenging and threatening of circumstances. Only after fighting for their survival could they reflect – could we all reflect – on what had happened and how our perspectives had changed, both personally and professionally. As occupational therapists we rethought our theoretical arguments and practical knowledge and reflected on the experience from the point of view of occupation and occupational therapy. We asked ourselves: What happens when abrupt and unanticipated changes in people's occupations are not self-motivated, when from one day to the next thousands of people's realities are transformed without them having participated willingly in these changes? And what does it mean to experience loss at every point of daily life as an individual, but have this experience shared by the devastated community around you? What happens to your sense of self and security when you thought it could never happen to you? And how could occupational therapy support recovery and preparedness on individual and community levels?

The painful experience of the floods, our involvement in emergency response and reconstruction, and our shared vision as occupational therapists motivated us to create a working group that would endeavour to link disaster and occupational therapy on theoretical and practical levels. Nobody we knew of had any previous experience in this area. As a group we began by doing some research, through the Universidad Nacional del Litoral (Santa Fe, Argentina), on the occupations of people affected by the floods. The title of the research was 'The change in habits and routines of those affected by the water catastrophe in Santa Fe in 2003'. It was our attempt to understand how disaster affected people's occupations, and how this in turn impacted upon their health and wellbeing.

Our study was the first systematic study in Argentina that was aimed at developing and validating the knowledge of occupational therapy related to the phenomenon of disaster. When we shared findings from the study among colleagues and students we were asked: How did you manage not to get emotionally involved when you heard such painful experiences being related? They wanted to know how we maintained that objective distance typically associated with research. We responded by saying that detachment did not feature in our investigation. On the contrary, we wanted to participate in the survivors' experiences and share in them as much as possible. We wanted to understand their experience – to be submerged in their words, and their silences. We felt honoured to have the privilege of being accepted as witnesses to that chapter in their lives. It gave life to our work and allowed us to understand, from their personal perspective, a phenomenon which shook all of our lives in Santa Fe. We later spent many hours going through each of their stories in the face of theories as a way of adding to the knowledge that exists within the field. Their experiences became the basis from which we reexamined and elaborated upon knowledge and theory in occupational therapy.

CONTEXT

The floods in the city of Santa Fe in 2003 were one of the biggest national catastrophes that had taken place in the last few years (Figure 6-1). They directly affected 130 000 people (one-third of the population) and occurred as a result of weak infrastructure and carelessness on the part of the government, which caused the Salado River to overflow.

'Nobody warned us, nobody said anything.'

There were no public warnings or orders to evacuate, and the situation was worsened by the authorities who publicly announced that people were to remain

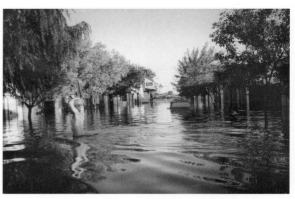

FIGURE 6-1 ■ The flood settles in, masking trauma.

in their homes. People were assured that nobody would get flooded. This announcement was made mid-morning and consequently people continued working and barely altered their daily routine in preparation for the floods.

> *'We went to the supermarket in the morning … the water kept rising … by that afternoon we stayed at home waiting and cooked for the children that would come home to eat.'*
>
> *'In case the water rose we built a small wall at our front door.'*
>
> *'We put all of our things off the floor: the mattresses, the refrigerator, our clothes, we put these on top of the table.'*

By nightfall 20 people had died. All of the western suburbs were flooded, the water level had risen to the city and all of the services had collapsed.

THE STUDY OF OCCUPATION AND THE STAGES OF THE CATASTROPHE

We started our study (Table 6-1) from the premise that the changes that occurred in the habits and routines of people affected began with the catastrophe. We soon decided to widen our study to include the occupational dimension of the catastrophe and categorized people's experiences into distinct but interrelated phases: pre catastrophe, catastrophe and post catastrophe/recovery.

TABLE 6-1
Overview of the Study

Type of Study: Descriptive.

Direction: Qualitative with ethnographic and phenomenological contributions. Triangulation of sources, researchers, theories and methodologies.

Time Frame: In accordance with the registration of occupational changes at different moments in time.

Population: 130 000 affected people.

Informants: 54 participants between 22 and 86 years old, of both sexes, from the most affected neighbourhoods, chosen intentionally and who volunteered to participate in the study.

Instruments: Narratives, in-depth interviews, and semistructured interviews.

Gathering Data: 20 months.

Processing Data: Three types of analysis content (especially thematic analysis), relationships, in particular of co-occurrence and of representation.

Internal Validity: Many researchers, the examination of external pairs, researchers as participants and the automatic register of data were used as criteria to increase internal reliability and reduce threats.

PRE CATASTROPHE

Pre catastrophe included the hours before the rise of the water in the houses, to the point of evacuation. People continued on with their normal occupational habits, despite the accumulating water around them. During our interviews with them they reflected on the fact that if they had known that there would be a flood, their (occupational) behaviour would have been vastly different – they would have done things differently.

The false information they received meant that they were not prepared for what occurred.

'Dad entered to carry sand bags to place on the door ... we ignored the tragedy that was about to occur.'

CATASTROPHE

'The water was so strong and so big in magnitude that we could hardly stand.'
' We didn't have time for anything.'
'We had our trousers rolled up, we held on to one another ... our eyes were glazed over, our mouths

BOX 6-1
OCCUPATIONAL DUTIES

'I kept washing clothes, drying clothes, cleaning and ironing.'
'I wasn't used to working so much, my body felt so tired.'
'Cleaning, drying clothes, documents, books in the sun, it was an all day task.'

dry ... we left our houses, our town, perhaps even leaving that life.'

Catastrophe began when the water burst into people's houses and began to wreak havoc on their lives. Nobody could keep doing what they had before. The rise of the water forced them to leave. The process of leaving was disorganized and people got repeatedly lost. Listening to their stories, from our perspective as occupational therapists, there was a complete imbalance in their occupations (Box 6-1). Their roles, routines and habits – so much a part of who they were – were suddenly inaccessible to them.

'We didn't know what to do, what things to save ... it was crazy. I can't tell you how I was but it felt as though I was in the air ... we were like ghosts, we walked randomly, as though we were lost, we were like living dead ... there were people wandering everywhere, with things in their hands, walking aimlessly, living on the street, anywhere they could find.'

Metaphors express the complex and profound nature of what was experienced:

'It was like a war movie ... the exodus.'

Some people did not want to leave their homes and they stayed on the roofs or terraces, determined to keep hold of those things that were important to them, the things that defined their lives and gave them a sense of security. The majority were men and one of them said:

'A canoe came past and wanted to take us ... I said "No! You won't take me from my house even if I'm dead!"'

Other people had to endure successive evacuations because the water rose to the places where they had taken refuge. Once people arrived at the evacuation centre or relatives' houses, they experienced what we consider an occupational phenomenon that was characterized by an imposition upon their habits and routines. Communal activities encroached upon any personal or private space, forcing people into a pattern of continuous adjustment of their personal habits and routines. On top of that a demand for new, and often foreign, occupations suddenly defined their everyday life, such as procedures for registration, vaccinations, census and all the necessary procedures related to housing, e.g. regaining electricity, gas, documentation, returning to their neighbourhoods, searching for and reclaiming things lost.

When the water subsided there was the immense task of cleaning, repair and reconstruction. For some people, asking for and receiving help, especially from the state, became a new and difficult role that conflicted with their previous occupations and sense of self.

'We were always used to living from the fruit of our labour … to ask for help was something new, difficult.'

Yet others were energized and inspired by a sense of solidarity and took up new roles involving social participation, reclaim and struggle.

'We organized activities with other groups: Black Tent, March of the Torches and human rights organizations … we created a congress of the flood affected … it was very important.'

These activities contrasted with the often mundane but necessary 'occupational duties', tasks such as washing clothes, appliances, objects and furniture.

People orchestrated themselves around the tasks that needed to be done, shifting their roles and interactions with each other to meet the demands of the situation. Families functioned as units around which routines were reorganized.

'My daughter's husband was in charge of cleaning the flooded house because she was

pregnant and she had to be careful of catching an illness.'

The distribution of occupations was done depending on the roles and responsibilities of each person in accordance with their characteristics and the context.

'We washed our clothes at my daughter's house because her house had not flooded and we had everything there.'

One mother, referring to her daughter's support, said that she delegated tasks to her in the first moments until she could return to her house, but that she 'didn't feel qualified'. The situation was foreign to many, if not most, and demanded adaptation, and with it, confidence in one's abilities. People had to draw on whatever knowledge and experience they had and cope with their new reality.

OCCUPATIONAL PLACES IN CATASTROPHE

There were two occupational places that were central and parallel to the experiences of participants: emergency houses or camps to which people were evacuated, and the flooded houses they had to leave. Emergency houses were places of transition that lasted approximately one to three months following the emergency. Some families, however, lived for over a

---

BOX 6-2
CHANGE IN HABITS

'I had quit smoking and then took it up again. I channeled my anguish into the cigarettes. I had never smoked as much as I did during those days.'

'All I wanted to do was sleep, to sleep deeply so I could escape all that had happened and would happen.'

'I didn't brush my teeth for about a week, until I realized it was because I didn't have a toothbrush.'

'I missed getting up in the morning and having my books to study and to prepare my classes, I always did this but after the flood I couldn't because there was nothing left.'

'I don't know if you can write down everything that you feel, I don't think you can, but this gives me the little push I need to carry on every day.'

'I needed to do something for others.'

year in emergency housing. The common experience of having to move from one place to another, sometimes once, or many times a day or week, was stressful, causing people to organize their occupations according to temporary parameters such as the duration of natural light (because there was no electricity in flooded houses) or the time that the state of emergency began during which they could not be on the streets.

During this period, many people mentioned that they had to change their habits (Box 6-2), due to absence and also excess. Examples included an increase in the number of cigarettes they smoked and changes to sleep patterns: difficulty getting to sleep, interrupted sleep due to nightmares to do with the flood or sleeping too long. There was also the abandonment or interruption of some habits due to the loss of objects. In these situations the lost object brought about the change in habit. However, the addition of new occupations helped people to cope with the situation. Participation in solidarity activities helped during the emergency, strengthening the bonds and connections between people, as well as creating opportunities for problem-solving, collaboration and shared responsibility. We highlight the value and function of the occupations, particularly collaborative ones, as effective support for coping with disaster and personal catastrophe.

We discovered changes in perceptions of time in people's testimonials (Box 6-3). The greater the level of urgency that was felt because of the flood, coupled with forced evacuation and a desperate search for a secure location, the greater the perception that time was passing more slowly:

'We spent five hours in the water. It was up to our chest, we didn't come out.'

'I had been at my cousin's house five or six days … we never imagined that it would go on for so long.'

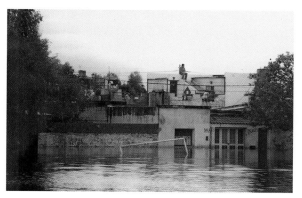

FIGURE 6-2 ■ Living on the roof.

For those who lived on the roof (Figure 6-2) or the terraces, the perception of time was even slower:

'I was on top of my house without eating. My dogs or I didn't eat. I couldn't wash, I spent all that time like that, it was never ending.'

'The water rose every two hours … but to us it felt like two days.'

For older people there was a profound sense of loss and perception that the future appeared to be limited, as expressed by the following statement:

'Imagine I am already older, what took a lifetime of sacrifice to create was gone.'

The continuous and transitory changes in occupational forms – people's habits and routines – caused considerable stress, and in some cases feelings of humiliation and contempt from others, as is illustrated in the following testimonial in regards to the routine of eating:

'In order to eat we had to queue in front of the army, … we had to stand in a queue in the rotten mud to get cold stew. They would throw it to me from above in the truck, they put the food in a plastic bottle that was cut in half, that is how I ate – like a bum.'

People had to endure incredibly difficult situations where their vulnerability was exposed, yet their strengths and resilience were also revealed through

BOX 6-3
PERCEPTION OF TIME

'We kept cleaning, the next day it was the same thing, because the water levels decreased slowly, it was only by millimeters.'

'The hours passed, it was midday, my parents left the house and the four of us siblings were left on the terrace. That is how our long stage of survival began.'

their responses to extreme circumstances. One of the clearest examples involved those who stayed on the roof of their house.

'Something unforgettable started in all of our lives, the story of the roofs … we lived on the roof for twenty days. We made tents and gathered things with which to live … When we woke up each of us would go to our own roof … we gathered together to eat … then we slept in the afternoon … We organized soccer matches and played with each other from one roof to the next.'

This affirmed to us one of the central assumptions of occupational therapy – that people are inherently occupational beings. Occupation is, in itself, a mechanism for adaptation, promoting health and wellbeing in the most difficult and limiting of circumstances and experiences. Through their stories we saw how people's capacity for adaptation was reflected in the organization of their activities on the roof tops. It revealed how, even in the most limited surroundings, people are not helplessly idle but attempt to take charge of their lives and the environments around them as much as is possible.

POST CATASTROPHE

'When the house was in order, my life was in order.'
  'Once I had my bed and a plate of food I was ok.'
  'We moved to a small house which immediately became a meeting place for the whole family and somewhere for us to feel safe and to slowly reorganize.'

In the accounts of disaster there were recurring experiences that marked the beginning of recovery: 'returning to the house' (flooded house) or to a place where people could live in stability and resume those occupations, for example work and study, that were important to them and had been interrupted by the flood.

The notion of home is a key point:

'We decided to return to our home even though it was a disaster zone … We didn't get used to living with strangers.'

Many people returned without having the basic services (electricity, gas, telephone) or with very precarious facilities. They explained the logic of this decision:

'I had to recuperate the image I had of my house …, we had to return to being with our family.'

Others did not return and decided to rent a house. The decision not to return was associated with pain, memories and loss.

'I felt as though it was no longer my house.'
  'My house is not my home.'
  'I couldn't, I don't know, until this day I can't, I hardly ever go, …. It's as though I am angry at my house, it is very bad for me.'

The return home, whether it was to the previous one or a new one, was associated with regaining control of their own lives and making decisions.

Paradoxically, this sense of control applied to a different life, as distinguished from the old one, because disaster had forever altered their lives that once were. Many people struggled with a sense of anger or resisted their changed circumstances, which was reflected in their actions and occupations.

'Once I was in my home I was angry, then I started my exercises again, but my mind was elsewhere.'
  'Now it has been more than four years that I have not painted the inside of the house, and I don't even feel like it, the house is not in a good state … that is not normal for me. Before, if the house needed a coat of paint I would do it on the first Sunday that was sunny and I would paint.'

For many families, the return to the flooded house was a cause for disagreement.

'This was, and continues to be, a topic of discord.'
  'We argue, we argue a lot, they wanted to return [refers to parents with whom they were living] and they just went … I stayed.'

Taking up work activities again was another strong focal point for recovery, and it revealed the significant

---

BOX 6-4
RECOVERY ASSOCIATED WITH OCCUPATIONS OF WORK AND STUDY

'The priority was for my father to clean up his workshop tool by tool ... so that he could start working.'

'My aim was to continue on with my studies, I have graduated and will now continue.'

'Work helped me to get on with my life.'

'I had to return to work in order to get organized and to return to the life that we had.'

---

material and symbolic value placed on work (Box 6-4). People related how:

'Two months later I was teaching again and continued with all of my jobs.'

'I was told at work that I should take as many days off as I needed, but I only took 15 days to be at home because not doing anything was the worst.'

Work appeared to function as the key organizer of routines, in some cases even during the emergency.

People regained their habitual roles of worker, student, housewife, and incorporated new roles into their lives. Others did not continue with occupations that they had previously been engaged in before the flood because those occupations lost meaning for them. Many stopped recreational or sports activities. Some continued with the activities but changed the way they did them.

For example, someone who was a reader and collector of books says:

'Now I read a book but I don't even keep it.'

For others, new occupations acquired new meaning.

'I started to go to the square, to participate in the rallies.'

OCCUPATION AND LOSS

'I felt anguish, my books, my work, my photos ... I had to throw out my furniture that took our

stories and history ... , a whole life of effort and sacrifice.'

'No, without the tools we couldn't do anything.'

'We used to put things away ... today, I use everything I have.'

The loss of objects and places of occupation, in particular houses and places of work, caused, in the majority of people, a sense of profound personal loss.

'She felt isolated and stayed at home ... she did not go out or speak to anyone again.'

That was how one participant described the moments before one of her relatives died. Many people mentioned in their stories the death of neighbours or people they knew. Their accounts were emotive and often people were crying or fell silent.

The reaction to the loss of material possessions was different. They can be grouped into two types of attitudes: to recover as much as possible, or to throw away and get rid of everything that remained. Some people clung to what was lost, while others responded to loss by redefining their occupations and discovered new meanings.

OCCUPATION AND THE POWER OF DECISION-MAKING

When people recover the sense of control over their own lives it is reflected in the decisions they make around occupations. Occupations forge a pathway to recovery – an opportunity to regain control, step by step, from the small, more manageable, things like eating, sleeping or buying something, to bigger decisions around occupation that have greater implications, like where to work and how to rebuild.

'Once I had my bed and a plate of food I was ok.'

However, the reorganization of occupations, and the power people were able to exert over decision-making, was directly associated with the opportunities that people had. Some people were able to recover more quickly than others because of available supports. For others, recovery has not yet ended. This illuminated the fact that people's occupations do not exist in isolation. They are inherently social, given that they are tied to the social context around them. A person's recovery was, to a large extent, influenced by his/her environment, including how supportive or restrictive it was in nature.

THE MOST EFFECTIVE SUPPORT AND HELP

'We were all saved here, we helped each other amongst the neighbours … A girl from the school let me stay at her house … Without being a member, the union helped me.'

Families, neighbours, friends and work colleagues worked together to support each other throughout disaster and recovery, giving material aid and affection. This forms an important piece of evidence when deciding how to prepare for and confront a critical situation such as disaster. It reveals that there are natural networks to tap into as a part of supporting recovery – networks that exist and function at critical moments and can be strengthened and supported as a point of intervention beyond individual occupations and decision-making. It reveals how efforts to cultivate solidarity are of potential value and can guide a more socially based intervention, or form of aid and assistance, and further to that, a more 'social' form of occupational therapy practice. The experiences of participants point to the need for such an approach.

Many relief and recovery oriented interventions underestimated the individual's ability and did not take into account their subjective needs:

'The policies made without considering the needs of people forced us to spend a lot of our time doing bureaucratic paperwork.'

Furthermore, the state and government's responsibility for the flood unleashed different reactions to the aid (Box 6-5). Some rejected it; others wanted to get the most out of it and to give to those who needed it the most. This brought on feelings of resentment, indignation and hate. Many resolved their needs without help from the state.

> **BOX 6-5**
> **CRITICISM OF OFFICIAL POLICY**
>
> *'They entered our houses and our lives and made decisions for us.'*
> *'What was given to us bore no relation to what we needed … we are not all the same.'*

OCCUPATION AND NEEDS

Needs arose in various forms during all stages of the catastrophe and continually changed, requiring a high degree of flexibility and responsiveness on the part of the government and humanitarian aid and development organizations. Yet there were many accounts of scarcity and inadequacy of resources and unjust assistance that was offered by the state, coupled with a lack of consideration for people's subjective needs. Socially attributed needs, finding no satisfaction, were seen as rights that were violated. Work, housing, secure atmosphere and justice were the needs that the majority of the participants said were not satisfied completely, and that they valued as priorities.

'I spent four days without food, and seven days without showering.'
'I was offered a mattress and blanket but what I wanted was a hug.'
'I didn't get what I needed.'

Largely, there is an absence of truth and justice surrounding the floods in Santa Fe (there is no accountable person who is in prison or charged), which has left people insecure and distrusting when it comes to the possibility of another flood.

'The next time I will leave the neighbourhood, the city.'
'My wife and I have already discussed it, we will probably sell.'

OCCUPATION AND CONTEXT

'There are people who did not return, people who died and who got sick, empty houses … the neighbourhood is no longer the same.'

The changes in the houses, the neighbourhoods and the city also determined the decisions made around occupations. Some people decided to return to the neighbourhood and they explained their decision like this:

'This is where I was brought up, I had my children here.'

' I needed to return to my house, my life is here, my daughter was killed on my doorstep ... for me, she is still here.'

This account was from a mother whose daughter was assassinated by the military during the dictatorship. They all expressed their attachment to place and the sentiment that neighbourhood and houses have in the stories about their lives.

OCCUPATION AND MEMORY

'The streets were deserted with sirens in the background, the shots and helicopters.'

'The sound of the water that shocks.'

'I will never again forget the screams.'

Occupational experience is a part of recurring sensory memories that are recorded as indelible marks on individual and collective consciousness. Memory emerges like a social phenomenon as a space of struggle and reconstruction:

'We went to the rally.'

'People go to the plaza every 29th of the month.'

In our country, to remember is to fight against forgetting and impunity and to engage in occupations collaboratively – to participate in activities in clusters, in our neighbourhoods, offices, streets and plazas – to take hold of our lives and futures and act as direct protagonists in the story after catastrophe (Figure 6-3).

What has been presented is a synthesis of life stories of which we have been a part, and represents four years of work and reflection.

CONCLUSION

We entered homes and places of work.

We shared histories, tears, silences, pain, memories and a few dreams.

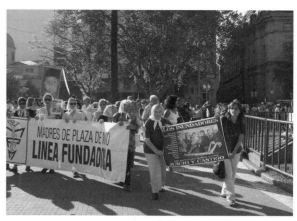

FIGURE 6-3 ▪ Marching to protest at poor flood planning and response.

We form part of the chain of narratives and accounts.

We are, above anything else, human beings convinced of the need to change the state of things.

We aim to understand the present within the framework of the past and the future, as a project and hope.

Injustice, poverty and disregard for human beings challenge our everyday professional work.

To make life more dignified is the goal. To fight for it is the path we are on.

FURTHER READING

Asaba K.M., 2005. "I'm not much different." Occupation, identity, and spinal cord injury in America. A dissertation presented to the Faculty of the Graduate School University of Southern California.

Bailey, D., 1997. Research for the Health Professional. A Practical Guide, second ed. F.A. Davis Company, Philadelphia, PA.

Balbi, J., 2004. La Mente Narrativa. Hacia una Concepción Posracionalista de la Identidad Personal. Paidós, Buenos Aires, Argentina.

Beck, U., 2000. Retorno a la teoría de la sociedad del riesgo. In: World Risk Society, Polity Press, Cambridge, UK. Boletín de AGE, Nro 30, pp. 9 a 20. Inglaterra.

Bericat, E., 1998. La Integración de los Métodos Cuantitativos y Cualitativos en la Investigación Social. Significado y medida. Ariel, Buenos Aires, Argentina.

Centro de Estudios Legales y Sociales, 2003. Derechos Humanos en Argentina. Informe 2002–2003. XI. Medio ambiente y derechos humanos. 3.2.2. Los efectos del agua. Situación de los refugiados ambientales en la ciudad de Santa Fe, CELS-Siglo XXI Editores Argentina. S.A, Buenos Aires, Argentina, p. 457.

CEPAL-BID, 2000. Un tema del desarrollo: la reducción de la vulnerabilidad frente a los desastres. Documento 12961. In: <http://www.cepal.org/publicaciones/xml/4/10134/l428.pdf>. México

Christiansen, C., 1999. The 1999 Eleanor Clarke Slagle Lecture. Defining lives: occupation as identity: an essay on competence, coherence, and the creation the meaning. Am. J. Occup. Ther. 53 (6), 547–558.

Clark, F., 2000. The concepts of habit and routine: a preliminary theoretical synthesis. Occup. Ther. J. Res. 20, 1235–1375.

Cohen, R.E., Ahearn, F., 1980. Manual de Atención en Salud Mental para Víctimas de Desastre. Editorial El Manual Moderno. OPS, México, D.F.

Cook, J., 2001. Qualitative Research in Occupational Therapy. Delmar Thomson Learning, Canada.

Fahrer, R., Pecci, M., Gómez Prieto, C., Besozzi, A., Garzarón, M., 1997. Salud mental y desastres: consecuencias psicológicas de las explosiones ocurridas en la Fábrica Militar Río III, Córdoba, Argentina. Acta Psiquiatr. Psicol. Am. Lat. 43 (3), 202–11.

Galheigo, S.M., 2006. Terapia Ocupacional sin Fronteras. Aprendiendo del Espíritu de Supervivientes. Panamericana, Madrid, pp. 85–95.

Jelin, E., Kaufman, S., 2001. Los niveles de la memoria: reconstrucción del pasado dictatorial argentino. In: Entrepasados, Revista de Historia, Año X, No 20/21. Buenos Aires, Argentina, pp. 9–34.

Kielhofner, G., 2002. Modelo de la Ocupación Humana: Teoría y aplicación, third ed. Editorial Médica Panamericana, Buenos Aires, Argentina.

Kondo, T., 2004. Cultural tensions in occupational therapy practice: considerations from a Japanese vantage point. Am. J. Occup. Ther. 48 (2), 174–184.

La Red. Red de Estudios Sociales en Prevención de desastres en América Latina, n.d.. Desinventar: Sistema de Inventarios de Desastres en América Latina. OSSO/ITDG, Cali, Colombia.

Larzon, R., Zemke, R., 2003. Shaping the temporal patterns of our lives. The social coordination of occupation. J. Occup. Sci. 10 (2), 80–89.

Levine, R., 1997. A Geography of Time. Basic Books, New York.

Losano Ascencio, C., 1995. La construcción social del medio ambiente a partir de los acontecimientos catastróficos que lo destruyen. In: Revista de la Facultad de Ciencias de la Información, UCM. Número extraordinario, Madrid, pp. 47–67.

Marcolino, T., Mizukami, M., 2008. Narratives, reflective processes and professional practice: contributions towards research and training. Interface – Comunic, Saúde, Educ. 12 (26), 541–547.

Médicos del Mundo Argentina, 2003. Inundaciones en Santa Fe. [Consultado en: www.mdm.org.ar, noviembre de 2005]

OPS-OMS, 1999. Asistencia humanística en casos de desastres, 2000. Los desastres naturales y la protección de la salud. OPS-OMS, Washington, DC.

Pichot, P., López-Ibor Aliño, J.J., Miyar, V.M., 1995. DSM-IV Manual Diagnóstico y Estadístico de Trastornos Mentales, fourth ed. Masson, Barcelona.

Polkinghorne, D., 1996. Transformative narratives: from victimic to agentic life plots. Am. J. Occup. Ther. 50 (4), 299–305.

Pujadas Muñoz, J.J., 1992. El método biográfico: el uso de las historias de vida en ciencias sociales. Cuadernos metodológicos. Centro de Investigaciones Sociológicas (CIS), España.

Rosenfeld, M.S., 1989. Occupational disruption and adaptation: a study of house fire. Am. J. Occup. Ther. 43, 89–96.

Sanahuja Rodriguez, H 1999 El daño y la evaluación del riesgo en América Central. Red de Estudios Sociales en Prevención de Desastres en América Latina, Costa Rica.

Santini, O., López, D., 1997. Desastres: Impacto Psicosocial. Alción, Buenos Aires, Argentina, Chapter I, pp. 11–23.

Silva P., 2010. Menos crímenes contra la humanidad. Publicado en ultranoticias. Available from: <http://ultra.com.mx>.

Simon, H., 1970. The architecture of complexity. In: Sciences of the Artificial. MIT Press, Cambridge, MA.

Subirats, E., 2005. Las catástrofes naturales no existen. In: Diario Página, 12, 20 September. Contratapa, Buenos Aires, Argentina, p. 32.

Sinclair, T.K., 2005. Disaster Preparedness and Response Project. Report of WFOT, Regional Workshop, Dec. 2005. World Federation of Occupational Therapists.

Townsend, E., 1997. Occupation: Potential for personal and social transformation. J. Occup. Sci. 7, 18–26.

Townsend, E., Wilcock, A., 2002. Occupational justice. In: Christiansen, C. (Ed.), Introduction to Occupation, Prentice-Hall, Upper Saddle River, NJ, pp. 243–273.

Wilcock, A., 1999. Reflections on doing, being and becoming. Aust. Occup. Ther. J. 46, 1–11.

Yerxa, E., Clark, F., Jackson, J., Parham, D., Pierce, D., Stein, C., et al., 1989. An introduction to occupational science: a foundation for occupational therapy in the 21st century. Occup. Ther. Health Care 6 (4), 1–17.

Young, J., 2001. Entre las historias y la memoria. Las misteriosas y extraordinarias voces de historiadores y sobrevivientes. In: Entrepasados, Revista de Historia, Año X, N° 20/21. Buenos Aires, Argentina, pp. 117–128.

7

REFLECTIONS ON HAITI

RUTH DUGGAN

LEILA'S* STORY

I had just come home from work and was standing at the gate in front of my house, talking with my neighbour. Then the earth began to shake. Everything was shaking and falling down. I watched my house collapse in front of my eyes. My father was inside the house. He was killed when the house fell on him. I couldn't do anything. ... I am thankful to come to work.

MY STORY

I had been to Haiti five or six times with Team Canada Healing Hands between 2006 and the time of the earthquake. I sat in shock when the news of the earthquake came on the TV the night of 12 January 2010. What else can happen to this poor country? I feared for my friends and their families, like Leila, who worked with our team as a translator over the years. Team Canada responded by making every attempt to get in touch with people we knew in Haiti, keeping our members as up to date as possible, and gathering names of volunteers who would be able to go to Haiti to provide rehabilitation support when we were needed. We thought that it would probably be a month or two before we would be called upon. The call came much sooner than that.

On 16 January a few members of our team, including me, were asked by Handicap International to go to Haiti as part of a small rehabilitation team to begin the long process of helping people who had been injured

*Name changed to protect identity.

as a result of the earthquake. Because of our experience in Haiti we knew the people, the landscape and some of the language. I arrived in Haiti via the Dominican Republic on 20 January, eight days after the initial earthquake hit.

Based on the news, I was prepared for the worst. At first glance it did not seem all that different than what I was used to seeing in Haiti, just exponentially *more*. There were more buildings falling down, more patients, more bumpy roads and more aid workers from more countries than I have ever seen in one place. Some areas of the city were totally demolished, while other areas seemed to be fine.

REHABILITATION POST EARTHQUAKE

Our job was to begin to assess the rehabilitation needs, to provide support to the field hospitals that had sprung up throughout Port-au-Prince and surrounding areas, and to train local community health workers who would both help us in our work and continue assisting people with disabilities after we left.

The first day of work we went to the large General Hospital. We had packed up a number of crutches and walkers in the van and were accompanied by two Haitian nurses that had been hired by Handicap International as community health workers. It took a long time to get there because roads were blocked with rubble, and there were UN vehicles guarding the area. This was new. Despite the years of unrest in Haiti, the last few years enjoyed relative freedom of movement and international military forces had been less visible.

The General Hospital consists of a number of buildings surrounding a large courtyard area. There had been a second earthquake on 20 January, and most of the patients were moved outside. The roadways and courtyard within the compound were crowded with beds, with patients and their families, with just a sheet or a tarp strung up over them to protect them from the sun. Most patients, and Haitian employees, refused to go inside a building even if it had been deemed safe. There were a number of different medical groups who had set up larger tents, providing medical care, including surgeries. The morgue was guarded by a lone soldier.

The number of people who had been injured was overwhelming, and this was just one hospital. We split up, each with a health worker/nurse who could help with translation, and went from bed to bed. We gathered information on each person about who they were, where they came from, where they thought they would go after they left the hospital, and types of injuries. There were people with injuries ranging from soft tissue wounds to multiple fractures, amputations and spinal cord injuries (Figure 7-1). Coming from a rehabilitation background it all seemed so acute to me. Where do we begin? We started with the basics to help the patients mobilize, from sitting up in bed to standing and walking with crutches, or giving them a wheelchair. We continued until the end of the day and had used all of our resources.

PSYCHOSOCIAL STRESS

I could see from that first day that people were suffering from overwhelming psychosocial stress. Many did

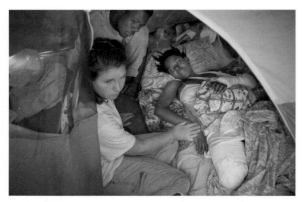

FIGURE 7-1 ■ Post-surgery assessment and treatment in tents requires flexibility and adaptiveness.

not know where their families or friends were or if they had survived. People would jump at the slightest aftershock or at a leaf falling from a tree. I remember seeing a woman trying to leave the hospital grounds on foot. She was wearing a night gown and had a long stick that she was using as a crutch. She was very nervous and screamed every time there was a tiny movement around her. She was clearly unsafe and so we stopped her to give her crutches. She did not want to take the crutches because it was taking too long for us to get them ready, but we persisted and then watched her teetering off with her friend. I wondered where she would go.

Over the next few days we were able to track down some of our old friends, like translators Leila, Lesly and Jide, and rehab technicians Shirley, Claiget and Sabine. Leila was one of the first people we found and brought to work with Handicap International. The first few days she was still in shock, and we understood when she told us her story.

EDUCATION AND TRAINING

With the growing national staff we decided to do a training day where we provided basic information about disability, expected long-term outcomes and basic education for people with amputations. We then split the group into two smaller groups: one occupational therapist (OT) did a session on how to fit and use mobility aids, and I did a session on psychosocial issues.

Who am I to talk about psychosocial issues that may arise after experiencing an earthquake? I am just an OT from Halifax who does consulting and goes to Haiti from time to time. Having studied client-centred practice for my Master's thesis, I thought about how to approach this and decided that I needed to have the group tell me what they were experiencing and how they could move through it. I would guide the discussion with a focus on occupation.

We started with a fun activity of juggling tissues. Just for a few minutes I showed everyone how to juggle with paper towel. They engaged and laughed as the tissues flew through the air and all over the place. They helped each other when a tissue was dropped.

Then we brought the group into a tight circle as I introduced how psychosocial issues are the thoughts and feelings that we have, and how we interact with people and the world around us. I acknowledged that the loss experienced by everyone in the group, and in Port-au-Prince, was enormous. We discovered that everyone in both groups had themselves – or knew of someone who had – been injured, lost their home, job, a family member or friend. We talked about how the patients they would be helping had probably lost all of these things, as well as becoming disabled by their injuries.

I asked each person to tell their story, their experience of the earthquake, while the others listened and acknowledged their experience, their pain, and sometimes their triumph. The stories ranged from very detailed accounts about what they were wearing and doing, and who they were with, to very brief: '... the earth shook and everything collapsed around me'. While some felt sadness, terror, weakness or nausea, others talked about increasing their faith in God, feeling strong to find their friends and family and having the courage to move on and help others. We then talked about how all of these feelings were normal and may change from day to day or week to week, and also that their patients would probably have these same feelings.

Pointing out that all of them had somehow managed to cope well enough to come to the Handicap International Office to get a job, we talked about different ways that each person coped with their own personal stressors. Of course, each person copes differently, according to their personality, surroundings, interests and abilities. Some of the things the group did to help themselves were to:

- Pray
- Play sports
- Keep busy
- Go to work
- Talk to friends and family
- Be close to people we love
- Play with children
- Think about other things
- Help others
- Make jokes
- Listen to music and dance
- Accept what had happened.

The theme of occupation, keeping busy, having a workplace to go to, being able to help others and

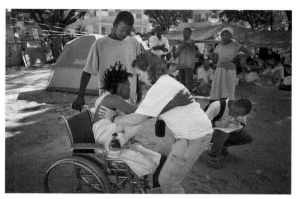

FIGURE 7-2 ▪ Mobilizing and educating – essential for ongoing functional capacity building and rehabilitation. Demonstrating techniques with clients, staff and family is a starting point for them taking forward good practice.

keeping a positive attitude was clear throughout the discussion. To most Haitians, having an injury that keeps them from walking means that they are not able to do anything, especially work to provide for their family. The hope that comes with having information about what to expect, what is possible, that they will have the opportunity to get a prosthesis and that they can get around now with crutches or a wheelchair is one of the best gifts we could offer to help people move forward (Figure 7-2).

We turned the discussion towards how each of the group members could use their experiences to help the injured people they would be seeing.

- Listen to individual stories with attention and compassion.
- Once the story is told and acknowledged, move on to coping and productive activity.
- Tell them what to expect in the process of recovery, getting a prosthesis, etc.
- Talk about and show them the things they will be able to do as they recover or get a prosthesis, like walking with crutches.
- Give information about how to care for themselves (e.g. wound care, prevention of pressure sores).
- Encourage as much exercise and activity as possible, including participation in daily activities such as helping to set up a new family home, helping others or getting back to work.

- Encourage sharing of things, ideas and emotions.
- Help regain confidence by making sure they are successful in the activities they asked their patients to do – take small steps.
- Breathe and relax – deep breathing helps you and your patients to stay calm and relaxed, which helps to manage pain.
- Keep a positive attitude and help to make people laugh!
- Encourage leisure activities – reading, watching a soccer game, playing dominoes.

We remembered that when we were juggling tissues, for that minute we forgot our stress and felt alive.

All but two of the group participants were able to engage in our group process. Those two women would not participate in the activities or the discussions. They were clearly not ready, and as a group leader, I talked about respecting each person's need to participate or not. We can set up the environment and show them that we are here and ready to help, and give information about what is possible, but do not push them and be present and available for when they are ready.

We talked about the importance of building a trusting relationship by not telling people things that they do not know for sure to be true, for example, that there will not be any more earthquakes, that the rain will not be a problem, or when their house will be rebuilt (unless you know for sure).

THE WORK

After that, at the beginning of each day I would pack a van with equipment and go with two or three national staff/community health workers to a different field hospital. They were all pretty much the same: patients outside in tents if they were lucky, or makeshift tents in the hospital grounds. One or two hospitals did have some patients inside, carefully positioned away from any major beams or walls. Makeshift hospitals were set up in tennis courts, a soccer field, car parks or any big flat spot that would accommodate them. It was both physically and mentally difficult working in such crowded conditions. We often had a photographer or film crew following us around, which

on occasion hindered our work. Reporters were looking for specific stories and asked us to assist in this. While it is important to get the true human stories out to the rest of the world, I sometimes found myself seeing one patient first just so I could get the reporter their story.

We had community health workers assigned more permanently to the larger hospitals where we knew there was a constant need. The number of expatriate therapists grew gradually, and so we were able to cover more ground, setting priorities and making plans to return to the different hospitals as needed. The goal was to get as many people out of the hospital as possible to make room for others. However, most people did not have a home to go back to, and many planned to move out to the provinces because they had lost everything. Being in hospital meant that they had shelter, water and food. It was hard for them to leave that comfort.

For the most part I was just going in, doing my job and trying not to think about the magnitude of the problem. Being an occupational therapist I could help people start to get mobilized, but I could also use what I learned from my Haitian counterparts in our education sessions to help begin to address the psychological stress of the patients. I sat and listened to stories and asked questions about families and where people would go, and what they would do after they left the hospital. The stories were appalling: watching their house crumble, having their whole family die, being trapped in rubble for many days, being only one of a few students who survived the university collapse.

OCCUPATION AS A HEALING POWER

The healing power of activity was clearly seen. In the field hospitals I saw and heard a father giving his sons music lessons on a bed under a tarp, discussed art with a painter who had all of his paints and brushes beside his mattress on the ground, and watched families and strangers working together to protect their dignity, doing the laundry or sharing a drink of water. On the streets I watched as people returned to their daily routines, marked out a space for their family on the street where their home used to be, or set up shop in a tent city, and started rebuilding their lives. Also the power of helping others: Haitians volunteering alongside the aid workers, helping us change our flat tyre and then giving us soap and water to wash our hands, patients helping and taking care of each other, all when they had their own tragedies to deal with. The shock on people's faces seemed to get less and less each day. I am humbled by the sheer strength I saw in so many.

Six months after the earthquake I had the opportunity to work with Leila again. She was doing better then, and had given me permission to tell her story. She continued to inspect any building that she entered, checking for cracks to see if it was safe. I remember how she delighted in having the opportunity to watch a baby being born.

LESSONS

Looking back on my experience of the response and recovery efforts in Haiti, there are a few key lessons that I have taken with me.

- Give space and time for people to tell their stories.
- Information and occupation give hope.
- Helping others is a good way for people to work through their own grief.
- Focus on what is in front of you.

USEFUL WEBSITES

Handicap International: http://www.handicap-international.org

Team Canada Healing Hands: http://tchh.org

8

LIVING WITH THE BONES

RACHEL THIBEAULT

'Kenbé mwen séré, Mamy. Kenbé mwen séré.' 'Hold me tight, Mamy, hold me tight.' Her screams wake me up again. Wide eyed, haggard, she is staring straight into her recent past. The cot we share was meant for one, so it is easy for me to reach over and hold her close. She truly awakes, leans against me and starts to cry. I can hear the rain pounding the tin roof, the wind shaking the banana trees, and just outside the two-room wood dwelling, goats bleating out in fear. Even the animals have been left traumatized by 'l'Évènement', the Event. A simple spring storm triggers it all over again. 'Who is Mamy?' I wonder.

I keep stroking her hair, tight braids dyed bright red at the tips, and along with the rain, Susana's sobs eventually recede. The silence of Ka Henri permeates the night. The mountain air is cool and filled with jasmine carried by the now-gentle breeze. 'Do you want to speak about the Évènement, Susana?' I ask, still holding her. 'Oui. Oui,' she whispers. And she then retells for the nth time her story of the earthquake, a story told by all Haitians I encountered. A story that could be summarized in a few words: loss of loved ones, loss of limbs, loss of livelihood. With the faint light of dawn, Susana drifts back to sleep.

Susana, a 20-year-old orphaned woman from Port-au-Prince, had been hired as our cook/helper for an evaluation mission at the earthquake epicentre. For about a week, a colleague and I travelled on foot along the fault line, a rather challenging set of 'mornes et plaines', sharp peaks and deep valleys unfolding in quick succession south of Port-au-Prince. Our mandate, given by the Association Québécoise d'Appui

aux Nations Unies (AQANU), was to review the earthquake's impact, both material and human, and to assess resulting physical and psychological disabilities along with avenues for sustainable livelihoods. AQANU has been involved in Haiti for over 30 years and has developed strong ties to local grassroots agencies. The journey provided us with an intimate look at life after the tragedy; no roads, only steep mountain paths connect the villages and so we walked from hamlet to hamlet, from house to house, sometimes up to 12 hours a day. The peasants – as they choose to be called – greeted us with boundless generosity and told their stories just as generously. They took us into their houses at night and, around the evening meal, shared all-too-fresh memories and concerns.

The first step, harsh but necessary, was to survey the obvious and ask who had died and how, who was maimed and in what ways, what was broken and what was lost. In the Mornes, it was an all-or-nothing proposition: the mountain sides either did not move or slid into the valleys, taking with them all living beings. There were few in between. Antonine lost four children, swept away with goats and boulders into the riverbed 300 metres below; Jean Baptiste did not lose as much as a hoe, but all mourn together the dead who will never be found, and all still live in fear. They sleep outside, despite sound wooden houses. They have nightmares and the roar of a rescue helicopter sends people scurrying in all directions. Women came to me after community meetings, speaking of the great fright in their heart that makes their mind so cloudy they cannot cook properly anymore. One showed me how she has been gnawing at her lips and cheeks since the Event. She can't stop, she said. She bled and cried, silently.

After some time, we tried to move on gently to the second step: asking about what remains, the strengths of the community, what they have achieved despite the tragedy. Without affectation, they described how they had coped, not even aware of their bravery, compassion and perseverance. They proudly took us to nurseries, carefully tucked in protected areas, where thousands of thriving trees will soon be ready to replant – blooming life in the midst of devastation.

When asked about their priorities, communities readily identified them as treating shock in a non-stigmatizing way, sowing the crops on time for the rainy season and rebuilding what had been destroyed. The villagers' expression blended strength, sadness and determination in equal measures, and by 5.30 every morning, men and women were toiling side by side in the fields.

Back in Port-au-Prince with the Petites Soeurs de Sainte-Thérèse, they too spoke of their fear and pain: six sisters died in the quake, 122 children were crushed in the school's collapse. Not all corpses could be recovered. Soeur Gisèle had not slept more than a few hours a night for the past month. She sighed: 'We will rebuild, you know. We're Haitians. We will rebuild. We always do. But living with the bones; it is so hard to live with the bones.' In shuffling steps, she walked back to the rubble left to be removed by hand.

CONCLUSION

From a therapeutic perspective, treating shock is clearly an urgent need after a major disaster and it would be tempting simply to give the label of post-traumatic stress disorder (PTSD) and tailor interventions to the dry definitions of the Diagnostic and Statistical Manual (DSM). But from an occupational therapy, client-centred perspective, doing so would distort the real nature of the situation: we would miss the courage and solidarity that are just as much a part of the survivors' psyche as their trauma. The human dimension, the very essence of who we are, is always lost in labels. Our labelling habit may point to our inclination for structure and clarity, but it may also expose our difficulty to meet with pain head on without the comforting veils of clinical discourse. We do not like much the intangible casualties of the heart, and yet our main role is often to enable others to live with the bones, a role that extends beyond the narrow confines of PTSD.

The last word goes to Annie Dillard, who does not resort to such veils:

> In the deeps are the violence and terror of which psychology has warned us. But if you ride these monsters down, if you drop with them farther over the world's rim, you find what our sciences cannot locate or name, the substrate, the ocean, or matrix, or ether which buoys the rest which gives goodness its power for good and evil, its power for evil, the unified field: our complex and inexplicable caring for each other for our life together here. It is a given. It is not learned.
>
> *Dillard 1982*

May we reach this field.

REFERENCE
Dillard, A., 1982. Teaching a Stone to Talk. Harper Collins, New York, p. 9.

9

CYCLONE YASI: THE EXPERIENCE OF QUEENSLANDERS WITHOUT A HOME

YVONNE THOMAS

▪ ▪ ▪ ▪ ▪ ▪ ▪ ▪ ▪ ▪ ▪ ▪ ▪ ▪ ▪ ▪ ▪ ▪ ▪ ▪

Have you ever wondered what happens to people who are already homeless during a cyclone? This case study is based on the voices of homeless people in Townsville, immediately following Cyclone Yasi in February 2011. It is presented as two collective narratives, highlighting and contrasting different experiences.

On Wednesday, 2 February 2011, Townsville prepared for a predicted category 5 cyclone to hit its shores. Cyclone Yasi had been forming to the west of Queensland for several days. Its size and strength were of particular concern, with at least 500 km of coastline expected to be affected. For Townsville the threat of a 6 metre storm surge, on top of the full tide, resulted in many parts of the coastal and low-lying city being evacuated. Evacuation centres were slow to be identified. The Mayor of Townsville declared that people should seek safety with friends and family; although some homeless people did this, many were left with few options. Most workplaces were closed and emergency supplies (batteries, water and food) had almost sold out. Everyone was told to stay off the roads after midday. The situation presented particular challenges for homeless people.

JEFF'S STORY

Jeff has lived on the streets for many years, and although he has family locally he decided to use the public evacuation centre.

Well I thought that the cyclone was going to be bad. It had been on the news at the drop in centre and the staff told me that South Townsville was going to get flooded. That's where I normally sleep out. So I thought it would be good to get away from there. The drop in centre was closed so there was nowhere to get meals. I heard that the council had opened an evacuation centre in the showground, well that is not too far to walk so on the morning of the cyclone I bought some food and went to the evacuation centre. I was pretty lucky because the shelter was full pretty soon.

When I got there I got some lunch. There were lots of people there just sitting and talking. It was good to sit and talk to people. It's good to meet different people, you know, just something new and different. Anyway it was OK at the showground. The next day at the crisis centre they provided three meals and coffee, and then we stayed a second night because there was a lot of damage and the wind was still going. Everything was wet and lots of trees had fallen down. It disrupted a lot of people's lives, they had lost electricity to their homes and they were worried because their food had gone off in fridges without power. After two days there I left and went back to the streets. It was wet everywhere and my clothes soon got drenched, but then the drop in centre opened up again, even though they didn't have power, but they had hotdogs on the barbecue. It has been a bit of an adventure really.

Jeff's story demonstrates how by presenting at the council's evacuation centre he was treated the same as everyone else and shared in a wider community experience. The cyclone provided a break from his life on the streets; it was an adventure and gave him an opportunity to chat to other people and get an insight into the anxiety of those who had homes.

TIM'S STORY

In contrast, Tim's experience highlighted his marginalized status and the negative perceptions of homeless people. He had been staying at a hostel the night before but it closed during the cyclone because the location was not safe. Tim and his friends were taken back to town with nowhere to go.

We were just walking the streets when the Police told us that we needed to go to the evacuation centre for the homeless. It was in a car park under the offices in town there. When we got there, there was a big crowd already. There were different mobs there. I stayed with the people I knew. You could hear what was going on outside but the car park was dry and we were going to be safe there. The Police Liaison Officers were there, they didn't want any trouble.

But it got pretty uncomfortable, it was concrete floors and walls, no mattresses or pillows, and it was hard to sleep. It was really hot too, humid and stuffy. There were a few fans at first but we lost power after a while and it became dehydrating there. And there was not much food either. We had vegemite sandwiches, and jam sandwiches, and noodles, but I don't like noodles. The thing that made me mad was that there were some that had meat on a barbecue but that was not offered to us, it was like we didn't matter. So we just stayed one night and then we walked the streets again. Everything was wet, and the police, they kept hassling us, they wanted us off the streets but there

was nowhere open and nowhere to go. Once the hostel reopened we went up there and got a shower, a decent meal and a change of clothes, but that was a few days later. People were pretty stressed really.

Tim and his friends left the evacuation centre as soon as they could, even though it was wet and there was nowhere open to take shelter. The experience was unpleasant and reinforced a sense of marginalization.

IMPLICATIONS FOR OCCUPATIONAL THERAPY

Cyclones occur frequently in tropical north Australia and residents are warned to prepare at the start of each cyclone season. Preparation for homeless people during cyclones and other natural disasters is rarely considered. During Cyclone Yasi there were insufficient evacuation centres for the general public to access, and the last minute arrangements for homeless people were clearly inferior to those provided to the public. Disaster management plans may fail to consider the needs of those that live on the margins, such as homeless people, who may be least able to prepare for themselves.

At an individual level people need help to prepare for, and access, the public facilities. Homeless people need assistance to plan what to do and to maintain some choice and control over where they go. The emergency homeless centre provided safety but few other human comforts, and those that used it felt that they were treated as second class citizens. People who are homeless have few physical resources to manage natural disasters. They often have no money to buy food and limited spare clothes, towels or bedding needed for the days following the disaster before services reopen. Occupational therapists can advocate for the needs of the homeless and disadvantaged before the crisis occurs. This will help to ensure that they have equal access to resources in times of crisis, and opportunities that enable their recovery.

10

AFTER KATRINA: STEPHANIE'S FOUR-YEAR STRUGGLE FOR SURVIVAL

EMILY F. PIVEN

S tephanie, a beautiful 51-year-old single African American woman, whose name has been changed to protect her identity (Figure 10-1), lived in uptown New Orleans when Hurricane Katrina destroyed her new condominium. Just three weeks before the hurricane, she spent her savings elegantly refurnishing her home and splurging on the most expensive new furniture. She had a good paying job as a funeral director, making $60 000/year, and then overnight it all changed.

The hurricane hit on 29 August 2005. The levee broke on 30 August 2005. Water started rising at about 4.00 pm in her two-storey condo. By 9.00 pm, there was about 9 feet of water on the first floor. She placed her Pomeranian puppy in the ice cooler, stood on her sideboard and punched a hole in her damaged roof with a broom handle. There was only a large can of tuna and a jug of water for Stephanie and the puppy that she could not forecast would need to last her seven days. On the third day, while she sat waiting on the roof, a soldier passed by and yelled from the helicopter, 'You have to leave the dog.' She yelled back, 'No! This is the only child I have.' The soldiers kept moving on to look for survivors without pets. On the fourth day on the roof she fell through, cracking her coccyx on the dining room table, an accident that would make it hard for her to work in the future.

VENTURING OUT

'I don't know how to steal,' she thought. 'I am not like them hoodlums that loot. I would be so scared that I'd get caught!' Still, she was so hungry. Pushing the puppy into the cooler, she found a store that had been looted.

There was a loaf of bread and some sausage that looked good to her, so she packed the items in the cooler. On the way home, she saw old people hanging out of the window of their home. Raised by her father, a Baptist preacher, Stephanie gave the bread and sausage to the elderly and went back to look for more food for herself. Much to her dismay, the store shelves were empty. 'I almost drowned coming back to my house that day. I held on to a light pole to roll my trouser legs up when I felt a pinch on my right leg. I kept going. I thought I felt a branch brush across my body in the water. When I looked back, there was a dead man who had touched me. I thought, Lord, you better save me or kill me. I can't take much more of this.' Almost at her house, a rescue boat from the TV station picked Stephanie and the puppy up on 6 September 2005. After that an army truck, helicopter and then a plane carried her to safety. She asked, 'Where are we going?' She kept hearing 'I don't know,' no matter who she asked. 'You must be taking us to Iraq to get killed!' As ridiculous as that statement sounded, she was scared and not much was making sense that day. Upon arrival at Fort Bliss, El Paso, Texas, she was immediately taken to William S. Beaumont Army Hospital to treat the snake bite she had on her calf.

Most of the almost 600 evacuees who fled Hurricane Katrina for shelter and assistance ultimately chose to restart their lives in El Paso and settled there permanently. Tens of thousands of others trickled back to New Orleans, the former tourist mecca.

I was later taken to the El Paso Judson F. Williams Convention Center where we were treated very nice. The 600 evacuees were divided with families and

73

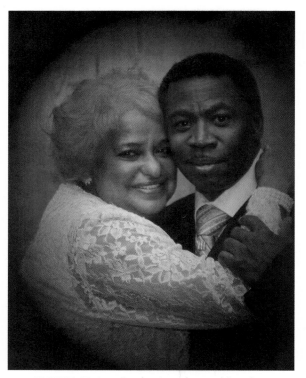

FIGURE 10-1 ■ Stephanie on her wedding day.

partners. I stayed three weeks. So many agencies helped us: the American Red Cross, police, fire department, Salvation Army, clothing and shoe stores, food vendors, hospitals, churches, civilians, the Sun Metro bus station, banks, apartments, restaurants, and the local animal shelter. The news media helped survivors link with family members. The NAACP and Black Chamber of Commerce provided Career Readiness Programs. I ate so much Mexican food; I thought I'd be able to speak Spanish. Even hotels opened their doors to help.

When I met Stephanie she was standing on the street trying to sell her clothing and shoes to buy the next meal. As ridiculous as it seemed, she was given only $10.00 of free food stamps per month. Stephanie took minimum wage jobs that did not work out. Often she would get late night shifts and the buses did not run, making it difficult to keep the jobs. Her lack of ability to speak Spanish was the largest barrier that kept her out of the job market in a primarily Hispanic

community. Though her housing was supported by the Federal Emergency Management Agency, she did not have a way of paying her utilities or eating. In her refrigerator there was a single can of opened soda.

Stephanie appeared depressed and despondent. Her face was pimpled from stress. She spoke of suicide. My heart went out to her. Before I knew it, I offered her a job cleaning my home. Thinking about her loss of important roles and relationships, I encouraged her to ask for what she needed from the local Baptist church, typed her resumé and practised with her to role-play job interviews. At first, she was resistant to asking for help. Gradually, her assertiveness increased and her true personality came out.

FINDING A JOB

With encouragement and $25.00, Stephanie renewed her funeral director's license and found a job at a funeral home two blocks from her home. The funeral home contracted a Spanish teacher to teach new workers conversational Spanish, but the teacher quit and Stephanie was told there was no further need for her services because of her language barrier.

A local vacuum factory offered a job on the night shift. Though hired as a technician in the plastic department, Stephanie would be asked to run errands for the supervisor during her lunch break. She was put on suspension when a public transport delay caused her to be late for work one night. She had her hours cut and was told by her supervisor, 'I don't do nice things for niggers.' This led to a $4500 settlement with the vacuum company president to avoid negative publicity and gave her 'survival money' for food for four months.

With growing confidence, Stephanie approached one of her fellow parishioners about a job with the Internal Revenue Service. Stephanie had previous work experience as a bank clerk and trained as an auditor. This job was very interesting, but without a car she could not take a full-time placement. She did audits of bank records and public officials on call. While working at this job for six months, she found a better paid job working at a local hospital emergency department filling out insurance forms, calling next of kin and working in the mortuary, but a layoff of 150 employees left her again without a job three months later.

This time Stephanie was able to obtain a job the next day as a photojournalist for a local TV station, preparing pictures for the evening news. One month later she received a promotion, making $18.00 an hour working for the meteorologist. Commenting on her rapid progress during a two-year period, Stephanie said 'It is easier to find a job when you have a job, and when someone believes in you.'

I believed in Stephanie. Though her situation was dire and had left her devastated simply trying to survive, she was tenacious, strong willed and resilient. I helped Stephanie to connect with that strength from within. I was not Stephanie's occupational therapist, I was her friend. I listened to her experience and the harsh reality of her everyday struggle. I connected to her on a human level and simply responded from the heart.

Stephanie's situation is very different today. She now has a 'mother and father' in her church and lots of friends. She now has a great job that she enjoys and a man who loves her (see her wedding picture - Figure 10-1). She survived because of her resilience. Given the continued support and friendship, she is getting back on her feet. It takes a long time to recover when a person is transplanted into another culture without formal education. Stephanie is making it now.

11

WILDFIRES: RESPONDING TO PSYCHOLOGICAL AND EMOTIONAL NEEDS OF THE COMMUNITY

ZOE EDMONDS

It was Saturday, 7 February 2009 when the fire began near my home. I live in Kilmore East, a small town in central Victoria, 85 kilometres north of Melbourne. I was involved in the Black Saturday bushfires, both in my private life and professionally as an occupational therapist.

After weeks of unprecedented hot weather with temperatures over 40° for days, a drought that had lasted for several years and humidity at only 6% on the day, all was tinder dry. Flammable gases releasing from the eucalyptus trees made the atmosphere highly explosive. Added to this, gale force winds from the north were assailing the land, turning it into a blast furnace. One spark was all that was needed to ignite the bushfire that was to cause one of the worst natural disasters in Australia's history, and that spark occurred just a kilometre from my home.

I looked out of the window and saw a huge plume of orange smoke over the ridge, opposite, and within 15 minutes the smoke plume had already moved several kilometres along the ridge, right into the middle of a large pine and gum tree plantation. When I saw the flames coming over the ridge, I left and drove north away from the fire to stay with friends.

THE FIRE

This 'small fire' was destined to join with others, eventually becoming a fire storm of unimaginable destructive power that caused catastrophic damage.

Fanned by the gale force winds, the fire moved at phenomenal speed, reportedly sending embers and fireballs up to 20 kilometres ahead of the fire front. So fast moving was it that it caught hundreds of people unawares, and with devastating consequences. For some there was literally no time to think.

The Victorian Bushfire Reconstruction and Recovery Authority, established two days after the disaster, reported on its website, 'The 2009 Victorian bushfires were the worst in Australia's history. The fires devastated nearly 80 communities across the state, destroyed more than 2000 homes and damaged about 430 000 hectares of land. By the time the fires were contained 173 people had lost their lives and many others were seriously injured.'

MENTAL HEALTH TEAM – FIRST FEW DAYS

On the Monday I went to work. I was employed as a case manager, occupational therapist (OT) in the mental health team for the Lower Hume area. Forty per cent of our area had been affected by the bushfire. The managers from head office were already there to support the team and work out strategies to manage the situation. Our first task was to attempt to contact all our clients in the area, not knowing if they had survived. By the end of the second day all clients had been located alive. Several clients had lost their homes.

Before we arrived back at work, we had all seen horrific images on the news. Many houses had been flattened to the ground, leaving warped tin roofs on top of burnt-out rubble. Everything was black and ash. Burnt-out cars, some alone, some smashed together in groups, were stark testament to the frantic flight of those who died there. It was easy to imagine what people must have gone through in the terrifying moments during their desperate attempts to survive, whether they were in their homes or on the road. One wife and mother said, 'We tore down the driveway, flames behind us, kids screaming; and my husband said to me, "Do we go left or right?" I had no idea, but I chose the right way. If we'd gone the other way we would have all died.'

I felt shocked and deeply upset, and I imagine everyone else in the team did, too. What we faced was an enormous emotional and practical challenge.

PREPARING TO GO TO THE AFFECTED AREAS

By the Wednesday after the fires, our service was making plans for the team to go out to support people in the affected areas.

I initially felt uncertain about how I would cope, about what people would need from me. Having never experienced anything like this before, I simply was not sure what I would need to do. I had had no training for this! In fact, none of us had. What sort of shape would people be in? How would I manage the sheer number of people involved, the level of their devastation, and their shock? What would their specific needs be? How would I be able to help? Would I even be able to help?

To get some guidance I spoke to two mentors of mine, both psychotherapists who are very experienced in working with traumatized people. They said, 'Do what we know you're already experienced at doing. Be there for people in an authentic way. In the beginning, too, don't be a counsellor or a therapist, just be a real person who's there to help out in any way that's appropriate. Being available to those who talk spontaneously about their experiences is important; and be prepared to do this leaning up against a fence post, walking along the street, standing at the door of a car – anywhere. As they talk, people will need you simply to hear and accept what they say about their experiences. Do your best to handle your own emotions while with them, and avoid jumping in and trying to reassure them and "make it okay" in some way (which often blocks people and what they need to do). And if they

fall silent just let time stretch out. They'll start again when they're ready.'

They added, 'You'll also find some people will be experiencing anger as a raw emotion. As a natural part of their trauma they may direct it at something or someone to which it does not belong. They need to express the anger, regardless of how rational or irrational it may be, in order to move through it gradually to talking in a more settled rational way about the issue and what they need to do. To help people with this it's important to meet their strength with strength in the way you talk with them so they experience you engaging with them, and also that you demonstrate you can handle the anger. This will often involve you talking firmly and directly.' I found often as I matched people's intensity, for example, saying, in effect 'Damn right you're angry! You've got a lot to be angry about, that this encouraged people to discharge the anger, just as a more soothing approach encouraged the release of distress.

MANAGING OUR OWN REACTIONS

In hindsight, I also certainly needed to process the emotional impact of what had just happened. My preference would have been for our team to have shared more of our thoughts and feelings about the horror in which we were involved, particularly on that first day at work. Expressing my feelings in order to digest and discharge them from my system usually works well for me. However, because I was in a work situation where many of my colleagues seemed to handle things differently, I thought I needed to keep my emotions in check; this seemed the 'professional' thing to do. The result was that I needed to manage a building intensity of feeling that was locked inside of me. This interfered to some degree with my normal level of functioning and ability to think clearly. I only experienced relief from this later that night when I expressed my pent up feelings with the friends with whom I was staying, and this made a big difference.

This need was also clearly relevant to people affected by the fires in the community. Some talked about their experiences and expressed their emotions, while others 'put on a brave face' and attempted to contain their feelings. One woman told me, 'I thought I was doing okay, then my grown-up daughter came up to help out and as soon as I saw her, I broke down crying. It all just came out.' It would become clear that the way people managed their responses affected their overall recovery. And understanding this led us to make sure that people had repeated opportunities to do things in the ways they needed to, although some well-meaning people missed this point at times.

Many people were stunned, bewildered, in shock, and finding it hard to think clearly or know what to do. Some people felt angry whereas some were feeling scared. Others were initially elated at having survived and some were still high on adrenalin. 'Survivor guilt' was a widespread issue, too. People thought they did not deserve support because they had survived when so many had not.

GOING TO FLOWERDALE

Our team members went to different areas when it was safe enough. Several days after the fire, my colleague Jane and I were sent to Flowerdale, a township towards the north end of the fire-affected area.

Our role there was to assess the mental health needs of community members and to support people in any way we could. In the early days this often involved providing practical help as well as emotional and psychological support. Jane was a wonderful model of how to act in an extreme crisis. She demonstrated by example how to get things done by being systematic, practical and well organized. People responded to her sense of order, helping them focus in the midst of extreme disorder, and this was exactly what was needed.

At the same time my occupational therapy background guided me to focus on how people were functioning and what they needed in order to recover following the disaster. I looked at people's needs, both physical and emotional, and their strengths and capacities to manage in a physical and social environment that was extremely disrupted and abnormal. Also, since qualifying as an OT I have engaged in extensive psychotherapy training, and my knowledge and skills in this area were important assets in my work to help individuals deal with the shock and process the emotional trauma, while also participating in the

setting up of effective support systems within the community.

Initially, we had to link in with the community and let people know who we were and that we were there to offer support. We did this by visiting the few public places where people had started to gather. As we did, we needed to adjust to working out of cars and dusty tents, all in a fire-blackened landscape with smoke and soot everywhere, and working in the midst of the very scenes we continued to see on TV news reports.

Flowerdale had been isolated for days before we got there. As one resident commented later, 'We were known as the forgotten town … we've not seen anyone but helicopters flying overhead.' The people of Flowerdale had shown remarkable adaptability, resilience and determination in coping without support in the midst of the fire and with its immediate aftermath. Ron, another resident, said, 'It was a characteristic of this place. We were absolutely determined we were all going to stay and occupy the places we had saved.'

Their isolation after the fire was due to the police roadblocks that cut off the area for several days because the roads were still very dangerous. Unfortunately, doing so limited the help that could get through to the town, delayed the arrival of many much-needed supplies and hindered the locals' ability to help themselves in their recovery. They needed to get food and water, and items such as generators, but were blocked in their ability to do so. For days, there was no power, telephone or running water, and many sewerage systems were damaged or destroyed. Fires could flare up again, houses even burnt down days after the main fire. Ron explained, 'It was a big problem. We knew we couldn't leave and we didn't want to abandon our homes, having saved them. There was the sense of being locked in with the problem.'

Understandably, having fought for their survival, people initially felt let down, hindered and abandoned by the wider community, and for some, this stuck to a certain extent as the weeks went by, although the army were in the area in the first few days, and many people told me they found the soldiers incredibly supportive and their presence in the area instilled a level of security in people.

Around 80% of Flowerdale's population of 1500 were homeless and 13 people had died. The majority of people were displaced and staying elsewhere. Even so, an estimated 200 people were still living in the area, some in their own homes, some with friends and neighbours. Six members of the Country Fire Authority (CFA) had lost their homes and were bunked down at the fire station. Groups quickly formed where people supported each other, two of which were highly significant: one at the CFA station and one at the pub. They were at opposite ends of the town. Meanwhile, other people remained significantly isolated, initially at least.

THE CFA GROUP

The CFA Fire Station became a place to get support and a safe haven for several people. Already an established group made up of local volunteers from Flowerdale with their own infrastructure, safety consciousness and peer support, the brigade was ideal for this. The following comments from Katherine, a new member of the CFA, show how important it was to people.

Knowing that I could call into the Fire Station or go and get advice from my brigade and other CFA members, without judgement from them, was of great help. I was in an absolute panic about fires returning for up to six weeks after February 7th.

The CFA brigade gave me a place to debrief what had happened to my partner, to our crews, and to me during the fires, including the fear when I was separated from my partner without communication until 7.30 am on Sunday 8 February – about 17 hours after the phone lines went down.

A physicality among brigade members arose – all of us touched each other on the arm or shoulder while talking, or hugged each other when we met, or just let each other cry.

The CFA members continued to be on call for two weeks to put out spot fires that continued to flare up (for about six weeks), until a fire crew from another area took over. Ian, another member of the CFA and resident of Flowerdale, commented as follows:

… congregating [there] … provided sanity … connectedness. During that week we all had breakfast together and meals together at night … it allowed us to wind down together before departing.

Those people going home were going home a bit more settled. We supported each other.

[Meeting like this] gave us a structure for the day as to what to do and how to do it. There was a lot of down time when we didn't do anything. We paced ourselves and we were focused. As a way of coping we really clung to each other, I guess. I went home every night but I was always back there the next day.

THE PUB AND COMMUNITY MEETINGS

The other main grouping to emerge centred at the pub. Steve, the owner of the Flowerdale pub, stepped forward right from the beginning. He and others in the community had spent all of Saturday night and Sunday fighting fires, including protecting a number of people who, fleeing the fires, had got marooned at the pub car park at the end of town, as fires raged around them.

By Sunday night Steve and a mate sat down exhausted and wondered about how to handle things the next day. Steve said, 'We'll get together in the morning, have a coffee and work out what we need to do.'

The next day a handful of people turned up. They needed to work out basic things like getting showered and comfortable. Each day more people turned up there in the morning. Steve recognized that people needed to know how to go about their day, they needed advice and help, and they needed food. This was the start of daily community meetings. Within a week, 200 people were attending this meeting at the start of each day.

Led by members of the community, these daily meetings became a focal point for people to come together, to be informed of the many developments that were taking place, to take charge of their recovery, and promote community cohesiveness. It also became the place where support agencies would share information.

Ian said, 'In terms of the morning meetings it was important for the community to have an understanding of the range of what was happening. [At] one meeting the police got a lot of heat for blocking off the roads, so there was the explanation of why and that diffused some of that, and that helped.'

It was also a venue for the community to have a voice with these agencies. Ian goes on to say 'When … what we've actually said is being heard, and therefore it's been done; it psychologically boosted our confidence and I think that was a major step forward.'

Having meals supplied was crucial in the early days when many people did not have access to cooking facilities, particularly for those who initially were finding it hard to function normally. The nutrition was essential, helped to keep up their strength and was nurturing. Within a short time about 150 people were being fed out of the pub at any one time. This was initially organized by the pub owners and community members. Later the Army provided catering as well as trained chefs, who came to volunteer their support.

COMMUNITY RESILIENCE

The resilience of people living in Flowerdale was obvious. Individuals had spontaneously stepped forward into positions of leadership and supporting each other. Morning meetings chaired by Steve quickly became an established start to the day. The day I arrived, the morning meeting was in full swing. They were discussing rigging up a laundry system by using the resources and skills they had available to them within the community.

Debbie, another community member, had taken charge of organizing relief supplies. Trudy, a friend of Debbie's, said, 'She's not looking for any credit; it's just in her nature. She's a doer. If there's something to be done she'll do it. And she's organized.'

Ron made line maps of the area, showing the houses left standing and who was living in the houses. These maps were eventually used by all officials coming into the area. Also, he organized a registration system to identify locals so they could move in and out of the fire-affected zone.

SUPPORT SERVICES

By Friday, six days after the fires, many professionals from different agencies were suddenly present in Flowerdale. However, while this was important, it had a downside to it. As Trudy said, 'It was overwhelming to start with. You looked at them and thought, who's this, and who's that, and where are they from?' At the same time, Ron said, '[At least] you had a sense that things are happening.'

It was clear that the professionals on the ground needed to get organized and word went round that we would have a professionals' meeting with several of the community members who had stepped into leadership roles. It was vital that we be informed by them to ensure that what the professionals did was aligned with what was needed to support the community in their recovery efforts and their sense of resilience.

At the same time it was clear that some of those in the community in positions of responsibility were themselves having to manage their own trauma and were overloaded by the demands on them. The support services needed to take the pressure off these people. So it was organized for the Army to take over the catering at the pub, and the relief supplies were moved from the pub to the community hall, where the Salvation Army then ran things.

A frustration was that support personnel were routinely taken off the job, often after one week and against their wishes, because of policies in their organizations about people not working in the affected area for too long. While this is understandable, many locals commented that the lack of continuity was a problem. Ron said, '[We] established relationships [and when they left] we were constantly starting back from scratch again' and Trudy said, 'When it's a totally different person you're absolutely gobsmacked … You've got to have consistency because people are going through enough turmoil.'

For several days we had a professionals' meeting after the community meeting. This was a crucial venue for discussing and coordinating responses to many existing issues. New challenges arose on a daily basis as well and had to be dealt with. The representative community members always played a key role in these meetings.

Once the recovery support infrastructure was in place, with an established coordinator, Jane and I, with the specialist trauma team from the Austin Hospital, Melbourne working alongside us, concentrated on providing help with emotional and psychological issues. As our role became more known, people started to come and see us for support. People often told us about others who they felt were struggling and needed input from us: 'Jonny up the road is isolated and I

REMEMBERING THE CANBERRA FIRES 2003 – GWYNNE'S STORY

It had been searing heat for days on end – there were bush-fires all around – smoke on the horizon. Mid-morning when my daughter and I emerged from a local shopping centre the whole place was covered in thick black smoke – seeing more than 5 m in front was impossible. The man on the radio announced that 'Canberra was in no danger!'

At home we started the preparations, laying wet towels along windows and doors – closing blinds, including the canvas out the front, and then we began wetting everything, filling drains with water and just trying to make everything wet – the man across the road threatened to report us for wasting water – he was to lose his home about two hours later.

We were so alone – no warnings, no police and no emergency services with warnings; a year earlier when fires threatened, we were placed on evacuation alert – this time nothing! My daughter who lives out of town called and asked me to come and collect her children – they had just been told that they were under threat. Soon after arriving home we made the decision to get the children and pets out of here – I called a friend and quickly took the kids over – this was about 1.00 pm and we still had had no warnings!

By 3.00 pm the fire was on us – roaring down the pathway across the road – sounding like a fleet of 747s preparing for take-off. Along with the roar of the fire we could hear explosions – found out later they were houses and the gas supplies exploding!

Our hoses melted, our buckets melted – we had no water! The front garden burnt but luckily the wetting of the mulch caused the fire to look for the easier option and it went around the side – it burnt the fences, the garage just melted and the backroom was burning. The decision to leave was made using the back roads.

The feeling of despair and helplessness was quite debilitating. I had not heard from my daughter – I didn't know if they were safe – I found out on Sunday morning that they were safe! We found out about the same time that our house had not burnt.

Going back was like being on another planet – everything was blackened – houses all around were burnt – nothing left, just a pile of rubble. The heat and intensity of this fire was incredible. I was left with a feeling of such anger – mainly because no one was given any warning or support – two people had died and nearly 500 houses within 5 km of us were destroyed.

We did not see any emergency services people until the Tuesday after the fire, when a fire truck pulled up and asked 'were there any people in that house?' About the best support we got in that first week was some people from one of the welfare groups who were handing out bottles of water!

I saw people totally destroyed – their confidence shaken and their despair at the lack of support – it really was soul destroying – politicians making excuses – the head of emergency services making excuses! Just a single 'sorry' would have made such a difference.

It was several months later that I sought out a psychologist to help me think through all that was in my head. I made a decision not to use the support/counsellors supplied – at the time all the emphasis, and rightly so, was on those who had lost everything. I felt that as I had not lost my home and my belongings, that this support wasn't for me. In fact we did not register for any help for the same reason. There were people in much more need than us.

My decision to seek help was thus a fairly arduous journey … It took several visits but eventually with the psychologist's suggestion of writing it all down, I wrote a poem. It has never seen the light of day, but it did help. I highly recommend it when anger overwhelms.

Today there are still times when I feel angry at what happened but it quickly goes. For a fleeting minute I panic when I smell smoke in the air. I watched and listened with horror at the terrible fires in Victoria and thought, 'they never learn' and I think this is my biggest fear.

My experience taught me:

- That I can operate under extreme stress – I won't panic. It's interesting on looking back that I seemed to operate on another level, in another zone where all thought was about how to manage the situation we were in.
- To trust myself – go with my 'gut instinct', this is rarely wrong.
- The importance of staying calm in circumstances like this – don't panic.

Gwynne Coughlin

don't think he's doing too well. He lives up such and such road, third gate on your left past the green shed.' Invariably it would be challenging and often time consuming to find the property and the person, but it was important that we did.

We developed a structured approach to make what we were doing organized and more effective. This was especially important as there were different people attending each day from the trauma team, recording referrals, who had been seen, the outcomes and identified need for follow-up with individuals. Relevant information was reviewed by the team at the start of the day and this informed many of our tasks for the day.

Within weeks the bushfire counselling service was also established in recognition of people's need for ongoing support to process the traumatic effects of the bushfire. Bushfire case managers were soon also in place to help people with the many practical demands of the recovery and rebuilding process: reconstructing a place to live, getting back into work, getting children in school again, and so on.

SUPPORT GROUP

By late March I was co-facilitating a bushfire support group in Flowerdale with Kate, an OT employed as a bushfire counsellor.

The group ran for 11 weeks. People told their stories, some more easily than others. There were tears and laughter and some heart-felt connections between people. Everyone was free to come as and when they could, so the numbers varied. The feedback generally highlighted the contribution the group had made: it was healing to share experiences with others, people got the sense of not being alone with their problem, and the mutual understanding and acceptance between people of what they were each going through had a strengthening effect.

LEAVING FLOWERDALE

My role in Flowerdale ended in late May, three months after the fires. We had been part of an emergency response to the initial emotional and psychological needs of the community. Jane and I ended the bushfire response work gradually so there was a smooth transition as others came in to take over.

Nine months after the disaster, the situation in Flowerdale is much more stable. At the same time people are still adjusting to the massive disruption to their lives. They know Flowerdale will never be the same. Ian said about the recovery, 'Different people have their own journey through the process … Some people are well advanced and some … have not even taken the first steps.'

And summer is again approaching rapidly. Kate, who continues to work as a bushfire recovery counsellor in Flowerdale, states, 'with the weather getting hot again, you can sense the fear in many people. They have barely learnt to cope with the Black Saturday fires,

and now they face the prospect of a longer, hotter summer than the last with all its risks.'

RECOVERING FROM WILDFIRES: KEY LESSONS FOR PRACTITIONERS

Establishing Safety and Order

The highest priority in a disaster and its aftermath is to establish safety and order as soon as possible. An increased sense of safety and security in the early days is immediately helpful to those affected and reduces the residual longer-term psychological and emotional trauma.

Organization

The rapid, effective response of the management teams in agencies helps to give backing and direction to their staff on the ground. The staff can then act more systematically with the people in the communities affected by the event. Likewise, it is important for those working on the ground to give feedback to the management teams organizing at a higher level in order to get what is needed into the areas.

Establishing an obvious supportive presence in the area, possibly with multiple agencies, is a high priority, so that people can access this as and when they are ready. When multiple agencies are involved, coordination of their efforts is essential. Also, the potential for overloading people with multiple offers of help from different agencies needs to be managed. Communicating promptly to community members what the services are and what support they provide is also essential. This could usefully include the establishment of a central hub where all agencies are based.

Linking in with the Community

It is far more effective for professionals to link with already established community structures and to support what was being done by locals. The latter often have important local contacts, knowledge and access to resources that the agency personnel need but do not have. Doing so also supports the resilience of local communities by backing the people who are taking the initiative.

Information

Making sure all community members have up to date information is crucial. It needs to include the most recent information about their safety, access to emergency personnel, availability of food and other essential supplies, the help on offer from different agencies, rebuilding, and all other ongoing developments. Effective ways of distributing this information include daily community meetings, large notice boards placed in public areas, local newsletters and, once electricity is re-established, websites and internet blogs. An innovative community radio initiative was set up which was itself an engaging, healing activity through which people gained information, told their stories and connected with those they had lost contact with.

Connectedness and Support

People who have lived through a disaster need to be able to connect with and support each other. This is obvious from the way people sought each other out in the aftermath of the bushfire disaster. At the same time, professional people need to stay alert for and reach out to those who are isolated. Opportunities for community activities are beneficial; for example, during the intermediate phase of recovery, people benefitted from participating in community events as part of their shared process, including attending memorial services, community dinners and other activities. While support is understandably directed towards those who have lost loved ones, homes and property, it is also important to consider the situation of others, like Gwynne, who felt they did not deserve the help and may therefore be invisible to registration systems.

Managing Trauma

Professionals and lay people working in the area are also liable to be deeply traumatized, even devastated, by their experiences. It is vitally important that they have external support to manage their reactions. Ideally, too, those brought in at short notice in particular need to be assessed for their capacity and suitability for the work that they will be doing.

Working with Traumatized People

Workers need to have knowledge about the effects of trauma and the most effective ways to support people through the recovery process. Survivors need opportunities to process their reactions and feelings. This is an unfolding process in which people will have different needs as time passes. Workers need to remain flexible about how they do their work because, particularly immediately after the disaster, there will be more natural opportunities to do this informally 'in the field' than in formal sessions. Generally, they need to stay practical, to be continually aware of the context and to deal with things simply and authentically. Counselling is often only appropriate some months after the initial events. As Gwynne concludes, 'I think this is a very challenging area – many people in the first few weeks just need to be able to come to a position where they can just get on with the day to day work. Sometimes people who mean well, coming in and intruding, will do more harm than good.'

FINAL REFLECTION

As an occupational therapist I am trained to think systematically and holistically, and this approach is useful in a post-disaster situation when there are a myriad of functional problems for people to manage. My role in Flowerdale was specifically to help people manage their emotional and psychological responses following the disaster and to promote recovery.

Basic occupational therapy training is not enough to equip people with the necessary skills and capacities to do this work effectively in a disaster zone. They will need further specialist training in how to help people through the trauma process. Also, people need to have a developed capacity to manage high levels of emotional and psychological intensity, both in themselves and in other people, and will need to be able to process their own responses well.

CONCLUSION

'Catastrophic' fire days are an increasing part of life in Australia, as they are in North America and Europe. The ability to prepare, respond and recover is a growing task that communities and professionals must share. As the capacity of authorities to control wildfires and protect lives and property is further stretched, individuals, families and community groups are being directed to 'prepare, act and survive' (Figure 11-1). So, in addition to assisting recovery in the aftermath of fire, helping to build mental and physical preparedness is a potential area for future involvement.

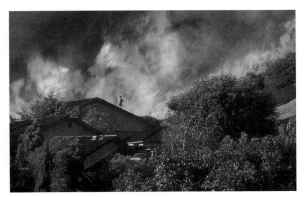

FIGURE 11-1 ■ Wildland fires: dangers and survival in the USA mirror experiences in Australia. In desperate actions to defend their homes, some people are ill prepared, such as this inappropriately clad and positioned man. Wind direction can change radically at any time, and this individual could have been incapacitated by a momentary blast of superheated air from the convection or radiant heat produced by the spreading fire. In the absence of any outside assistance, this would then have left him vulnerable to burning by direct flame contact along with his home. Fortunately for this person, shortly after the photo was taken, an air tanker dropped a load of fire retardant near the advancing flames and effectively nullified the fire's spread and intensity. *(Reproduced from Auerbach, P. 2007. Wilderness Medicine. Elsevier Health Sciences, St Louis, MO. © Elsevier.)*

Acknowledgements

I would like to acknowledge the members of the Flowerdale community who feature in this chapter, all of whom in their own way contributed very significantly to the recovery effort of their community: Ron Ross, Debbie Shultz, Steve Phelan, Trudy Goudge and Ian Charles.

I also want to acknowledge the great work of my colleagues, Jane Douglas and Kate Lewer (both mentioned in this chapter), who shared the journey of working to support the recovery effort in the days and months following the disaster. (Kate continued to work as a bushfire counsellor in Flowerdale for several years.)

To all of my colleagues at the Goulburn Valley Area Mental Health Service who worked together during this challenging time to support the recovery effort in several communities across the region.

I would also like to express my deep gratitude to Ken and Elizabeth Mellor who provided a high level of professional mentoring and personal support to me during this time.

REFERENCE

Auerbach, P., 2007. Wilderness Medicine. Elsevier Health Sciences, St Louis, MO.

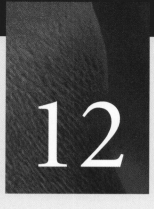

12 TERRORISM: A SURVIVOR'S STORY

SUE HANISCH

INTRODUCTION

The miracle is not to fly in the air, or to walk on the water, but to walk on the earth.

Chinese Proverb

There are times in all of our lives when the music stops, doesn't it? And there is little or nothing we can do on our own to get it going again. For me the music stopped at ten to eight on a Monday morning, 18 February 1991, at Victoria Station, London, England. I was making a quick telephone call to my mum and was only in London for the weekend, as I was living in Holland at the time.

Suddenly, and shockingly, an anonymous face with evil in their heart ripped my life apart. With the devastating blast of an IRA bomb, it meant that nothing was the same. Nothing could ever be the same again.

As I lay on the floor of Victoria Station and tried to get up I could see that I had lost my right foot and had severe injuries to my left leg. My right hand was injured and my hair was burning; still I couldn't understand why I couldn't get up. There was chaos everywhere. Shouts went up that there were two further unexploded bombs within the vicinity, according to the IRA warning which had been received and ignored several hours earlier. A kind fellow human being held my hand and reassured me for the 60 minutes I lay there before I was stretchered away to Westminster Hospital.

The man next to me died instantly and probably saved my life, but for the next 60 minutes the paramedics rigorously tried to resuscitate him, to no avail.

Some losses were immediately obvious then and in the months to follow, but some I only realized and faced years later.

My physical losses took priority, which of course they had to; the injuries to both my legs were severe and permanent. At night I would wake up screaming in hospital, begging for the nurses to come and rock me. I had no sense of where I was or who I was in this world any more. I was in and out of London hospitals for three years for the necessary surgical repair. But years on, when my physical disability had become a daily reality, the enormity of the changes to my self-identity was truly disabling.

By this I mean the things which I felt made me, me. I had lost all sense of location, stability and identity and had become completely detached from my former feelings, hopes and dreams. I did not know what was wrong with me, but felt like my soul was no longer inside my body, that I had detached from my violated body and that I was no longer engaging with anyone or anything around me. Trying to live life as if stuck behind a glass wall is very perplexing as you can be seen and heard, despite not actually sensing or feeling anything in relation to your immediate surroundings.

I knew that I was not well. After 11 years' experience working as an occupational therapist around the world, advising other people with disabilities on how to cope and teaching them ways to adjust to and accept their change in body and circumstances, I realized I had never had a true understanding of disability at all.

How arrogant I had been! How could I start to rebuild the person I had been with what was left?

Nothing around me was recognizable or familiar, I felt like I was an alien on the wrong planet and that I did not want to stay.

My body wasn't the same any more, my relationships weren't the same any more, and at that point my husband of 16 years left. If only I could have had the choice of leaving me and my disabled life and disabled thinking behind.

Then, five years after the bombing, I wished, for the first time, that I had not survived at all. What a lonely, frightening time that was. The survivor's guilt and shame after a violent incident is well recorded but impossible to explain away. As a Christian, how can one continue living without a sense of gratitude for life itself, especially if one feels neither alive nor dead? All my rehabilitation had been completed, my limb fitting service established and I had endured years of 'person centred counselling' which only made me feel worse. The legal profession involved in my case only focused on the losses to my life and all the things I was no longer able to do. When one is in a state of trauma (a hypnotic trance state), the worst possible approach is for a professional to embed suggestions which the survivor is unable to question or defend. The sense of victimhood was profound and totally disabling, but I was so traumatized and so vulnerable that I could not defend my position or see the bigger picture. This situation, as an occupational therapist, made me feel even worse: with all the knowledge and experience I had, why could I not find a way to adjust to and accommodate my altered circumstances? Self-blame, self-hatred and shame made me withdraw even further into confusion, and my absolute terror was that this might be a permanent state that stopped me from sharing this unbearable distress with any other individual. There is a history of suicide in my family and I was constantly reminded of this option during this lonely journey into hell.

I am certain that it is harder to survive than it is to die. At the time of the bombing I had felt a sense of serenity, dignity and time expanding. I knew as I lay on the floor of Victoria Station that it was safe to let go and die, hence I now started to come to the realization that this near death experience had left me with an out of body experience which was causing me great discomfort in trying to live on the earth again. This is a classic example of how dissociation begins. I felt that there had been a terrible split between my body and soul, yet had no idea what to do about it. I resumed work and went through the motions of my life like a cardboard cutout, repeating daily routines, never having any fun, never looking forward to anything and feeling enormous resentment for anyone who could engage in fun. Celebrations were things to be avoided as I became ashamed of my limited outlook and lack of hope for the future. The sense of being different from those around me was intense and led to even further isolation, withdrawal and self-loathing.

When, ten years post bomb, I was in the South of France with some friends and the cannon in Nice fired at 12 noon, I found myself on the ground kicking, screaming, rocking, crying and unable to work out what was wrong. I recognized at last that I would have to pursue some effective form of trauma treatment before it really was too late. We are so hardwired for health that the body will keep yearning for another avenue of healing at a visceral level; such ancient wisdom of the body needs to be heeded.

From that point onwards I intuitively started tapping into my forgotten knowledge of what makes me human, what a child needs to know when he arrives in the world, as well as the deep well of my occupational therapy experience with dyspraxic children, patients with cerebrovascular accidents (strokes) as well as conductive education, leprosy, etc. Intuitively I started to create therapy sessions for individuals and this began to have the most profound reciprocal benefits for me too. The children started to reawaken to their daily experiences, and in unison my body responded. We developed ways in which we could control our internal responses to external influences. Following the effects of frostbite to a limb it is recorded that using the heat of another's body, not one's own, is of most benefit in the process of thawing. The phrase 'no man is an island' becomes more and more apposite when we can appreciate how connected we are to one another through our shared common humanity and remember that we are more alike than we are different.

THE EFFECTS OF TRAUMA ON THE MIND, BODY AND SOUL

The physiological effects of stress on the body are well documented and these are all perfectly normal responses to life. These responses are automatic and are made without conscious thought or consideration, immediately as an event takes place.

Walter Cannon first described the 'fight, flight, freeze' response in 1923. Nature provides us with all the mechanisms to survive dangerous situations without any judgement of the method employed to survive. When the body perceives a threat it will automatically behave in a certain way, which sets off a sequence of events within the body/mind system. The body gets into a state of readiness for fight, or flight, or death, using various strategies: the muscles tense, the heart beats faster, the rate of breathing increases, the brain becomes sharp and focused. This stress response is designed to be activated by the perceived threat and then worked off physically by the body in order to return to a state of rest. The amygdala is a part of the limbic (reptilian) brain, which is the gateway from our outside world to our inner world and keeps guard subconsciously to monitor our safety at all times. It uses past memories to gauge how safe or unsafe stimuli and situations might be, and in turn our bodies are put into a state of awareness for action, or remain calm. In my case I believe that my body had the expectation of death and went into a state of complete surrender. I was unable to defend myself and my body in the bombing and I believe in that moment I relinquished my right to life and 'gave up my soul'.

Following a traumatic event, a vicious circle is established whereby acute states of vigilance can turn into chronic states of discomfort in various forms:

- Physical symptoms – the body is tense, trembling, restless, jumpy, sweating, breathless, nauseous, etc.
- Emotional symptoms – loss of confidence, mood swings, irritability, intolerance of others.
- Mental symptoms – poor concentration, poor executive skills, inability to make good decisions, poor memory, vagueness, lack of awareness.
- Spiritual symptoms – despondency, lack of interest in self and others, loss of hope for the current situation, lack of interest or belief in any future.

After a traumatic event where the experience had been so overwhelming that the individual thought death was inevitable – as I did – the mind stays vigilant, ever on alert, which in turn keeps the body and

mind in an unnatural aroused state without any relief. If the body adopts the 'freeze' response to the trauma, in which it acts as if it were dead to the world, the body is trapped in a state of reaction as though the danger were still present and that it had not ended. When a cat is playing with a mouse, the mouse may 'play dead' in order for the cat to give up the game. There is a sense that the soul surrenders itself at this stage, as if it no longer needs or trusts the body to hold it as a safe vessel within such a hazardous environment.

BLOCKS TO THE SENSES AND RESOURCES

All people dissociate in many ways throughout the day in order to focus on a subject, engage in a hobby or to just switch off from their present environment. This is a natural feature of brain activity in order for us to survive and learn, and for the brain not to become overloaded with too many stimuli at the same time and become overwhelmed. We all 'check in and out of our bodies' many times throughout the day with little or no awareness, or detrimental consequences. In the case of trauma, the overwhelming happens too quickly without any preparation, and the effects on the amygdala can be devastating.

The neocortex (rational brain) is so powerful and complex that through fear and over-control it can interfere with the subtle restorative instinctual impulses and responses generated by the reptilian core (Levine 1997). When the neocortex overrides the instinctual responses that would initiate the completion of this cycle, the organism will be traumatized. The immobility response in animals is normally time limited: they go in and they come out. The human immobility response, however, does not easily resolve itself because the supercharged energy locked in the nervous system is imprisoned by the emotions of fear and terror.

The senses have been put into a state of such overwhelm that no more feeling or sensing can be tolerated, so the mechanism for reading these is blocking any further input.

The sense of safety is greatly diminished and the detachment can lead to lack of care, as well as a lack of hope and meaning, and great disconnection from the world. For ten years I went through the daily motions of 'living my life' even though I was on automatic pilot and felt disjointed, disconnected and disenfranchised from my surroundings. From the outside others would not have recognized or identified my internal agony and my lack of desire to live. What made things worse was that I knew there was no one around who could appreciate these feelings, but within the therapy sessions with my clients I felt huge degrees of connection and meaning.

Dissociation as a concept has been in use for a long time, but exactly how it occurs is not yet known, despite several theories. It is possible that dissociation is the mind's attempt to flee when flight is not possible. There is a sense in some people that as their body was violated by someone else, it no longer belongs to them. Many feel unsafe and unprotected within their body structure and turn to coping mechanisms such as addictive behaviours, self-sabotaging behaviours, avoidance and self-harming in order to try to destroy feelings or create an illusion of escape. The body has literally 'forgotten how to live': it has lost trust in itself and its surroundings, and little self-belief or self-trust remains. There may also be an element of self-blame for not managing to get out of harm's way, in addition to the survivor's guilt for having lived when others died. In my case I spent hours in rumination questioning why I had lived when others had died. These questions with no answers are futile and waste energy, but they remain in place and continue the persecution.

Our outer circumstances are but a reflection of our inner thoughts.

Various authors

The meaning we attach to our circumstances has great significance for how we think about them and ourselves, as well as the meaning we give to life itself. It also affects how we heal. Following trauma there is much rumination, introspection and confusion due to unrealized expectations. Things did not work out how we had expected; the world has turned into a different place.

In my own case I found it pivotal to go through a process called 'the rewind technique' which was delivered to me by a 'human givens' practitioner. With this technique I was put into a relaxed state during which I watched a tape in my imagination of the bombing at Victoria Station and my reactions to my situation. In my mind I ran the tape backwards and forwards in order to reduce the emotional arousal and reprogramme the memory with a different emotional tag, in order that it could become a much safer memory for my amygdala to store. Once the event had been recontextualized for me, and a healthier emotional tag assigned to the memory, the energy was diffused. In my mind I was able to run away from the scene where I was immobilized in 1991 and my legs trembled vigorously during the experience. The events of me falling to the floor in Victoria Station (and then again in Nice ten years later) at the sound of an unexpected loud explosion have not been repeated. I still jump out of my skin at the sound of a loud bang, such as a balloon or a firework, which is unexpected, but I have never again been out of control. This process has informed and enlightened how I now work with others who have experienced forms of trauma.

GENTLE METHODS TO WARM THE BODY BACK TO LIFE

When working with traumatized individuals, it is vitally important to understand the function of the amygdala and to normalize what is happening within the body on a day to day basis. It is important for all of us to understand the normal reactions of the brain to dangers, so that we can recognize our reactions to certain stimuli and accept that this is a normal response for our survival. In this way we can gain control of our body's reactions and begin to feel much safer and less threatened. I need to create the expectation within my clients that they can regain some control over their reactions to what they are feeling. I often give examples to my clients of how certain situations influence how I feel and what I need to do in order to regain a sense of safety. It is then up to the client to attempt different ways of coping and to practise what works and to dismiss what does not work for them.

For the benefit of the children with whom I work, I call the amygdala 'the run away brain'. I explain to them that certain things might make them feel like they want to run away, e.g. the smell of a certain perfume, the way someone looks at them, the atmosphere in a room or in class, or even the season. I let them recognize how they are feeling when they are feeling threatened and uncomfortable, and then we work out different strategies to deal with these situations. The children very often make their own suggestions and find their own solutions about what they need to do in order to reduce their emotional arousal.

The element of surprise should never be used with a person who has experienced trauma; the reaction may well be unexpected and unbearable. I plan interventions with some pauses for quietness and stillness. If the individual is not ready for what is planned, then perform the activity while they observe you; for example, if they do not want a hand massage, I first let them do it to me, and they get the reciprocal benefits due to the neural feedback and mirror neuron activity. It was in Australia when observing the work of occupational therapists with Aboriginal wheelchair users, and watching how the therapists helped them to the ground to sit on the earth or to put their feet into the creek, that I appreciated how much I had missed my connection with the earth and my sense of knowing where I am in space.

With the intense forces associated with a bomb blast, the vestibular and proprioceptive sensory apparatus of the inner ear is subjected to massive sensory input, and indeed the crystals within the semicircular canals may be dislodged, causing further complications with balance and feeling grounded. The linking of vertigo, dizziness, balance disturbance and nausea can recur under conditions of arousal, and craniosacral work may need to be sought in order to restore some sense of balance within the head. In my case I found craniosacral work of profound benefit. Over the years my brain had automatically made huge vestibular adjustments to how I balance and now I am over-reliant on visual cues for stability.

Establishing a safe environment that is quiet and undisturbed, and allowing the individual to sit in a position where there is no activity going on behind them, will increase their sense that nothing unexpected can happen without prior warning. By using gravity and balance to establish a good body position of stability, I often work with clients on the floor, and if necessary I also use cushions or beanbags to help the client feel more supported. When working on the floor, if the body's sense of stability or safety would be increased by using a weighted blanket, then I use one. This has

FIGURE 12-1 ■ Familiar old comfort patterns, ancient wisdom for the body to recognize at a cellular level.

the effect of calming the 'run away' element and also gives the body some proprioceptive feedback of where it is in space.

I use safe, gentle language at all times and am very guarded about using words such as 'triggers' or 'bullet points'. I use images that create expectations of feeling better and the body learning to feel safe again (Figure 12-1). This prepares the individual with the hope and expectation that their body will soon be feeling better again. This is often enough to bring about a sense of relaxation. Metaphors for healing, and use of imagery for warning or protection against danger, can be brought in as appropriate. For example, with the children I invite them to tell me about their hero from television or film, and we adopt ways within their imagination whereby they are able to protect themselves from danger. I also often use as many of the physical senses as possible, using a multisensory approach and bringing awareness to the body during this experience, so they can feel the connection between their feelings and their body. By keeping the approach gentle and playful, and allowing for fun, I allow the individual to proceed at their own pace to maintain a sense of wellbeing and control. I use language of resilience and strength and help the individual to learn and practise new skills to develop more choices. The use and knowledge of neurolinguistic techniques is useful in order to strengthen the experience. Use of nonviolent communication is also beneficial in order to identify what the specific needs are in the current instant: for example, if an individual is feeling distressed or overwhelmed in a certain situation, they may think that they are upset for a certain reason, but by identifying exactly what they need in that moment, it might well be revealed that they need something else.

Often, within an individual's experience of trauma, something will have 'gone wrong': they will have been unable to complete something due to the traumatic event, or somehow there has been an unexpected outcome or an unfulfilled expectation. In my sessions with my clients, we create situations in which a different ending can be created in order to arrive at that different ending. Story telling is of vital importance with many people who have experienced trauma. In my own case the story of the Odyssey and being shipwrecked on the rocks brought to life the idea that being shipwrecked on the rocks did not necessarily mean the end of the journey homeward. The images of the Ice Queen waking up when winter had passed, and the flowers breaking through the frozen earth, were powerful for me to reawaken to a potential change of season, using all the senses.

POST-TRAUMATIC SENSORY REAWAKENING

Establishing a well-rounded profile of who this person was before their trauma is important to the process: what made them tick, what were their passions, what were their qualities, values? Pay specific attention to detail if the person is from a very different background, culturally. Do not forget that they have lost touch with this person, so may need time and gentle questioning to find the answers. Tapping into the senses can help to unlock blockages and reconnect body, mind and soul.

Olfactory: Smelling carries with it the most evocative, powerful memories. Create situations where you can sit around a campfire smelling the different types of wood burning. Use essential oils carefully to stimulate various moods. Use aromatherapy products that nourish the body/soul experience. Use smells that were enjoyed as a child – certain flowers, soaps, farmyard smells and so on – there are infinite possibilities. The various seasons bring their own smells, which can be very evocative of certain memories.

Auditory: Following trauma an individual often hears very acutely. Certain composers (Mozart, J.S. Bach, etc.) have written music that has been identified as having profound benefits on brain waves. I try to use music of a healing nature, of the person's choice, recognizing that different types of music resonate differently with individuals, and in time and place. Language is not always necessary if sharing an auditory experience created from an external source. Try raku pottery where firing can take place in a crackling sandpit outdoors. Try to sit next to someone at the cinema and create a situation where you can whisper to them or speak quietly only to them. Some male youngsters have never been spoken to in such a way.

Visual: We often 'see' what we expect to see. By using many different colours and textures we can use observational skills to bring immediate awareness to the experience of seeing the fine details and noticing the surroundings around us. Build on spatial awareness and use many prepositions: how things fit together, on top of, behind, as well as 'How far away do you think the horizon/biggest tree is?' I use phrases such as 'I wonder' and 'just notice' in order to invite the individual to awaken the imagination.

Vibration, touch, proprioception, movement: So many activities can be used to stimulate these senses. I use various massages using slightly exfoliating creams, drumming while sitting on the floor, listening to music while sitting on the floor resting one's back against speakers. Emotional freedom technique is a method of tapping quickly on the meridians to bring some balance and equilibrium back to the body. Clapping games and tapping rhythms can be used to sequence movements and develop new patterns in movement as well as cross the midline. Feldenkrais is also a useful therapy in which the body is trained to move in alternative patterns to those already developed. Kinesiology can be used to locate and reduce cellular memory, which can bring huge relief.

Oral: Many different activities can be used, such as singing, humming, whistling, screaming and whispering. Gently blowing on a candle flame or humming against a balloon can bring sensory feedback. Musical instruments can also give oral feedback.

Taste: Using a variety of textures and foods reintroduces the subtlety of various tastes. Discuss comparative qualities and enquire about personal preferences.

CONCLUSION

Helen Keller said, 'A happy life consists not in the absence but in the mastery of hardships.'

In hindsight it is no surprise that the treatment I received in hospital, and subsequent counselling, was of no lasting benefit. Only 'talking therapies' or medication were on offer back in 1991 and there was no provision of treatment to nurture the physical senses. Thankfully, as an occupational therapist I eventually created my own therapeutic working environment in which my body started to heal itself. By working with traumatized children within the care system, and by using games and activities in which the senses are stimulated, I put myself in situations where I shared experiences with children at the same time and thereby also gained the benefits.

There is still a sense of resistance within my body that I have to monitor and manage on a daily basis. It does not frighten me anymore. The cellular memory throughout my body structure remains in place, but manageable. My body locates and identifies what it perceives as unsafe behaviours in other people, and unsafe situations, and I recognize my 'pattern match' to historical events which have left some mark on me but no longer dictates to me how I should be or how to react.

An altered awareness to life and the universe eventually emerges and one is left with a stronger sense of being, both animal and spiritual. I have no fear of death as I feel I have already looked into the face of God and chosen to live. I have one unresolved conflict and that is to work within my survivor's guilt, to help people to have the courage to survive and to find the courage to hang onto life. The risk of suicide following trauma is enormous and often unrecorded. Survivors of traumatic events need assistance in living, not assistance in dying. The expectation of death that was activated at the time of great danger needs to be altered by working off the freeze response and by using all the senses. One can be brought back to experiencing life once again, the expectation to live can be restored and the survivor can begin to interact with the world once more following the agony of being an unwilling spectator.

REFERENCES

Cannon, W.B., 1923. Bodily Changes in Pain, Hunger, Fear and Rage. Appleton & Company, New York.

Levine, P., 1997. Waking the Tiger: Healing Trauma. North Atlantic Books, Berkeley, CA.

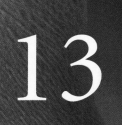

13 SEEKING ASYLUM IN THE UK

NICK POLLARD

A 25-year-old has recently been told that he has been granted leave to remain in Britain after eight years of living in the country. Immediately, because he is no longer an asylum seeker, his benefits stop and he can no longer pay the rent on the room where he lives. Social services tell him he is now a new claimant and it will take some weeks for his benefits to be processed. For three weeks he has no money, cannot pay his bills and lives on the charity of friends and workers at the small project he attends so that he has some social contact. He has lost touch with his family in Eritrea, and although there are other Ethiopians in the city there is no sense of community between them. People from that part of the world tend to avoid each other, after the war.

This chapter describes some of the experiences of asylum seekers in Britain, based on narratives, some fictional and some published witness accounts. It would have been preferable to have an asylum seeker tell their own story, and the original intention was to do so. I began working with an asylum seeker who agreed to contribute to this book in order to do something to enable other people to offer help to those who have had something similar happen to them. However, the process was very challenging for him and is an illustration, in itself, of the problems people can face. After so long living in poor housing and without much money, having endured considerable hardships to get to the UK, he was in very poor health, physically and mentally. At times it was very difficult for him to

concentrate, and at others, thinking about his experiences caused him emotional pain. He experienced frequent problems with the benefits system and had to attend interviews so that he could continue to receive his allowances. He was often very tired or ill, and he had to move home several times to different addresses around the city. Finally, despite having written a narrative, he was reluctant to commit it to print, which has to be understood given his experiences.

As a reader you may need to imagine yourself in his situation, after many years of being unable to settle, being allowed a little money, then denied it, finding a place to live, then finding you have to move on. This may follow the loss of your father and siblings, the rape of your mother by soldiers, and an uncertain journey that cost most of your family's wealth. It is possible that some of your family is still alive – unlikely, but still possible – and if you publish your story it might get back to them. It might also get back to someone else who knows where they are. I have therefore taken some portions of his story, but removed any reference to specific events, place or identity. Where I refer to him, he has been given an arbitrary Tigrean name, Abraha.

Although, unfortunately, we were not able to work as planned, similar stories are available and they fit the same details. Books such as Refugee Boy by Benjamin Zephaniah (2001), who based his narrative on the accounts of Ethiopian and Eritrean refugees, or Mahi Binebine's (2003) Welcome to Paradise, which describes the stories of a group of people waiting to be trafficked into Europe, are easily found. Some of the other texts I have drawn on are refugee witness accounts produced through community publishers in the UK.

There are over 70 tribes in Ethiopia. Eritrea was a region of Ethiopia but fought a 30-year war of independence that ended in 1991. When Eritrea separated from Ethiopia the official language changed from Amharic to Tigri. The calendar in Eritrea was European, not Coptic. The currency also became European. When Ethiopia and Eritrea went to war again in 1998, people from different tribes who had intermarried found themselves in the middle of the conflict in which family members belonged to opposing sides. People were being forced to go back to their original countries. The family of Zephaniah's character, Alem, find themselves in this predicament. With a mother from one community and culture on one side of the conflict and a father from the other, it becomes clear that such a family will be regarded with suspicion by both sides. The violence was brutal. Alem's mother is hacked to death by soldiers.

According to Abraha, in the areas where the Ethiopian government invaded Eritrea, people's property and houses were confiscated. Where possible, people sold everything they had to avoid this before the invaders came, and fled to the neighbouring countries. In Zephaniah's book, Alem is taken to England by his father, where he leaves him to become a refugee. Abraha reported that life was very cheap and many people died in Eritrea. Often, Ethiopians beat refugees without any preamble, randomly kicking out straightaway. Even now, he remains afraid that he might be caught and has no contact with other people from the region. While he is physically safe, his mental condition remains unstable due to depression. He does not go to bed before three or four in the morning.

In Binebine's account of people gathering in Morocco to get across to Spain, the characters come from several countries around the Sahara. Abraha had to pass through countries where the local soldiers were hostile to the refugees. This was a difficult journey, taken with 80 or 90 other people. There were constant demands for money. Even across the border it was not safe and the soldiers, recognizing the refugees as foreigners, arrested them, beat them up and took their money. Abraha rang his mother, who told him that it was not safe for him to return and she would try to arrange somewhere else for him to go. After two weeks,

a man met Abraha and said that he could take him to somewhere safe in Europe. He prepared a travel document for him to catch a plane, although Abraha had no idea where he was going until he got aboard. He found himself heading for England.

Zephaniah's Alem is a boy of school age who is picked up from the bed and breakfast where his father has left him by workers from the Refugee Council. The experience he has is difficult, but the workers enable him to find a secure place to live. Refugee Boy, written for children and young adults, contains some idealized elements in the process Alem goes through in his progress to being given leave to stay. Abraha met immigration officials at the English airport who asked him in a screening interview why he had run away. He was sent to a hostel and given some money, but after a day he was sent to an asylum screening unit (ASU) in another city, where a solicitor presented his case for asylum. When this was refused, Abraha had to represent himself in an appeal because there were no more funds for a solicitor. The appeal was also refused and he was moved to a hostel in another town.

The people living in the hostel were from several other countries, all of them places that were experiencing conflicts and political violence, but none of them from Eritrea. Abraha was moved to another hostel. The experience was very difficult as previously he had always lived with his family, and here he was in a house with strangers. Most of them had been in the city for a year or so and began to show him around and explain how to survive. Hostel staff instructed him in how to collect his benefits from the post office, and a social worker took him around the town centre to show him the shops and to get him onto a college course. He had £30 a week on which to survive, which at first was difficult to manage. It was not enough to buy clothes, but could be eked out carefully at some of the cheaper supermarkets.

After a few days Abraha began to go out alone. It was very cold and he had pulled his jumper tightly around himself, walking with his hands in his pockets. Three people 'wearing silver' showed him that they were police and asked to check his pockets. Abraha was very scared but agreed. They asked him if he was selling drugs, though he didn't know what drugs were at that time. They asked him for his ID and allowed him to go. After this experience, which terrified him, he did not go out for a week. The other people in the house said that in England if you cooperate with the police when they stop you there is no problem.

This description indicates the terror arising from an experience that would not be unusual for many young people in the UK. A young person who looks a little anxious and is perhaps out of place is going to attract the attention of a street patrol. To a person fresh from a civil conflict, and a situation of great hostility, an encounter like this might promise to end in beatings and imprisonment, perhaps arbitrary killing, though in the UK casual meetings with the police are cordial.

Zephaniah's Alem speaks good English and is able to get by, but Abraha had difficulty. Living in a European setting was very different to anything he had previously experienced and it was difficult to find food that he was used to. Alem, being of school age, is initially placed in a social services home and encounters not only strange food but also the brutalized institutional culture of the other boys. A substantial part of the story concerns the experience of adapting to and learning to live alongside the perplexing diversity of British youth cultures and attitudes. Alem is studious but finds himself among children who regard school irreverently; he tries to fit in but is often conscious of his differences.

After a year Abraha became sick. At first the doctor said he had a cold or flu, but he developed cold sweats and a cough. He went to hospital, where following blood tests he was diagnosed with tuberculosis. Abraha was in hospital for five or six months, during which no-one visited him and he lost contact with the people he had met. Because tuberculosis is a very dangerous disease, other people in the Eritrean community in the city did not want to know him or invite him home. Abraha was discharged and accommodation was found for him through a disability team. He received an increased allowance for his disability of £39 a week, but once he was no longer ill this money stopped and he had to leave the house.

Abraha was now a guest, living at the home of a friend of a friend. He rarely left the house and eventually was referred to the community mental health services. They informed him that his benefits would stop, though a social worker asked for a reassessment. Abraha walked out of one meeting in frustration and

a further reassessment was asked for. He was also referred to a community project, where one of the volunteer workers found him some accommodation where he could stay until his money was sorted out. Abraha has continued to have difficulties with benefits, which are often stopped, so he has to attend interviews at the benefit office to have them reinstated. The problems with his benefits create difficulties with keeping a steady place to live. Abraha's engagement with the community project has enabled him to learn more about life in the UK, to improve his English and to develop some social contacts. He has, through a social worker, had some short courses in cooking and using a computer. Abraha regards himself as lucky, despite all the difficulties he has had with the culture and the language, because he has had learning opportunities and he has found people friendly. It is too early to know what the future will bring: 'Sometimes I wake up in bed wondering where I am – but it is safe, you can walk out.'

ASYLUM IN THE UK

Abraha's story suggests that many refugees from the Eritrean conflict may not have been able to leave neighbouring countries. The narrative is typical of the experiences of others from this region: travel to the UK is a very expensive process, assisted by the support of relatives, which often involves a middle man taking a substantial amount of the money raised (Papadopoulos et al 2004). To have survived and to have negotiated a path to the UK, and to have attained the status of permanent residency is, itself, a testament to his resilience and courage.

Telling Abraha's story was difficult and had to be negotiated in stages. He explained that once you have forcibly been made to leave your home, have lost your family, and find yourself living in a strange country with a different culture, you can never forget why you are there. For the narrator it is not easy to repeat your story, as you must do frequently to explain your status. Authoring this chapter, listening to, reflecting on and supplementing the text of this story has also been hard emotional work. There are silences while you struggle with the enormity of what the other person has experienced, and is trying to make sense of, spaces that few words in any language can fill. Engaging with people who have experienced such problems requires resilience, good support and time for both parties to reflect on how their work together is progressing (Mitchell 2008).

The number of people living in the UK who have fled oppression, civil war and violence is not accurately known. Many of them are in fear of being returned to these situations and are avoiding the authorities. Because of policy issues, including a lack of detailed research (Aspinall & Watters 2010, Connelly et al 2006, Davies 2008), it is not always clear in some communities whether migrants have taken up opportunities to come to the UK or are escaping violence.

Ethiopia is a country of many different ethnic groups and a complex history of political violence and conflict (Papadopoulos et al 2004). Even a small number of people from this country might represent a considerable diversity, which is often not understood in the West where people lack detailed knowledge about the countries that refugees and asylum seekers come from (Temple & Steele 2004).

If definitions with regard to nationality and culture may be complex, status is also unclear. While 'refugees' and 'asylum seekers' would outwardly appear to be coterminous, in fact asylum seekers are treated differently from refugees in the UK because they have usually arrived in the country independently of any recognized refugee programme (Phillips 2006). The United Kingdom Border Agency (UKBA 2010), a department of the Home Office, defines asylum as 'protection given by a country to someone who is fleeing persecution in their own country … under the 1951 United Nations Convention Relating to the Status of Refugees'. Home Office figures record around 23 000–24 000 applications for asylum in each year since 2005, though this is a reduction from the previous four years' figures of 70 000 or even 80 000 (Aspinall & Watters 2010). Nineteen per cent of the people applying for asylum in the UK in 2007 were accepted as refugees. A further 9% did not qualify for refugee status but were given temporary permission to stay for humanitarian or other reasons under the European Convention on Human Rights, 'which prevents us sending someone to a country where there is a real risk that they will be exposed to torture, or inhuman or degrading treatment or punishment' (UKBA 2010). In 2007 there were as many as 450 000 old asylum applications to be processed in the UK (H.M. Government 2010).

Having been accorded refugee or humanitarian protection status, a refugee is given a five-year 'leave to remain'. If this permission is granted a person can claim the same benefits and rights as other UK citizens and obtain advice and limited assistance in building a life in Britain. After a four-year period, a further application can be made for permission to settle in the UK. Up to 750 refugees a year can enter the UK through the Gateway Protection Programme operated through the United Nations High Commissioner for Refugees (UNHCR) without going through this process. Only 10% of the people applying for refugee status actually do so at the ports of entry to the UK, even though most will be given temporary admission, pending a decision on their asylum application (Aspinall & Watters 2010). Perhaps this is because they may fear that they will not be allowed to stay, but if they apply for asylum later, they have to go to a UK Border Agency asylum screening unit to do this in person. There are four in the UK, at Croydon, Liverpool, Glasgow and Belfast. The UKBA will then allocate the asylum seeker a 'case worker' who manages every aspect of that person's application through to the conclusion of their case.

The UKBA has had a policy of concluding cases within a 6-month period since 2007. Despite having case workers, 13% of the applicants do not receive a final decision within this time (H.M. Government 2013). This group are regarded as asylum seekers, but the term also applies to people who do not have refugee status or have already been denied it and may be staying illegally in the country (Aspinall & Watters 2010). Earlier figures for Ethiopian refugees showed that only 7% of those who had lived in the country for five years had been granted leave to remain (Papadopoulos et al 2004). Some limited support is still available after refugee status has not been granted, but people may not accept this because it entails an agreement that they will return to their country of origin. At this point they can fall outside the system. The Refugee Council (2007) has found many asylum seekers living in destitution because they have run out of opportunities to appeal against deportation. Other people who have been smuggled into the country have no official status and would not want to be visible to a system that would question their right to be in the

UK. Although being discovered may lead to them being able to apply for asylum, this can result in being held in detention for some time. UKBA figures suggest that most such people are eventually scheduled to be deported back to their original country. Nonetheless, a number of these are able to evade deportation and remain in the UK but without any national status. Recently it was thought that as many as 250 000 denied asylum seekers might be living in the UK without any official status. Abraha had to wait seven years before he found out eventually about his status. He had several assessments and, despite being a young man of only 17, had had to represent himself. He had at times become exasperated with the process of obtaining benefits, and it is easy to see from his account that an asylum seeker might choose to disappear.

The shifting global geography of oppression is a significant determinant of the nature of asylum applicants, and of their reception. Groups such as the Ugandan Asians who came to the country in 1972 as Commonwealth citizens, Chileans who fled the Pinochet coup and military crackdown of 1973, and the Vietnamese arriving in the early 1980s had very different – welcoming or begrudging – receptions determined by government policy at the time. While these groups could be described as 'refugees', they are now mostly settled with subsequent generations living here. A rule of thumb is that the person has been living in the country for less than 10 years, but this does not mean that the memory of their traumatic experiences, or their guilt at their survival when others did not, is necessarily diminished (Connelly et al 2006).

Historically, the UK claims to have received many different waves of asylum seekers and refugees (O'Neill & Spyby 2003), something the Border Agency alludes to in its description of asylum and refugee status (UKBA 2014). Taking a small sample of community publications produced by various groups in the UK, covering the latter part of the twentieth century, reveals accounts by Basques in 1937 fleeing Franco's fascist army (Marshall 1991), Greek Cypriots fleeing the 1947 civil war (Kyriacou & Papathanasiou 1990), Iranians during the 1980s (Rouhifar 1989), Polish war refugees (Kyriacou & The Polish Reminiscence Group 1989, 1994), Somalians (Deria 1994, Fozia 1993, Gatehouse 1997, Karim 1994) and Ethiopians (Jama 1994). The UK has the second highest number of asylum applications in Europe, after France (Aspinall & Watters 2010), a figure that is partly due to its occupational narrative as a nation, i.e. its history as a colonial occupier. The legacy of this is in the network of international relations through which Britain seeks to uphold an interventionist role. In 2008 many of the asylum applicants came from Afghanistan and Iraq, countries in which the UK has been engaged in conflict. Other significant groups came from Nigeria, Zimbabwe and Pakistan, former UK colonial possessions, but the fourth largest group have the same origins as the narrator (Aspinall & Watters 2010).

SURVIVAL AND OCCUPATION

The numbers of people who may be unofficially living in the UK suggest that there are significant numbers who feel that to return home would probably result in their torture or death and further persecution for their families. They may be denied health services, cannot obtain work and often find it very difficult to access other occupational opportunities independently (Davies 2008, Smith 2005). State health workers who offer them services may find themselves disciplined (Davies 2008), but in other countries occupational therapists have developed their own agencies to address these needs (Wilson 2008). As Abraha has described, the everyday occupational experience of asylum seekers in the UK is often about simple survival, living well below the minimum sustenance level in the UK. A threshold for poverty offered by the Poverty Site (Palmer 2010) is £119 for a single adult after housing costs. For clothes, cooking utensils and other than basic appliances, a person living on £36.62 per week (current level of benefit for a lone person aged over 18 (UK Parliament, 2013)) is going to be dependent on charity handouts, even though the UKBA will provide furnished and rent free accommodation with electricity, gas and water. There is no choice about where the agency will locate a person on arrival in the UK if they are destitute (UKBA 2014), and the cost of living varies considerably between regions, depending on access to supermarkets and public transport. Purchasing food in economic quantities for one person can be difficult. A small loaf of bread usually costs more than £1.20. A cheap can of tomatoes is around 36p. The use of public transport, at £1.50 for a reasonably short journey, is a decision which might impact on whether a person can eat later in the week. Like other people from the region (Papadopoulos et al 2004), the narrator describes some of the difficulties he has with finding culturally acceptable food which is also affordable.

For asylum seekers, social participation is a significant problem, not only because of lack of money but because it may make a person visible as vulnerable, with the risk of becoming a target for other people for further persecution and exploitation. Frequently this is because the housing provided is in areas where the levels of poverty are high and the social fabric already precarious (Phillips 2006). Refugees can be understandably reluctant to depend on other people. Much of British life is based in an individualistic culture, whereas the previous experience of asylum seekers may have been more family centred (Papadopoulos et al 2004), but individual needs should not be ignored (Temple & Steele 2004). Abraha is unable to establish friendships with other people from the same region because of the raw nature of the hostilities between groups in the civil conflict of which he is a victim, and for Alem in Zephaniah's novel this has tragic consequences. Many of the basic coping strategies other people from the region might have developed through having a social or family group with whom to share emotions and socialize (Papadopoulos et al 2004) have been unavailable to Abraha.

Previous refugee accounts (Kyriacou & The Polish Reminiscence Group 1989, 1994, Marshall 1991) tell how they developed networks to offer various forms of support, including loans to enable them to settle and guide them through the process of obtaining work. Some aspects of these population movements remain transnational as people try to maintain contacts with their relatives, while for others, such as the narrator, ties are disrupted. Transnational networks can be positive in enabling new migrants to survive among familiar cultural communities, but they can also be oppressive. Al-Ali et al (2001) suggest that Eritreans in the UK have continued to organize social actions around supporting their government (despite a reluctance to return) but this is understandably not evident in the narrator's account, which is the result of more recent changes in the political situation. Al-Ali et al describe some of this action as having the characterization of 'enforced transnationalism' (2001, p. 596) because those who have

escaped persecution were shamed by others in their community into contributing funds to the continued conflict between Eritrea and Ethiopia. Currently Abraha belongs to a social network, composed of both local people and others with a migrant background, in which he has been able to feel welcomed and accepted. It is clear that this is precarious given the instability he experiences with his health, interruptions in his benefits and having to change address.

Given the diversity of asylum seekers, many of whom come from minorities within their own cultures, language is a significant problem (Connelly et al 2006, Mitchell 2008, Temple & Steele 2004). Few of these cultures are represented in the staff of health and social or other public services, and there are problems in trying to negotiate sensitive health care issues or other needs without trained interpreters. Fozia (1993) is one of a number of people whose narrative has been transcribed and translated by her school-age child in a publication that was produced to illustrate the linguistic capacities of children who did not have English as a first language. Her story is one of several traumatic narratives in a volume describing parents' experiences of coming to the UK, an example of how often children are called upon to explain sensitive issues. Other publications from the same Sheffield school (Earl Marshall School 1992, 1993, 1994) reveal children coming to terms with violent and horrific experiences of conflict and abuse. The position in which refugees may find themselves in trying to articulate their needs is made worse by the problem that often occupational therapists and other health workers cannot have direct involvement because the status of the individual is in doubt (Davies 2008).

Asylum seekers may not be legally entitled to a service: a professional who offered services to someone without entitlement could face disciplinary action; many other asylum seekers do not know what they are entitled to (Connelly et al 2006). Abraha went directly to the Home Office officials on arriving in the UK, and in the processes that have led to his case for asylum eventually being accepted, he was able to register with a GP and so receive treatment through the health system. He identifies a number of health issues in his narrative: loss of, and loss of contact with family and difficulty in establishing social contacts, particularly with people with whom he may share a culture (Derges

& Henderson 2003, Whiteford 2004), prolonged uncertainty about legal status and accommodation (Connelly et al 2006, Phillips 2006), inadequate diet and clothing, a continual pressure of not understanding everything that happens around him (Scott & Bolzman 1999). His physical and mental health problems include tuberculosis and being unable to concentrate sufficiently to follow classes, possibly a symptom of stress. Refugees sometimes have a faster ageing process due to such combinations of previous lack of health care, multiple health problems, traumatic experiences and subsequent poor housing (Connelly et al 2006, Sundquist 1995).

The needs of asylum seekers and refugees change with their circumstances. Although there are signs that he has increasing personal confidence, the narrator faces considerable challenges to his social inclusion, having waited seven years before he has had indefinite leave to remain, during which much of his interaction with the social world around him has been within a framework of threatening uncertainty and impermanence. However, workers at the voluntary project in which he is involved support him in accessing health care. The project offers gardening activities two days a week and access to other community groups, such as a conversation club to enable speakers of English as a second language to gain confidence.

Abraha enjoys the groups he now attends but remains isolated from other people from his own culture. While education may offer some means to overcoming his isolation, he has often been unable to concentrate, which would make attending college difficult. Projects involving horticulture and low key encounters with nature have proved significant in enabling other asylum seekers to connect present with past experiences and bridge some of the cultural differences they are experiencing (Rishbeth & Finney 2006). As a consequence of the social activity around this group, Abraha has been able to make friends and enjoy some of the other novel cultural experiences of being part of the local community, visiting at Christmas and attending football matches, as well as learning to cook.

CONCLUSIONS

Each experience of seeking asylum is different, a deeply personal journey of discovery mixed with loss and survival, with difference and uncertainty. The influence of these conflicting tensions has a considerable impact on individual health and the capacity to engage in basic occupations of daily living. This requires far more than a merely technical understanding of the transitions asylum seekers have to make; it necessitates the negotiation of rapport and empathy, and a lot of time to navigate the communication, the necessary reflective silences and withdrawals. This careful process of encouraging people to nurture their capacities in new environments is often shaped by larger processes determined by policy or the communities in which asylum seekers are located. A significant aspect of Abraha's experience has been the connection with the groups he attends and their focus on engaging activities which allows him to adjust and discover his potential at his own pace. Abraha's previous experience has been arduous; his future is quietly positive.

REFERENCES

Al-Ali, N., Black, R., Koser, K., 2001. The limits to 'transnationalism': Bosnian and Eritrean refugees in Europe as emerging transnational communities. Ethn. Racial Stud. 24, 578–600.

Aspinall, P., Watters, C., 2010. Refugees and Asylum Seekers: A Review from an Equality and Human Rights Perspective. Equality and Human Rights Commission, Manchester.

Binebine, M., 2003. Welcome to Paradise. Granta, London.

Connelly, N., Forsythe, L.A., Njike, G., Rudiger, A., 2006. Older Refugees in the UK: A Literature Review. A Refugee Council Working Paper for the Older Refugees Programme, Refugee Council, London.

Davies, R., 2008. Working with refugees and asylum seekers; challenging occupational apartheid. In: Pollard, N., Sakellariou, D., Kronenberg, F. (Eds.), A Political Practice of Occupational Therapy. Churchill Livingstone/Elsevier, Edinburgh, pp. 183–189.

Derges, J., Henderson, F., 2003. Working with refugees and survivors of trauma in a day hospital setting. J. Refug. Stud. 16 (1), 82–98.

Deria, A., 1994. Journey from Burao. In: School of the World. Earl Marshall School, Sheffield, pp. 78–79.

Earl Marshall School, 1992. Valley of Words. Earl Marshall School, Sheffield.

Earl Marshall School, 1993. Lives of Love and Hope, A Sheffield Herstory. Earl Marshall School, Sheffield.

Earl Marshall School, 1994. School of the World. Earl Marshall School, Sheffield.

Fozia, 1993. Lives of Love and Hope, A Sheffield Herstory. Earl Marshall School, Sheffield, pp. 127–131.

Gatehouse, 1997. A Song for Carrying Water and Other Stories from Somalia. Gatehouse, Manchester.

H.M. Government, 2010. UK Border Agency: Follow-up on Asylum Cases and E-Borders Programme – Home Affairs

Committee, Available at: <http://www.publications.parliament.uk/pa/cm200910/cmselect/cmhaff/406/40603.htm> (Last accessed 16.10.2014).

H.M. Government, 2013. Immigration statistics: January to March 2013, Available at: <https://www.gov.uk/government/publications/immigration-statistics-january-to-march-2013/immigration-statistics-january-to-march-2013> (Last accessed 16.10.2014).

Jama, N., 1994. Nabat's journey. In: School of the World. Earl Marshall School, Sheffield, pp. 80–81.

Karim, A., 1994. So many places. In: School of the World. Earl Marshall School, Sheffield, p. 82.

Kyriacou, S., Papathanasiou, T., 1990. Xeni: Greek Cypriots in London. Ethnic Communities Oral History Project, London.

Kyriacou S and The Polish Reminiscence Group, 1989. Travelling Light: Poles on Foreign Soil. Ethnic Communities Oral History Project, London.

Kyriacou S and The Polish Reminiscence Group, 1994. Passport to Exile. The Polish Way to London. Ethnic Communities Oral History Project, London.

Marshall, O., 1991. Ship of Hope. Ethnic Communities Oral History Project/The North Kensington Archive at Notting Dale Urban Studies Centre, London.

Mitchell, A., 2008. Reflections on working with south Sudanese refugees in settlement and capacity building in regional Australia. In: Pollard, N., Sakellariou, D., Kronenberg, F. (Eds.), A Political Practice of Occupational Therapy. Churchill Livingstone/Elsevier, Edinburgh, pp. 197–205.

O'Neill, M., Spybey, T., 2003. Global refugees, exile, displacement and belonging. Sociology 37 (1), 7–12.

Palmer, G., 2010. UK: numbers in low income, Available at: <http://www.poverty.org.uk/01/index.shtml> (Last accessed 16.10.2014).

Papadopoulos, I., Lees, S., Lay, M., Gebrehiwot, A., 2004. Ethiopian refugees in the UK: migration, adaption and resettlement experiences and their relevance to health. Ethn. Health 9 (1), 55–73.

Phillips, D., 2006. Moving towards integration: the housing of asylum seekers and refugees in Britain. Housing Stud. 21 (4), 539–553.

Refugee Council, 2007. Social Exclusion, Refugee Integration, and the Right to Work for Asylum Seekers. Refugee Council, London.

Rishbeth, C., Finney, N., 2006. Novelty and nostalgia in urban greenspace: refugee perspectives. Tijdschr. Econ. Soc. Geogr. 97 (3), 281–295.

Rouhifar, Z., 1989. In Exile: Iranian Recollections. Ethnic Communities Oral History Project, London.

Scott, H., Bolzman, C., 1999. Age in exile: Europe's older refugees and exiles. In: Bloch, A., Levy, C. (Eds.), Refugees, Citizenship and Social Policy in Europe. Macmillan., Basingstoke, pp. 168–186.

Smith, H., 2005. 'Feel the fear and do it anyway': meeting the occupational needs of refugees and people seeing asylum. Br. J. Occup. Ther. 68, 474–476.

Sundquist, J., 1995. Ethnicity, social class and health. A population-based study on the influence of social factors on self-reported illness in 223 Latin American refugees, 333 Finnish and 126 South European labour migrants and 841 Swedish controls. Soc. Sci. Med. 40 (6), 777–787.

Temple, B., Steele, A., 2004. Injustices of engagement: issues in housing needs assessments with minority ethnic communities. Housing Stud. 19 (4), 541–556.

UK Border Agency, 2014. Immigration leaflet for asylum applications, Available at: <https://www.gov.uk/government/publications/information-leaflet-for-asylum-applications> (Last accessed 16.10.2014).

UK Parliament, 2013. Standard note. Online. Available at www.parliament.uk/briefing-papers/SN01909.pdf Last accessed 17.4.2013.

Whiteford, G., 2004. Occupational issues of refugees. In: Molineux, M. (Ed.), Occupation for Occupational Therapists. Blackwell, Oxford, pp. 183–199.

Wilson, C., 2008. Illustrating occupational needs of refugees. In: Pollard, N., Sakellariou, D., Kronenberg, F. (Eds.), A Political Practice of Occupational Therapy. Churchill Livingstone/Elsevier, Edinburgh, pp. 191–195.

Zephaniah, B., 2001. Refugee Boy. Bloomsbury, London.

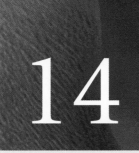

14

SOLOMON'S STORY

RACHEL THIBEAULT ■ MARIE CLAUDE BERNARD ■
SOLOMON PATRAY

The Lord is my shepherd, I shall not be in want.
He makes me lie down in green pastures.
He leads me beside quiet waters.
He restores my soul.
He guides me in paths of righteousness for his
name's sake.
Even though I walk through the valley of the
shadow of death, I will fear no evil, for you are with
me; your rod and your staff, they comfort me.
You prepare a table before me in the presence of
my enemies. You anoint my head with oil; my cup
overflows.
Surely goodness and love will follow me all the
days of my life, and I will dwell in the house of the
Lord forever.

Psalm 23, New International Version

I wrote the whole psalm on a piece of paper I had
found. Folded it and put duct tape all over it. Hid it
under my bandanna. It was my protection, nobody
knew but me. It was my protection. I would think
about it and it helped me go through rough times.

Solomon Patray, 10 April 2010

Solomon Patray needed all the help he could get. Raised by a caring aunt in Liberia's Bopolu District, Solomon had enjoyed a good family life, a lively group of friends, education at the Mission School and his chores on the farm. To his not quite 3000-soul community, the civil war that had torn the country apart for three years felt distant, almost unreal. Monrovia was so far away. Or so it seemed. But Solomon's

peaceful existence came to an abrupt end in 1992 when he was kidnapped by a Liberian rebel group. Against his will, the then 9-year-old joined the ranks of the more than 300 000 children engaged in over 30 conflicts worldwide (Amnesty International 2003, Coalition to Stop the Use of Child Soldiers (CSC) 2008, Machel 2001). In Liberia alone, 21 000 children were conscripted by government or opposition forces, often under the guise of protection (Kaplan 2005). The then president, Charles Taylor, had endorsed the creation of a 'small boys unit' with commanders sometimes barely 12 years old. He justified the move to the *New York Times* in these terms: 'Most of these boys are orphans of the war. Some of them saw their mothers wrapped in blankets, tied-up and burned alive. We keep them armed as a means of keeping them out of trouble.' (cited in Kaplan 2005).

For two years, Solomon led the life typical of children associated with armed forces or armed groups, children formerly referred to as 'child soldiers'. This was a life of deprivation, fear and violence. Among other tribulations, Solomon was forced into combat, hard labour and drug use, a trajectory common to most of his peers.

Nonetheless, astute and quick-witted, Solomon managed to escape in 1994, only to be kidnapped again in 1996. Respite had been brief. He was now part of an even bigger league, The United Liberation Movement of Liberia for Democracy (ULIMO), a group of dissidents dedicated to overthrowing Charles Taylor. A strategic ally of the Sierra Leonean army against the Revolutionary United Front (RUF), ULIMO had gained extensive war experience in the neighbouring state before coming home in 1991. It deserved every bit of its reputation as a merciless force perpetrating a broad range of human rights violations. To seize diamond mines in Lofa and Bomi counties, ULIMO had burnt entire villages, committed countless murders and rapes, mutilated survivors and looted anything of value.

When war waned in 1996, Solomon left the front and was informally adopted by an ex-commander and his family. They earned a modest living through a small taxi business and Solomon was treated as a real son: he was well cared for and got to resume school. But war broke out again shortly thereafter, marking the family's downfall. The cab was lost and Solomon found himself fighting again until 1999. He was homeless, slept on the street and went from one government office to another to seek help. Although he knew of rehabilitation services available for ex-child soldiers, he feared the stigma attached to such programmes and, instead of joining, chose to search for his family of origin. In his village, he discovered strangers living in his childhood home, and there was no trace of his mother who had fled the rebel invasion. Acting on vague clues, Solomon wandered through Sierra Leone, Liberia and Ghana, and in 2003 he finally tracked her down in Côte d'Ivoire. With war still raging in Liberia, they got to speak over the phone, but could not meet. Their hope was to reunite after the ratification of peace accords that were already underway. But when the time came Solomon's mother had vanished, and despite his search of refugee camps, he could never find her again.

In 2004 his grandfather, a New York City resident, convinced him to go to the United States. Solomon (Figure 14-1) now lives in Providence, Rhode Island, where he has taken health care training: he works for a foundation that assists people with physical and psychological disabilities. 'This work helps me cope, too,' he says. In the meantime, Solomon has launched his own nongovernmental organization (NGO), Veteran Child Soldiers Association of Liberia (VECSAOL). The 300-member organization aims to 'encourage the ex-combatants to live in the present and to not have their future dictated by the past' (Hoffman 2007). VECSAOL supports veteran child soldiers in identifying and addressing issues characteristic of their situations, while raising awareness around children associated with armed forces or armed groups. It also promotes their involvement in

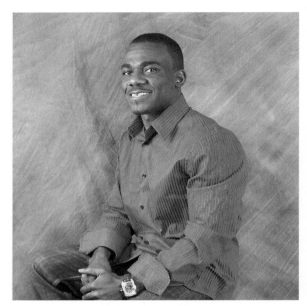

FIGURE 14-1 ■ Solomon.

community development initiatives to enhance self-esteem and shift social perceptions of former child soldiers from collective liability to valuable citizens.

CHILD SOLDIERS AND SECTION 7 OF THE PARIS PRINCIPLES: OCCUPATIONAL THERAPY'S POTENTIAL CONTRIBUTION

Nearly 20 years after Solomon's first kidnapping, most armed conflicts still take place in sub-Saharan Africa. Although child soldiers are a global phenomenon identified in more than 86 countries, 120 000 children between the ages of 7 and 18 are estimated to be currently fighting on the African continent (CSC 2008, Fafo 2002), with West Africa having the largest number (Landry 2006).

Through the United Nations, the international community has reacted to the problem by adopting, in 2007, the Principles and Guidelines on Children Associated with Armed Forces and Armed Groups, called the Paris Principles (UNICEF 2007). Seventy-six member states, including a number of conflict-affected countries, adhere to these principles to oversee disarmament, demobilization and reintegration of all child soldiers, male and female. The Paris Principles focus mostly on acknowledging the diversity and complexity of issues, providing children with safe environments, preventing recruitment, ensuring gender equality and involving the families. They are divided into 10 sections that span a wide array of concerns, including legal matters, operational guidelines, the situation of girls, monitoring and follow-up. Section 7, Release and Reintegration, is of more immediate relevance to occupational therapists. It specifically addresses planning and preparation for reintegration, material assistance, support for families and communities to which children return or integrate, family reunification and family-based care arrangements, supporting children in finding a role in their community, children with a disability and others requiring particular support, children who were not separated from family or community, interim care, prevention of re-recruitment, general reintegration, reintegration of girls, health, psychosocial aspects, education, vocational skills training and livelihoods.

Ideally, children associated with armed conflicts would undergo a seamless process from demobilization to reintegration. They would be interviewed in transition centres where their social context and physical and mental status would be carefully assessed. Generally, the main physical conditions encountered relate to abuse, torture (Human Rights Watch 1994) and addictions (Amnesty International 2006, Honwana 1998, International Bureau for Children's Rights 2009). Gunshot wounds, blows to the head and body, amputations (Chrobok & Akutu 2008), mutilation, malnutrition and the multiple consequences of rape and sexual violence (Human Rights Watch 1994, Humphreys 2009, Muwonge 2007) are also prevalent. Psychologically, children report mostly flashbacks, nightmares (Annan et al 2008), suicidal ideations, and unrelenting fear and anxiety (Cohn & Goodwin-Gill 1995). Post-traumatic stress disorder (Bayer et al 2007, Derluyn et al 2004, Pham et al 2007, Twum-Danso 2003), hallucinations (Albertyn et al 2003), behavioural problems (Hill & Langholtz 2003) and lack of adequate social roles (Kostelny 2004) are frequently observed. For numerous children, the severe abuse translates in learning disabilities (Gislesen 2006).

Depending on the initial evaluation's outcomes, the children would be directed to medical services, rehabilitation facilities or community programmes. In a broad sense, most interventions would unfold under three basic clusters: acute treatment, rehabilitation and reintegration, each cluster coming with its own set of challenges and strategies.

Central challenges associated with acute treatment have been outlined above and are targeted under Section 7. It is worth mentioning that although occupational therapists do not, as a rule, intervene in medical emergencies, they can still play an active role in this cluster, especially around questions of traumatic shock, amputations, depression and suicide. However, their expertise would be mainly put to use in the two remaining clusters: rehabilitation and reintegration.

The rehabilitation cluster encompasses physical and psychosocial care. Occupational therapists can help decrease stigma around physical disabilities while providing appropriate services, such as orthotics, positioning, activities of daily living training, mobility or any other modality deemed suitable for each individual case. In conflict or post-conflict settings where staff turnover is high and monitoring often neglected, meticulous documenting of interventions and progress is paramount for successful follow-up. From the onset, policies, programmes and their related documentation should be designed in a spirit of social inclusion, community participation and advocacy for people with disabilities. With regards to psychosocial care, occupational therapists would focus chiefly on the development of safe and supportive environments, social skills, problem solving and conflict resolution abilities, healthy leisure choices (Michael 2006, Hamakawa & Randall 2008, Ravizza 2008, Verhey 2001) and peer support networks.

The reintegration cluster presents challenges of a more socioeconomic nature. Reintegration is often marked by resistance at the community level and triggers rejection and ostracism (Charchuk 2007, Gislesen 2006). In response, children exhibit poorly controlled aggressive behaviours (Muwonge 2007). Poverty compounds the problem, with the unskilled ex-child soldiers being perceived as economic burdens. To foster self-sufficiency in the long term, reintegration strategies would rest on schooling (Chrobok & Akutu 2008, Women's Commission for Refugee Women and Children 2000), vocational training (Bernard et al 2003, Boothby et al 2006, Chrobok & Akutu 2008, Deng Deng 2001, Landry 2006, Muwonge 2007) and income generating activities, with vocational training being initially reserved for those children with no interest in going back to school (Williamson & Carter 2005). In some situations the use of local rituals could also facilitate the transition (Women's Commission for Refugee Women and Children 2000). Given the skill set required, occupational therapists could provide a considerable share of essential reintegration services or enable their provision through the training of local trainers.

In all three clusters, occupational therapists would work according to the principles of normalization, social role valorization, meaningful occupations and gender equality. Doing so, they could contribute significantly to the children's healing and the mobilization process of communities and families towards full reintegration and sustainable livelihoods.

CHILD SOLDIERS AND SECTION 7 OF THE PARIS PRINCIPLES: SOLOMON'S PERSPECTIVE

Reality, though, is vastly different and the comprehensive therapeutic sequence described above has yet to be devised and implemented. The Paris Principles have been created to help close some of the existing gaps, and Solomon's story has underscored a few.

Comfort and Safety

First, as mentioned before, Solomon avoided the rehabilitation programmes offered to him because of the stigma they carried. Instead of being located in the community and structured in non-stigmatizing ways, such as home- or family-based services, programmes often replicate rigid institutional practices. Child soldiers can be readily identified as such by the surrounding community, increasing their sense of shame and vulnerability. 'If you were an ostracized child soldier, do you think you would like to be associated with a centre specifically catering to child soldiers? This is the best way to be found out, to have the whole community pointing its finger at you.'

Relevant Approaches

Ex-child soldiers who have been in a position of authority and have known extreme danger resent being patronized by treatment personnel they see as weak civilians. 'They think: you don't know man … you just don't know what's going on there.' Ishmael Beah, an ex-child soldier who recounts his involvement in Sierra Leone's civil war in his memoirs, makes the same observation (Beah 2007). Faced with condescending attitudes and expectations to behave and play like regular children, his group reacted violently, murdering a member of a rival gang and battering a staff member.

Accountability

Child soldiers have to survive by their wits, and most become shrewd observers. They learn rapidly to analyse systems and read power differentials. As a result, they are quick to notice discrepancies between official statements and reality. When an agency's resources do not match services offered, children recognize underlying mismanagement or corruption and feel cheated. 'Child soldiers are not receiving the help of those organizations. DDR [Disarmament, Demobilization and Reintegration, the body coordinating aid and therapeutic programmes for demobilized adult combatants and child soldiers] programmes are not well accomplished and need a good monitoring system.'

Aware of DDR shortcomings, Solomon opted for a more solitary path and charted his own course. Of the strategies reported in the literature, Solomon spontaneously applied three, even outside any formal rehabilitation programme.

Schooling

Solomon eloquently speaks of school as a pivotal factor for his self-esteem and reintegration. 'My mom sent me to a good school before the war. I had the foundation of school before the war, of playing, of praying, of reading the Bible … I knew I wanted to be a doctor or to have a good work for my future.' The fact that he had attended school before being kidnapped also allowed him to understand and frame some of the events he was subjected to. '[When people harmed me], I knew it was wrong. Because I had education I knew it was wrong.' And resuming life after the war was made more achievable because of his previous education: in New York City, Solomon could register into a variety of educational programmes. 'Education saved me. Education was the key.'

Social Skills and Retraining

With his adopted family, an informal mentor and other social contacts, Solomon set to rebuilding adequate relational skills through dialogue, reflection and practice. 'It was not easy, I'm telling you, it was not easy. [When you are a soldier] everything you take is free, you don't ask, you take, you order: do that, ok, do this … you don't have any patience anymore, it makes you dangerous. After you get back, you have to ask, you have to be polite: "Yes ma'am! Thank you ma'am! Can I? Sorry." It's not easy. You need patience.'

Belonging. When asked how he managed to survive his years as a child soldier, Solomon laughs and says: 'I'm African!!! And an African child is not the same as an American child.' He goes on to describe a fundamental difference between the two societies: the importance of roles and responsibilities even at a tender age. In most of Africa, children as young as three already have small chores they perform with pride. Solomon was no exception, and when caught in the web of war he came back to the life-sustaining strategy of solidarity. 'We were five … five of us were friends. We were the youngest … I was maybe 9-10-11 years old. I was not alone, they were there with me. We kept each other's spirit, we talked about escape, about surviving, protecting ourselves.'

CHILD SOLDIERS AND RESILIENCE: OCCUPATIONAL THERAPY'S POTENTIAL CONTRIBUTION

The issue of resilience is obviously at the core of the recovery process, and specific therapeutic interventions are needed to maintain or enhance coping skills. How could occupational therapy enable these competencies? An emerging framework has been proposed that explores occupational strategies conducive to happiness and resilience (Thibeault 2011). Based, among others, on the works of Seligman (2002), Ricard (2003, 2008, 2009) and Lutz et al (2004, 2008, 2009), this framework focuses on six universal, positive virtues that can not only improve psychological wellbeing but also modify neuronal pathways (Seligman 2002, Ricard 2003, 2009). They are:

- Wisdom and knowledge
- Courage

- Love, humanity, compassion
- Justice
- Temperance
- Spirituality and transcendence.

Increased resilience occurs when one chooses to consistently embody some, or all of these six virtues, even in the face of adversity. Recent research confirms that positive change is not a matter of happenstance, but the product of a mostly conscious and steady reframing of perceptions and attitudes around these values. Although simply evoking them and shaping positive intents already alters neuronal pathways for the better, these virtues fully unleash their transformative power when given occupational form through action. Five occupational strategies are suggested that appear to influence happiness and resilience, if approached in a spirit of love, courage, gratitude, forgiveness, justice, etc. These strategies are (Thibeault 2011):

Centering: Occupations that foster presence, awareness and calmness through releasing nervous energy. They are often repetitive tasks, productive or 'nonproductive', such as jogging, vacuuming, pounding the grain.

Contemplation: Occupations of a reflective, spiritual nature that induce a sense of beauty, of awe, of gratefulness, such as praying, meditating, taking a stroll in a natural setting.

Creation: Occupations that meet the need to create – even if only for oneself – such as painting, cooking a meal, making music.

Connectedness: Occupations that deepen the sense of belonging to one's community, to life, such as doing sports, having friends over for a meal, snuggling with a pet.

Contribution: Occupations that allow one to give back, to be a valued, productive community member, such as volunteering to clean riverbanks with an environmental group, mowing the lawn for a sick relative, doing one's work with dedication and care.

Most partners and participants who shared the narratives that yielded these five strategies used three or four of them to build their own resilience. Solomon is no different.

CHILD SOLDIERS AND RESILIENCE: SOLOMON'S OCCUPATIONAL STRATEGIES

To live through shock and suffering, Solomon has explicitly cultivated over time three out of the five occupational strategies highlighted above. They remain current in his life today.

Contemplation: Occupations of a reflective, spiritual nature that induce a sense of beauty, of awe, of gratefulness.

I learned the Bible. I grew up with Christian people. I'm not religious like my mom. At school, if you failed religion you failed school. But I believe in a path. [...] I feel good now ... I feel more compassion for my peers, I focus on the positive ... I consider that I'm lucky, very lucky.

Connectedness: Occupations that speak of belonging to one's community, to life.

When you talk about that [your story] it can only make you feel better. It helps to talk. Sometimes, I sit down with friends and we talk.

Contribution: Occupations that allow one to give back, to be a valued, productive community member.

To tell about my story makes me feel better because I know it can help others ...

As someone told me: You didn't die in the war, you lived for a reason. I think it's true.

I'm happy to be alive but I'm sad to be alone ... houses were burned, people had nobody to turn to ... when I think about all of this, I want to see a change, a difference. I'm free and I could live the American dream, it's easy to do that ... I want to go back there and do something for people that stayed there.

CONCLUSION: FOOD FOR THOUGHT

When asked about what hindered or enabled his healing, Solomon offers insightful remarks and brings into focus many elements, positive and negative. Throughout this chapter he has identified events and factors that have significant impact on the reintegration of most ex-child soldiers, and also coping strategies that are more personal. His comments were well thought out, the fruit of several years of reflection. One such comment was especially troubling and unexpected: an observation on our own reductionism and voyeurism. Weighing his words, Solomon strove to render accurately his experience:

When people approach us [ex-child soldiers], they want to know if we have killed, how we have killed, how we have been kidnapped, what we did in the rebel armies. They're looking for thrills. They are not really interested about what we are going through right now. Nobody asks how we're doing, what's becoming of us, how we cope with these traumas ...

Although health care workers speak of strength-based models, normalization and social inclusion, theoretical discourse and actions sometimes diverge. While claiming to help build these survivors' future, are we trapping them in the past? Solomon's story illustrates the remarkable resilience of the human spirit: he has travelled a road strewn with pain and death and reached a place of compassion and solidarity. In the partnership that links a child soldier to the health team, honouring his path, and where he is now, could be a worthwhile first step.

REFERENCES

Albertyn, R., Bickler, S.W., van As, A.B., Millar, J.W., Rode, H., 2003. The effects of war on children in Africa. Pediatr. Surg. Int. 19 (4), 227–232.

Amnesty International, 2003. Children and Human Rights (Online). Retrieved January 2009 from: <http://www.amnesty.org/>.

Amnesty International, 2006. DRC: Children at War, Creating Hope for the Future. London: AFR 62 / 017/2006. Retrieved November 2008 from: <http://web.amnesty.org/library/Index/ENGAFR620172006?open&of=ENG-COD>.

Annan, J., Blattman, C., Carlson, K., Mazurana, D., 2008. The State of Female Youth in Northern Uganda: Finding from the Survey of War Affected Youth. Feinstein International Center, Somerville, MA.

Bayer, C., Klasen, F., Hubertus, A., 2007. Association of trauma and PTSD symptoms with openness to reconciliation and feelings of revenge among former Ugandan and Congolese child soldiers. JAMA 298 (5), 555–559.

Beah, I., 2007. A Long Way Gone: Memoirs of a Boy Soldier. Sarah Crichton Books, New York.

Bernard, B., Brewer, B., Dharmapuri, S., et al., 2003. Assessment of the Situation of Women and Children Combatants in the Liberian Post-Conflict Period and Recommendations for Successful Integration. Development Alternatives, Maryland.

Boothby, N., Crawford, J., Halperin, J., 2006. Mozambique child soldier life outcome study: lessons learned in rehabilitation and reintegration efforts. Glob. Public Health 1 (1), 87–107.

Charchuk, S., 2007. An assessment of the current community-wide system for rehabilitation and reintegration of child soldiers in Northern Uganda. Royal Roads University, Victoria, BC.

Chrobok, V., Akutu, A., 2008. Returning home – children's perspectives on reintegration: a case study of children abducted by the Lord's Resistance Army in Teso, eastern Uganda. Coalition to Stop the Use of Child Soldiers, London.

Coalition to Stop the Use of Child Soldiers, 2008. Child Soldiers: Global Report 2008, London.

Cohn, I., Goodwin-Gill, G., 1995. Child Soldiers: The Role of Children in Armed Conflict. Claredon Press, Oxford.

Deng Deng, W., 2001. A survey of programs on the reintegration of former child soldiers. Government of Japan. Retrieved March 2008 from: <http://www.mofa.go.jp/policy/human/child/survey/index.html>.

Derluyn, I., Broekaert, E., Schuyten, G., De Temmerman, E., 2004. Post-traumatic stress in former Ugandan child soldiers. Lancet 363 (9412), 861–863.

FAFO, 2002. L'utilisation des enfants dans les conflits armés en Afrique centrale: Manuel pour l'évaluation rapide. Retrieved January 2009 from <http://www.reliefweb.int/rw/rwb.nsf/db900SID/OCHA-64DDQL?OpenDocument>.

Gislesen, K., 2006. A childhood lost? The challenges of successful disarmament, demobilisation and reintegration of child soldiers: the case of West Africa. Norwegian Institute of International Affairs, 712. Retrieved October 2008 from: <http://scholar.google.ca/scholar?hl=en&biw=1240&bih=598&nfpr=1&bav=on.2,or.r_qf.&bvm=bv.79189006,d.aWw&um=1&ie=UTF-8&lr=&q=related:aLiqKAw1QLKPFM:scholar.google.com>.

Hamakawa, T., Randall, K., 2008. Measuring the unmeasurable: community reintegration of former child soldiers in Côte d'Ivoire. Save the Children UK, London; Harvard Kennedy School, Cambridge. Retrieved July 2009 from: <http://resourcecentre.savethechildren.se/library/measuring-unmeasurable-community-reintegration-former-child-soldiers-cote-divoire>.

Hill, K., Langholtz, H., 2003. Rehabilitation Programs for African Child Soldiers. Peace Rev. 15 (3), 279–285.

Hoffman, L., 2007. Available online at: <http://www.catalystforpeace.org/voicetovision/blog/the-veteran-child-soldiers-association-of-liberia/> (Accessed 7 April 2010).

Honwana, A., 1998. Okusiakala ondalo yokalye: Let us light a new fire. Local knowledge in the post-war healing and reintegration of war-affected children in Angola. Retrieved March 2008 from <http://www.child-soldiers.org/resources/psychosocial>.

Human Rights Watch, 1994. Easy Prey: Child Soldiers in Liberia. Human Rights Watch Children's Project.

Humphreys, G., 2009. Healing child soldiers: childhood injuries and violence. Bull. World Health Organ. 87, 330–331.

International Bureau for Children's Rights, 2009. Connaître les droits de l'enfant. Retrieved December 2009 from: <http://www.courteechelle.com/connaitre-les-droits-de-lenfant>

Kaplan, E., 2005. Council on Foreign Relations. Available online at: <http://www.cfr.org/publication/9331/> (Accessed 10 April 2010).

Kostelny, K., 2004. What about the girls? Cornell Int'l L. J. 37 (3), 505–512.

Landry, G., 2006. Child Soldiers and Disarmament, Demobilization, Rehabilitation and Reintegration in West Africa: A Survey of Programmatic Work on Child Soldiers in Côte d'Ivoire, Guinea, Liberia and Sierra Leone. Coalition to Stop the Use of Child Soldiers, London.

Lutz, A., Slagter, H., Rawling, N., Francis, A., Greischar, L.L., Davidson, R.J., 2009. Mental training enhances attentional stability: neural and behavioral evidence. J. Neurosci. 29 (42), 13418–13427.

Lutz, A., Slagter, H.A., Dunne, J., Davidson, R.J., 2008. Attention regulation and monitoring in meditation. Trends Cogn. Sci. 12 (4), 163–169. NIHMS # 82882.

Lutz, A., Greischar, L.L., Rawlings, N.B., Ricard, M., Davidson, R.J., 2004. Long-term meditators self-induce high-amplitude gamma synchrony during mental practice. Proc. Natl. Acad. Sci. U.S.A. 101, 16369–16373.

Machel, G., 2001. The Impact of War on Children. UNICEF-UNIFEM, London.

Michael, S., 2006. Assistance à la réintégration des ex-combattants: bonne pratique et leçons pour le MDRP (Dossier de Travail No. 1).

Muwonge, M., 2007. Community based reintegration of ex-combatants: a case study of the Lords Resistance Army in northern Uganda. Presentation and discussion during the 4th International Institute For Peace Through Tourism African Conference: Educators Forum. Retrieved May 2009 from: <http://www.iipt.org/africa2007/PDFs/Muwonge.pdf>.

Pham, P., Vinck, P., Stover, E., et al., 2007. When the war ends: a population-based survey on attitudes about peace, justice, and social reconstruction in northern Uganda. Human Rights Center, University of California Berkeley: Payson Center for International Development, Tulane University & International Center for Transitional Justice.

Ravizza, D., 2008. At play in the fields of young soldiers in northern Uganda: the use of sport in armed conflict settings. Washington Network on Children and Armed Conflict. USAID DCOF. Retrieved May 2009 from: <http://www.sfcg.org/programmes/children/pdf/ravizza-sport-conflict.pdf>.

Ricard, M., 2003. Plaidoyer Pour le Bonheur. NIL, Paris.

Ricard, M., 2008. L'Art de la Méditation. NIL, Paris.

Ricard, M., 2009. The Skill of Happiness. Audio CD. No Mud No Lotus.

Seligman, M.E.P., 2002. Authentic Happiness. Free Press, New York.

Thibeault, R., 2011. From unsung heroes: occupational gifts for a meaningful life. In: McColl, Mary Ann (Ed.), Spirituality and Occupational Therapy. CAOT Press, Ottawa.

Twum-Danso, A., 2003. Monograph 82: Africa's Young Soldiers. The Co-Option of Childhood. Institute for Securities Studies, Pretoria. Retrieved May 2008 from: <http://www.issafrica.org/publications/monographs/monograph-82-africas-young-soldiers.-the-co-option-of-childhood-afua-twum-danso>.

UNICEF, 2007. The Paris Principles. Retrieved March 2010 from: <http://www.unicef.org/emerg/files/ParisPrinciples310107English.pdf>.

Verhey, B., 2001. Child Soldiers: Preventing, Demobilizing and Reintegrating (Africa Region Working Paper Series, No. 23). World Bank, Washington, DC.

Williamson, J., Carter, L., 2005. Children's Reintegration in Liberia. USAID, Washington, DC.

Women's Commission for Refugee Women and Children, 2000. Untapped potential: adolescents affected by armed conflict: a review of programs and policies. Women's Commission for Refugee Women and Children, New York. Retrieved June 2008 from: <http://www.unicef.org/emerg/files/adolescents_armed_conflict.pdf>.

15

THE DADAAB REFUGEE CAMPS AND THE VOICES OF PEOPLE WITH A DISABILITY

SIYAT HILLOW ABDI ■ BRIAN MATTHEWS

This chapter is the story of one man's attempts (the first author) to grapple with a severe disability (vision impairment) in the African context and then to go beyond his own disability and explore the impact of a range of disabilities on people living in, arguably, the most deprived of circumstances, that is, African refugee camps (see Abdi 2008 and Abdi & Matthews 2009 for more details of this journey).

MEETING SOLOO

Dr Abdi met Soloo* in the Dadaab refugee camp in November 2005 while he was interviewing people with a disability as a part of his studies. The focus of his study was to examine the situation of Somali refugees with disabilities in Kenya. Dr Abdi wanted to clarify and describe the concept of disability as it relates to the Somali community in the refugee camps, as well as to develop suggested plans for community rehabilitation and recovery.

Soloo was 23 years old at the time he was interviewed. He was a single Somali man with a primary level class 8 education and was one of 200 people with a disability that were interviewed. The themes running through the interview with Soloo were reflected, in their own individual ways, by many of the others with whom Dr Abdi spoke. Their experiences are also woven into this chapter to help describe the realities that people with a disability face in refugee camps.

*Name changed to protect identity.

My name is Soloo. I was 9 years old when the war came to Mogadishu where I was living. We did not leave immediately. However, the fighting intensified and life became unbearable. So many people were killed. I stayed up to 2000 when I lost my limbs as a result of gun shots which paralysed both my legs. I was forced to seek assistance and treatment. My mother assisted me greatly and I was taken to Keisanne Hospital in Mogadishu.

It is my view that traditions and customs that discriminate against people with a disability are not good. They are not of benefit to the community nor the disabled. People who have a disability feel neglected by the same community which raised them. The best thing is to change the attitude. Disability is a natural phenomenon and we must all accept it.

Currently, the efforts are not adequate. The disabled members are marginalised and the majority are unemployed. I am now in school and I hope I will continue up to university education if I get the opportunity. I strongly believe that education can change my life and the community attitude. Since I cannot do any manual work, I must achieve high academic excellence.

REFUGEES AND DISABILITY

To be a refugee is to be seen as vulnerable, powerless and a stranger alienated by both the public and the media. 'Refugees stop being persons, but are reduced to pure victims of the worst type in mankind. They are stripped of the particular characteristics of their person, place and history; left only with humanness of the most basic sense' (Horst 2003, p. 11). Once labelled as such, refugees are excluded from the normal life of the host communities. This adversely affects their dignity, worth, rights and self-esteem.

To be a refugee with a disability adds another layer of complexity to the alienation already experienced. Disability, especially in developing countries, is not very well understood. Social and cultural myths surrounding disability limit proper awareness about it, leading to isolation and underestimation of certain forms of disability. Most attention on disability in refugee camps is focused on mobility and physical rehabilitation, which is only the beginning of relevant disability related interventions.

In January 2005 the total population of persons with disabilities in the Dadaab camps registered with the local refugee agencies was 3073, including male and female children and adults; 1687 people were male, representing 55%, and 1386 were female, representing 45% of the total number of persons with a disability. The most prominent disability group consisted of those people with a physical disability (43%). The age group containing the largest percentage of people with a disability (43%) was the 18–59-year age group, 38% were 17 years old or younger, and only 19% were 60 years and above (Abdi & Matthews 2009).

It must also be noted, though, that there were many persons with disabilities in the camp who were not identified as such because parents, neighbours and relatives feared exposing them to discrimination and stigmatization. In fact, discrimination and stigmatization were often reported by the refugees with a disability interviewed. Due to a culture of fear, it seems very likely that the United Nations High Commissioner for Refugees (UNHCR) database underestimates the number of people with disabilities living in the camps.

THE MAJOR CAUSES OF DISABILITY AMONG THE SOMALI COMMUNITY

War in Somalia was seen as the main cause of disability for most of the people interviewed. Many persons obtained physical injuries during combat and were left traumatized, as reflected in the following responses:

I lost my sight in Somalia due to hunger and hardship. Our home was attacked and gangsters beat me up when I was only 11 years old. I was tortured and we had to walk long distance to escape without food and enough water. I suddenly felt sick and lost my sight.

Cumer

I became partially blind in 1991 when I was at my village where I was a farmer. One day some militia men came to me and disappeared with all what I had as property. They looted everything. They also violently raped my dear wife in front of me. I could not bear the pain and shame. I tried to save her. Unfortunately, I was overwhelmed by the gangsters – one of these was smoking and he pushed the burning cigarette into my left eye.

Abdi

Although disability is a plan of God, my disability was directly caused by the civil war in Somalia. It was caused by gun shots, as well as hardships and hunger associated with the war.

Nastexo

I am physically handicapped and also visually impaired so I have multiple disabilities. I became disabled during the civil war. In my own house, my brother was killed. My husband was also killed in cold blood in front of me and my children. I was also violently raped in front of my children.

Xawa

Diseases and poor diet also cause disability within the camps. However, disability was culturally explained as a result of curses. Most people interviewed associated bodily malfunctioning and certain disorders with curses. Certain groups of people, especially those born with certain unique characteristics, were also believed to possess powers to curse, and evil spirits were also believed to cause disability.

THE QUALITY OF LIFE OF REFUGEES WITH DISABILITY

Generally, the quality of life of refugees with disability was reported to be poorer than that of refugees without disability. This was due to the stigmatization of disability in the Somali community. The refugees with disability were discriminated against and thus disadvantaged, economically and socially. They did not adequately access the resources that were available in the camp, such as education, food and employment, nor were they fully involved in decision-making.

According to people with disabilities in the camps, nondisabled refugees regarded them negatively and used terms detested by people with disabilities. Negative descriptions reported included 'Naanaays', nicknames referring to the type of disability of individuals such as 'Dhadol' (deaf), 'Indhool' (blind) or 'Doogon' (fool), the last referring to individuals with intellectual disability. The negative attitude was reflected in the humiliation, demoralization and isolation of people with disabilities in the camps. The derogatory names used were socially and historically embedded within the degrading depiction of disability in many Somali oral narratives, sayings and proverbs.

Seventy-eight per cent (78%) of those interviewed stated that, generally, neighbours, family members and fellow refugees isolated people with a disability. One would expect that these groups of people would be the very ones to provide moral and material support. This is typically not the case because such isolation emanates largely from the fear experienced by families. Not only do they fear the stigma and perceptions that their family member is 'cursed', but they too may experience direct consequences of this stigma, and in the struggle for scarce resources people with disabilities (and their families) risk being left behind.

COMMON NEEDS IN THE CAMPS

The struggle for scarce resources within the camps relates to basic needs for nutrition, health care, safety and security, and livelihood. People with disabilities share a common set of needs with the rest of the population but may have specific considerations to ensure they have access and can utilize the resources optimally.

Nutritional Issues

Since 1991, refugees in the Dadaab camps have largely depended on rations provided by the international community through UN agencies and nongovernmental organizations (NGOs). As Verdiram (cited in Horst 2004, p. 67) observed, any organization that

forces refugees to depend on rations is obliged to ensure the distribution of sufficient food. Refugees in the Dadaab camps are under the care of the UNHCR (the main funding body) and the food ration is distributed under the World Food Programme (WFP) every 15 days. However, the rations are insufficient and effective food distribution in these camps is often lacking. Nutritional surveys commonly indicate that the general ration distribution is deficient in micronutrients such as vitamins A, B_2, C and niacin, and absorbable iron (SCF 1999).

Security Concerns

Somali refugees, having fled from countries that have experienced protracted and very brutal forms of armed conflict, find themselves with no viable livelihood. Without freedom of movement, with few economic or educational opportunities, with insufficient and declining assistance over time, the Somali refugees have almost no immediate prospect of finding a solution to their plight. The UNHCR (2006) defined a protracted refugee situation as 'one in which refugees find themselves in a long lasting and intractable state of limbo. Their lives may not be at risk, but their basic rights and essential economic, social and psychological needs remain unfulfilled after years in exile. A refugee in this situation is often unable to break free from enforced reliance on external assistance.'

This definition accurately describes the condition of many Somali refugees in the Dadaab camps. In addition, the location of these camps (a few kilometres from the borders of Somalia) neither provides protection nor offers any viable livelihood for the refugees. The prevalence of idleness, aid dependency, a legacy of conflict and weak rule of law are potential factors that can induce fresh cycles of violence. Security in and around the camps is problematic and clan conflicts and personal intimidation were regularly reported.

Income Generation and Employment

The activities of international NGOs in the camps provide most of the job opportunities to the refugees and are, in most cases, a source of refugee livelihood. For example, CARE employs 1200 incentive refugees and these individuals have considerable purchasing power in the camps (CARE USA 2006). 'Incentive' refers to the money paid to refugees employed directly by the UNHCR or by one of its implementing partners in the camps. The incentive refugees are employed in a variety of jobs with different levels of responsibility and work, such as teachers, loaders, community development workers, auxiliary nurses, secretaries, school inspectors, cooks, cleaners and doctors.

From the survey done in the Dadaab camps, the majority of people with a disability (78%) were unemployed, and an insignificant number (3.5%) were employed permanently or on contracts. People with a disability in the Dadaab camps find it hard to generate supplementary income to support their families, and depend heavily on relief support. Remittances that are often received by nondisabled refugees, and which form a major source of income in the camps are, generally, not available to refugees with a disability because they are 'invisible' and have no, or limited, contacts in the countries to which other refugees have emigrated.

Furthermore, refugees with a disability were disadvantaged in relation to marriage prospects, and even a relatively high level of educational achievement in the camps (secondary level of literacy) did not influence their employment opportunities. Women with a disability were even more marginalized and vulnerable in this area.

Health Care Services

The health care needs of the refugees with a disability need to be given adequate consideration. In order to achieve this, refugees with disability need to be carefully identified and their specific forms of disability documented. Medical needs, in particular, must be identified and addressed promptly. Just a few of the pressing health requirements in the camps are: curative health care services against influenza, high blood pressure, diabetic management, HIV/AIDS and malaria; improvement of immunization opportunities; early disease detection and intervention; and provision of appropriate preventative education and protection against sexually transmitted diseases. In addition, there is an urgent need for more nurses and therapists.

REHABILITATION ISSUES IN THE DADAAB CAMPS

It is clear that both international and local organizations operating at the Dadaab camps need to improve

their response to the needs of refugees with a disability from a more holistic perspective. Increased coordination, systematic exchange of information and a better working relationship could help reduce the negative effects of discrimination and marginalization experienced by refugees with a disability. Therefore, organizations need to readjust and streamline their policies and practices to meet the challenges.

In situations such as those in the Dadaab camps, emergency rehabilitation needs to encourage the provision of relief and rehabilitation based on the individual's entire needs – physical, social, economic and psychological – while at the same time providing rehabilitation and sustainable recovery in the longer term. Livelihood-based approaches to support improved relief, and rehabilitation interventions for people who have experienced brutal civil wars and post-war hardships, seem to have much potential value. However, continued distress causes disruptions that last for years, and this may create permanent changes in people's lives. Recognition of individual differences, and factoring these differences into rehabilitation programmes, remains a challenge at the Dadaab refugee camps.

The cultural and religious backgrounds of the Somali refugees play a significant role in causing and/or perpetuating disability. Some cultural and religious beliefs and practices condemn persons with disability as evil, lazy, burdensome and helpless. These fatalistic and pessimistic attitudes deprive persons with disability of dignity, self-esteem and the motivation to strive and thrive in society. However, a careful examination of the dominant religion (Islam) does not suggest that the religious teachings are prejudiced against people with disabilities (Bazna & Hatab 2005). Prevailing rehabilitation efforts do not seem to address these cultural and religious impediments.

The prevailing rehabilitation efforts in the camps are mainly external initiatives that tend to be implemented using a top-down approach. This does not provide the refugees with adequate opportunity for participation. Given the entrenched stigmatization and discrimination against persons with disability among the refugee community, it becomes extremely difficult, if not impossible, for many Somali refugees with disability to determine their destiny. Poor representation and participation of persons with disability remains a challenge in all rehabilitation programmes.

Education

Although education may be one viable way of rehabilitating refugees with disability in the camps, many children with disabilities are not taken to school. The formal schooling system merely places pupils with disabilities and nondisabled pupils together, and subjects both to the same curriculum. This passes as 'inclusive' education. The child with disability is then left to adapt to the needs of the school.

Vocational Training Programmes

Vocational training attempts to empower persons with disabilities to become economically self-reliant. Vocational training institutions need to liaise with other stakeholders to ensure that persons with disability graduating from these institutions receive financial support to initiate income-generating projects. It is our contention that providing quality vocational training for persons with disability can help foster work-ready attitudes and values in refugees with a disability.

Provision of More Opportunities for Resettlement

The role of resettlement is recognized as an important instrument of protection within the framework of the UNHCR's supported three 'durable solutions'. Often, countries that are involved in refugee resettlement, in close cooperation with the UNHCR, carry out assessment of existing resettlement needs and priorities, and allocate their resettlement quota. The UNHCR also encourages countries to take refugees with a disability through its special programme called Ten Plus. Countries are encouraged to take only 20 refugees with a disability, and their families, for resettlement. However, very few countries sign up for this programme.

As a result of these strict immigration rules, tragic situations have occurred. For instance, it was reported to the first author that some families have left behind, and even disowned, their members who have disabilities in order for the rest of the members to be resettled. Refugee families, including people with a disability, have been affected by 'Buufis' (a disease produced by

the notion of resettlement which affects the psyche of many refugees; see Horst 2006a & b, for extensive discussion of the 'Buufis' phenomenon).

COPING STRATEGIES

Refugees with disability adopted various strategies to enable them to cope with refugee life. Soloo, who was quoted earlier, pursued education vigorously, believing that it would help him cope better in life. Another person, Abdi, adopted reflection as a coping strategy. He focused more on his strengths than on weaknesses and disability. He also chose to ignore negative comments made in relation to him. One of the female refugees with a disability, Xawa, on the other hand, preferred to withdraw and attend to her business. She worked very hard to prove to those who looked down upon her that she was as capable and dignified as any other person in the camp, despite her multiple disabilities.

Even those interviewees who presented examples of resilience under difficult circumstances reported that one great challenge in their lives was 'shattered dreams'. Soloo, for instance, had hoped to be a professional footballer, but during the Somali civil war both of his legs were destroyed. Abdi witnessed with horror the raping of his own wife and had his vision damaged when he tried to intercede. Xawa was raped in front of her children, her husband was killed and she lost her vision and suffered physical disabilities in the violence. However, it is important to stress that this study also found some people with a disability who retained self-respect and determination to succeed in life, in spite of the prevailing negative view in the community.

LOOKING AHEAD: COMMUNITY-BASED REHABILITATION (CBR)

Community-based rehabilitation (CBR) may be used as a central reference for guiding interventions in the camps. CBR is a community development strategy distinguished by its focus on the rehabilitation, equalization of opportunities, and social inclusion of all people with disabilities. It is implemented through the joint efforts of people with disabilities (including their organizations and families), NGOs, communities, government institutions and the private sector.

Community-based rehabilitation promotes close collaboration among the various stakeholders to provide equal opportunities for all people with disabilities in the community (ILO, UNESCO, WHO 2004).

According to UNESCAP (2006), and from the perspective of the International Disability and Development Consortium (IDDC 2003), the advantages of CBR are that it:

- Promotes respect for human rights as well as participation of persons with disability.
- Enables persons with disability to access equal opportunities, irrespective of age, sex, type of disability and socioeconomic status.
- Aims at enabling people with disabilities to identify, develop and use their physical and mental abilities, and thus become responsible agents in society.
- Sensitizes communities with regard to the rights of people with disabilities. The community is encouraged to respond empathically to the needs of persons with disabilities and to recognize their strengths and capacities, thus social integration and harmony is fostered.
- Aims to alleviate poverty and expand the role of persons with disability in community life.
- Perceives disability broadly, to include barriers to participation, which is a violation of human rights. It thus addresses attitudes, practices, systems and policies that contribute to disability.
- Perceives rehabilitation as holistic attempts to enhance the quality of life of persons with disability, as well as other members of the community, which are not imposed but are formulated, implemented, monitored and evaluated with the active consent and participation of the beneficiaries.

Given the merits listed above, the WHO (2004, 2010) has identified CBR as a viable strategy for rehabilitation since it equalizes opportunities, reduces poverty and advocates the active involvement of persons with disability in community life. However, the WHO acknowledges that people's needs and concerns are diverse and no one CBR intervention can be universalized. Instead, innovative interventions need to be formulated that adhere to the general principles of CBR, as outlined above, and adapted to local contexts. This involves building upon existing resources and networks (e.g. families, disabled people's organizations, self-help groups), strengthening individual and community capacities, and 'raising the voice' of refugees with disabilities to influence policy and practice, and ultimately quality of life in the camps. This requires a concerted effort from all the stakeholders, and in this case, namely the government of Kenya and the international community, the refugees without disability, refugees with disability, the NGOs, organizations representing people with a disability, religious organizations, educational institutions and other relevant institutions.

THE VOICE OF THE PEOPLE

When asked for recommendations about what to do for people with disabilities, six of the people who agreed to longer interviews answered as in the excerpts below. These concluding words contain messages of hardship and inequity, but also focus on the things that could bring about positive changes in the quality of life of people with disabilities who live in the Dadaab Refugee Camp Complex.

My recommendations are: Give them opportunities whenever such opportunities occur, e.g. scholarships, employment, training and resettlement. Also the education sector should note that the disabled are marginalised and should not treat them like the non-disabled in relation to secondary cut-off points for entry.

Soloo

Get organisations' experts in disability issues and development.

Abdi

I would recommend these institutions to increase their resources and provide better education. This is a powerful asset that can uplift their life.

Nastexo

I would say that the disabled people are vulnerable and this is even worse in refugee life. Let the international community stop resettling the Somali community by their tribes. This will only increase ethnic fighting and dominance. Let them consider the real vulnerable groups, especially the children, women, the aged and the disabled. These groups need care and rehabilitation as well as vocational training for employment.

Cumar

Let them appreciate our feelings and treat us equally. The services are for all refugees. For example, we all run away from wars and face common hardships but some organisations favour certain people for resettlement and neglect us disabled mothers because we have disabled children. This is not fair.

Sahar

CONCLUSION

Refugees with disabilities face stigmatization and discrimination; their specific needs are not met for shelter, nutrition, safety and security, employment and income-generating opportunities. Rehabilitation services in the camps are inadequate. But even more poignant is the damage to the dreams and aspirations they previously held dear. Explicit moves need to be taken to address each of these areas to ensure that refugees with disabilities are treated with dignity and included in all aspects of community life. Somali refugees with disability aspire to achieve self-reliance, recognition of their potential by the rest of the community, fulfilment in life, despite disability, integration in community life and participation in the life of society. Guided by such aspirations, some refugees with disability have been proactive and assertive with positive results, but opportunities for promoting self-reliance need to be further identified and developed.

In order to address the needs of people with a disability, and build upon their strengths and capacities, cultural constructions about disability need to be carefully evaluated and transformed. Towards this aim, a participatory approach is necessary in which members of the Somali community, together with their leaders, reexamine the prevailing attitudes and beliefs about disability and consider their implications and the consequences on human wellbeing.

We would like to conclude with the words of Xawa, a woman living in the Dadaab camps, because they illuminate a way forward towards a more inclusive society.

Come close to their needs. Understand them and their emotions. Open the doors for them. Integrate them. Give them equal opportunities and services just the way you help the non-disabled refugees …

This is our dream for the future.

REFERENCES

Abdi, S., Matthews, B., 2009. The Journey of Somali Refugees with Disability in Kenya: Voices of Refugees with Disabilities in the Dadaab Camps. VDM Verlag Dr. Müller GmbH & Co. KG, Saarbrücken, Germany.

Abdi, S.H., 2008. Evaluation of approaches to disability and rehabilitation, in the context of Somali refugees in Kenya. PhD Thesis, Flinders University, Adelaide, Australia. Available from: <http://theses.flinders.edu.au/uploads/approved/adt-SFU20080904.150115/public/02whole.pdf>

Bazna, M.S., Hatab, T.A., 2005. Disability in the Qu'ran: The Islamic alternative to defining, viewing and relating to disability. J. Religion Disabil. Health 9 (1), 5–27.

CARE USA, 2006. Annual Report. From: <http://www.care.org/newsroom/publications/annualreports/index.asp> (Retrieved 19 December 2007 – no longer available electronically).

Horst, C., 2003. Transnational Nomads: How Somalis Cope With Refugee Life in Dadaab Camps of Kenya. PhD Project, AGIDS, University of Amsterdam.

Horst, C., 2004. 'Money and Mobility: Transnational Livelihood Strategies of the Somali Diaspora' in Global Migration Perspectives. No 9 October 2004. Amsterdam Institute of Metropolitan and International Development Studies, Amsterdam. Available from: <http://www.iom.int/jahia/webdav/site/myjahiasite/shared/shared/mainsite/policy_and_research/gcim/gmp/gmp9.pdf>

Horst, C., 2006a. Transnational Nomads: How Somalis Cope with Refugee Life in the Dadaab Camps of Kenya. Berghahn Books, Oxford.

Horst, C., 2006b. Buufis amongst Somalis in Dadaab: the transnational and historical logics behind resettlement dreams. J. Refug. Stud. 19 (2), 143–157.

IDDC, 2003. Reflection Paper on CBR. IDDC CBR Task Group. Dutch Coalition on Disability and Development (DCDD) April 2003.

ILO, UNESCO, WHO, 2004. CBR: A Strategy for Rehabilitation, Equalization of Opportunities, Poverty Reduction and Social Inclusion of People with Disabilities Joint Position Paper 2004 Geneva: WHO, ILO, UNESCO, Switzerland. From: <http://www.ilo.org/wcmsp5/groups/public/---ed_emp/---ifp_skills/documents/publication/wcms_107938.pdf> (Retrieved 6 December 2006).

SCF, 1999. Food Economy Updates of Dadaab Camps: Ifo, Dagahaley and Hagadera, Save the Children Fund (UK) for WFP and UNHCR. Kenya Refugee Study Final Report 25 September 1999 pp 1–29. Dadaab, Garissa District, Kenya.

UNESCAP, 2006. Asia Pacific Disability Forum Second General Assembly and Conference 2006, Bangkok. Available from: <www.worldenable.net/convention2006/slidespurpose.htm> (Retrieved 20 December 2006 – no longer available electronically).

UNHCR, 2006. The State of the World's Refugees. From: <http://www.unhcr.org/cgi-bin/texis/vtx/template?page=publ&src=static/sowr2006/toceng.htm> (Retrieved 10 December 2007 – no longer available electronically).

WHO, 2004. Meeting Report on the Development of Guidelines for Community Based Rehabilitation (CBR) Programmes (1 and 2 November, 2004, Geneva, Switzerland).

WHO, 2010. Community Based Rehabilitation: CBR Guidelines. WHO, Geneva.

16

DISABLED PEOPLE'S ORGANIZATIONS (DPOS) IN DISASTER: LEARNING FROM THEIR EXPERIENCE

NAZMUL BARI ■ BROJA GOPAL SAHA

INTRODUCTION

Cyclones Sidr and Aila hit the coastal belt of Bangladesh in 2007 and 2009, respectively. Many people, including people with disabilities, were severely affected. After these cyclones the Centre for Disability in Development (CDD) with the support of CBM had supported its partner organizations in the coastal belt to undertake emergency relief, rehabilitation and inclusive-development programmes for persons with disabilities. This chapter is based on CDD's experience and the real life accounts and views of persons with disabilities and one of their local DPOs from Barguna, Bangladesh. The authors collected information from the people with disabilities and the local DPO of Barguna in October 2009.

SURVIVING SIDR AND AILA

We weren't prepared for such a disaster, I don't know how I cheated death, I was at my home, no one imagined that the winds will be so strong, that sea water will rise so much, I am lucky to be alive to share my experiences today! That day I heard from people about the cyclone Sidr, but I did not go to the shelter considering all the difficulties I will need to experience. Besides, a few months back there was a tsunami warning but nothing happened; this time I thought it will be the same. I stayed back. At first I placed myself on the bed, but the water soon rose above that. I clung to the ceiling and then climbed on top. I was scared to

death; if the water rose any further I will have no place to go.

Monirul Islam is a person with physical disability, who uses a wheelchair

We had no prior warning that the water was rising so fast. My uncle informed my parents. My parents were undecided what to do. They immediately sent my younger sister to a safe location, and then we waited, but the water was rising quickly. When my parents finally decided to leave with me, the water rose up to my throat level; it was difficult for my parents to walk through the rising water, in a windy condition, carrying me all the way to a safe building for shelter. On the way I was scared, very, very scared. I thought I will drown; such an event never occurred in my lifetime! At the building I was carried up to the second floor; my father was exhausted carrying me. There I faced many problems; it was a new world for me; it was crowded, and there were no latrines that I could access. It was a hell-like experience. I was there for nearly two days!

Sharmin is a 14-year-old girl with mild cerebral palsy

I was left alone at home with my sister. She fought against the roaring forces of nature and took me to the shelter, carrying and swimming. It was extremely difficult. At the shelter I was carried up by three men; I did not feel comfortable being

119

treated like a sack of goods. The shelter was overly crowded. There was not enough space to sit. There was absolutely no privacy for women. I felt worse as a woman with disability. The toilet of the shelter was outside the building. It was another challenge and a painful mission to try to use the only toilet of the shelter, the same toilet used by a thousand others. I tried desperately not to use the toilet.

Halima is a young lady with physical disability

These are only three of the thousands of real life experiences of persons with disabilities who survived two of the deadliest disasters to strike the coastal districts of Bangladesh in 2007 and 2009, causing colossal destruction and loss of lives. The Government of Bangladesh, along with the private sector and the civil society, with its limited resources, had tried with maximum effort to recover from the loss. People living in poverty were the most affected; women, children and the elderly were especially vulnerable, and if they had a disability, this vulnerability was manifold.

CYCLONES: THE IMPACT ON PEOPLE WITH DISABILITIES

Disasters such as Cyclones Sidr and Aila are especially devastating to the lives of people with disabilities on multiple levels, extending beyond the emergency itself to include their recovery. An inaccessible toilet in a crowded shelter presents major challenges and reduces a person's sense of dignity and confidence; being 'treated like a bundle of goods' can also affect a person's sense of security and self-esteem.

Most of the houses of the persons with disabilities were made from materials that could not resist the strong wind and the surge of water from the sea. They had to take refuge on dam banks, in temporary shelters made of plastic sheeting and bamboo sticks, or in cyclone shelters, living an inhuman life. For most of the people, food was not available for the first few days; many survived drinking green coconut, or eating some dry food, the little that they could salvage, but all were inadequate. There was a severe dearth of safe drinking water, with the water sources polluted and filled with saline sea water.

Persons with disabilities suffered the most, reaching the shelter and safe locations under duress, often having received the warning late, their normal path to the shelter submerged under water and blocked by fallen trees and the debris from destroyed structures dangerously lying around. Alone, or with family members, they had to cross all these hurdles to reach the shelter. Lives were endangered. Many were injured. Many others did not make it at all.

The cyclone shelters were located some distance away. At the shelters there was no space; bodies were pressed against each other. Many took refuge downstairs, and during high tide they had to stand in water and wait it out. Toilets were few and often unusable for people with disabilities; they had to defecate on their clothes, which were washed by family members at night. Other people detested this and wanted them to leave. Security was another concern, especially for the young girls and women with disabilities.

The cyclones destroyed people with disabilities' sources of livelihood. This loss drained them emotionally as it had taken a lot of effort, perseverance and resources to start a livelihood, to earn an income and contribute to the family. This income and contribution to the family expenditure played a part in enhancing their status and recognition as a valued member of their community. With the cyclone, they not only lost their income but were fearful of losing their position in the family, and once again being dependent. They also experienced mental stress and anguish worrying how they could access resources again to restart their livelihood.

The descriptions above, including the harrowing experiences of Monirul Islam, Sharmin and Halima, highlight a broader and important issue: people with disabilities are not being adequately considered in disaster response, recovery or preparedness policies, plans and practices. This translates into limited access to relief and support to rebuild livelihoods and recover from disaster. More specifically, people with disabilities are mostly left out of disaster preparedness identification processes, resource and risk mapping; early warning systems; search, rescue and evacuation; emergency relief and health services; and reconstruction programmes.

Many shelters are located at a distance; the structures and toilets are frequently inaccessible

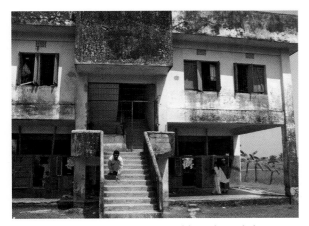

FIGURE 16-1 ■ An inaccessible cyclone shelter.

(Figure 16-1), and negative attitudes held by others often compound the problems people with disability experience. There is also a lack of security and threats of exploitation in shelter environments. Furthermore, persons with disabilities often lose their assistive devices during disasters, which make them even more vulnerable during emergency and crisis periods. During resettlement the needs and issues of people with disabilities are also overlooked in the construction of new houses, in livelihood and food security programmes, and also in education.

The survivors in the stories shared all faced barriers to accessing relief. They also experienced some form of psychological stress and described a feeling of helplessness when depending on others for food, relief, care and safety. But people with disabilities need not be helpless victims or passive recipients of relief and assistance. They can help themselves and others in their community to generate solutions and play a key role in 'building back better'.

Disabled people's organizations are an example of people with disabilities coming together, supporting one another, and strengthening their voice in the context of the broader community to effect change and influence policy and practice. They have a key role to play in mainstreaming disability into disaster management and risk reduction in collaboration with local communities, governments and non-governmental organizations, donors and other key stakeholders.

DISABLED PEOPLE'S ORGANIZATIONS (DPOS)

Not long after Cyclones Sidr and Aila, local self-help groups (SHGs) and DPOs joined forces to support the people with disabilities who were affected. Self-help groups are informal groups of people who come together to address their common problems. While self-help might imply a focus on the individual, one important characteristic of self-help groups is the idea of mutual support – people helping each other (CBR Guidelines 2010). SHGs not only educate, empower and encourage persons with disabilities in the community to develop and be aware of their rights but also build a network among other social groups such as women's groups, youth groups, groups of elderly persons, and so on, to solve their problems and work for sustainable development in the community (APCD Newsletter Volume 17, October 2006).

DPOs in Bangladesh are different to SHGs in that they are registered and have a minimum of 51% of people with disability as members of an executive council. They are led by a person with disability and are organized to enable them to advocate for their own rights (as opposed to someone doing this on their behalf) and to influence decision-makers in governments and all sectors of society.

BEGINNING OF A DPO

Many DPOs in Bangladesh are formed by persons with disability who have experienced barriers in their lives. Their intention was to support other people with disabilities to mobilize and lead a process of bringing positive changes to society, and hence to all people with disabilities. The local DPO in Barguna had a similar intention. Mr. Habibur Rahman, the Executive Director of a local DPO* in Barguna, was affected by polio at a young age. He experienced many challenges in his own life due to his own impairment and barriers in society. He interacted with other people with disabilities in his community and realized that their conditions were much worse than his, that many of them were leading a life

---

*The local DPO is named Southern Socio-Economic Development Programme (SSDP). From 1 January 2012 CDD does not have any partnership or working relationship with the organization.

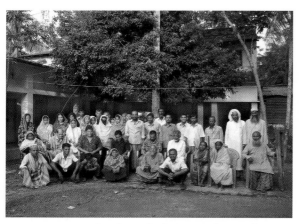

FIGURE 16-2 ▓ Southern Socio-Economic Development Programme (SSDP) with its members and beneficiaries.

without self-esteem and dignity. Persons with disabilities were excluded from the rehabilitation, development and social affairs of their community. He was saddened that many people with disabilities had accepted their condition as their fate, but at the same time was encouraged that there were a few who had the courage and determination to challenge the discrimination, neglect and ignominy that they faced. He, a few people with disabilities, and some of his friends were determined to act against all of these injustices.

They formed the local DPO with the goal of creating a society where persons with disabilities would enjoy equal rights and dignity with any other member of society (Figure 16-2).

In October 2009 this DPO had 67 staff members, including volunteers. They formed SHGs with local people with disabilities. In total, 250 persons with disabilities (information correct as of October 2009) are part of these SHGs and their DPO network.

The work of the local DPO included community mobilization, raising awareness and sensitization, advocacy, networking, organizing people with disabilities into groups, and developing their capacity, inclusion of people with disabilities into education, health, livelihood programmes, emergency relief and disaster preparedness, and also issues such as gender, child rights, HIV/AIDS, etc. They believe in empowering people with disabilities so they do not remain passive recipients.

DISASTERS AND DPOS

DPOs and SHGs provide a critical, preexisting community-based network to support people with disabilities in times of emergency. It is through DPOs and organizations working on disability inclusion that national organizations, such as CDD, with its connections through to international disaster and development funding agencies, can help galvanize emergency response and recovery efforts. Local DPO and SHG involvement in Cyclones Sidr and Aila is an example of how this works.

Immediately after the cyclones the first priority of local DPOs and SHGs was to locate the whereabouts of their members. It was near impossible, initially, for their members to move from their locations, as the surroundings were typically changed and made impassable by the cyclones and associated tidal surges.

CHALLENGES FACING LOCAL DPOS IN THE AFTERMATH OF THE CYCLONES

Immediately after the cyclones, finding out about the situation of the people with disabilities who are members of my DPO was a big problem; the telecommunication network was not working – even mobile phones weren't working; the road communication was blocked, and while the army with special equipment worked tirelessly to clear the roads, it took time. And during this time the people were appealing for food and water, which was not there. Limited relief was distributed in the inaccessible areas from helicopters, but it hardly reached the vulnerable, let alone the people with disabilities. The strong were getting more and the weak hardly any.

We saw health conditions deteriorate, especially the children, elderly and the people with disabilities. Their physical and mental health was weak and not prepared to endure so much hardship. Fever, diarrhea and skin diseases were a common complaint. But the condition of local pathways, filled with thick mud and worse when it rained, made moving to get help, even with assistive devices, almost impossible.

Chief Executive of the local DPO

LOCAL DPO'S INITIAL RESPONSE

Within days, those people with greater mobility came out and started to enquire about others. Grouping under the leadership of the local DPO, they approached the District Disaster Management Committee, the local media, civil society, the rescue agencies and the security forces to mobilize help for persons with disabilities.

The DPO had a list of members who are persons with disabilities. They took the list to local government offices so that persons with disabilities could be included in the emergency and survival interventions. They also highlighted that this list only included the DPO's and SHGs' members. There were many more persons with disabilities who needed help now!

At the same time the local DPO started sending emergency appeals to different international and national NGOs with whom they had connections. They also started communicating with local NGOs, especially those that work on disability issues, to coordinate their efforts. They participated in the local disaster coordination meetings organized by the District Commissioner's Office, and through this were able to inform everyone about the situation of persons with disabilities and to lobby that the issues of persons with disabilities not be overlooked.

They also started emergency relief operations with the limited resources they had, or could collect locally. This mainly included water, medicine, utensils, clothes and dry food. As more relief started coming into their area they maintained regular communication so that persons with disabilities were not left out.

Unfortunately, despite all of these efforts, the majority of the persons with disabilities were still not taken into account or reached through the relief operations. Besides, the relief agencies were mostly reaching the easy to access areas; the difficult and distant areas received little attention.

SITUATIONAL ASSESSMENT

The DPO intensified its communication with different organizations for support. Some of these organizations responded positively and agreed to undertake an emergency response and rehabilitation programme.

These organizations first requested an emergency damage and needs assessment of the affected persons with disabilities.

The DPO noted:

This was a challenge and a very difficult task for us to undertake, as comprehensive information on the situation of persons with disabilities was hardly available, and whatever information was accessed, there were questions regarding its accuracy and reliability. We went to the local government offices, disaster focused-NGOs and disaster management committees, but adequate and appropriate information was not available. So, this became our first task. On our own we collected information from our beneficiaries, SHG members, the community people and the local Union Councils. This information was then sent to the agencies who had agreed to provide support.

RELIEF WORK

Immediately following both cyclones, the DPO supported persons with disabilities and their families with survival packages.

Based on the results of the assessment we made an initial list of persons with disabilities in different affected communities to receive the 2 weeks survival package. This list was then scrutinised to ensure eligibility and to prioritise. The selected beneficiaries were provided with a slip and asked to bring it on distribution day. The packages were distributed on a particular day in the presence of local administration and media, where each recipient had to deposit their slip and sign on receiving the package.

We also formed different committees with our staff, board members and local people to ensure that accountability and transparency were maintained. There was also monitoring from the agencies supporting us.

Executive Director, local DPO

In total, approximately 6000 persons with disabilities were reached through the initiatives after cyclones Sidr and Aila. Despite these efforts a large number of persons with disabilities remained unattended.

PLANNING FOR RECOVERY: WHO TO HELP?

During this emergency response period the local DPO, in consultation with the persons with disabilities and the SHGs, identified rehabilitation, reconstruction and mitigation needs. Among the different needs identified, there were three broad categories: needs specific to disability, such as assistive devices, therapy and counselling services; needs related to safe shelter, including housing, sanitation and clean water; and inclusion in development initiatives, notably livelihood, education and social safety nets.

However, the DPO noted:

The resources that we could access or receive from supporting agencies were limited and not everyone could be supported. It was extremely difficult to decide whom to support, especially as most persons with disabilities had suffered and all had needs after the cyclone… Finally, in collaboration with CDD it was decided that vulnerability criteria be used, and that our efforts will be a pilot initiative for learning, and as a model for possible replication in the future by organizations working on disaster preparedness and response.

REHABILITATION AND RECONSTRUCTION

There are two understandings of 'rehabilitation' in Bangladesh. Within the disaster management cycle, rehabilitation is an integral part of the recovery phase and includes social, economic and psychological rehabilitation. Specific to people with disabilities, rehabilitation refers to assessment, therapy, referral and assistive device services. According to the Bangladesh Government's Standing Orders on Disaster, April 2010, reconstruction means 'the process of restoring affected infrastructure to pre-event condition', preventing its further deterioration or making it better.

GETTING MOBILE AGAIN

In identifying the most vulnerable persons with disabilities for rehabilitation and reconstruction support, the DPO first assessed people who had lost or damaged their assistive device during the cyclone, and also those who had new requirements resulting from the effects of the cyclones. Assistive devices, including wheelchairs, tricycles, crutches, white canes, etc., were procured and provided as feasible with the available resources. This enabled people to move out of their shelters and homes, to go to the bazaar and community places where they could interact more widely with different people – activities that were very therapeutic, emotionally and physically. The trained Disability Rehabilitation Worker of the DPO also extended therapeutic and counselling support to people, as and when it was sought.

SAFE, ACCESSIBLE SHELTER

Because people with disability tend to be among the poorest in affected communities, it is not surprising that their houses, made mostly from bamboo and corrugated tin, were not strong enough to withstand the cyclonic winds and water surge. Many were either destroyed or significantly damaged.

Following Cyclone Sidr the DPO was able to help a few people with disabilities acquire well-constructed, accessible houses with toilets. Criteria for selecting beneficiaries included, most significantly, that the land where the house was to be constructed be allocated in the name of the person with disability. This was done to ensure that the persons receiving the house were not later evicted by others, including family members. Nor could the house be constructed on Government land. It was further agreed that these homes would be used for SHG meetings if required.

During the second cyclone these houses survived and the families did not lose valuable possessions as they did last time. In addition, some of these houses were used as 'safe shelters' by other persons with disabilities living in that community, especially where the nominated cyclone shelters were difficult to reach.

At a later stage these houses were fitted with solar panels. This has allowed children to study at night and given many persons with disabilities the option of working at night in their homes on handicrafts, making fishing nets, etc. They have also saved money as they need not buy kerosene or candles for light.

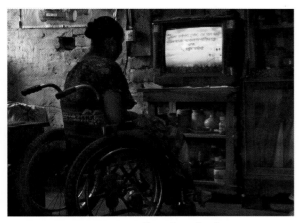

FIGURE 16-3 ▪ Sharmin at her home.

In Sharmin's house* a television was installed, which ran from the electricity generated by the solar panel (Figure 16-3). Sharmin was very happy that she could watch TV; she said, 'I can now remain updated on news around the world; I have also made new friends, as children of my age come to my house to watch TV, we watch different programmes together and have lots of fun together.'

GENERATING AN INCOME

Prior to the cyclones some people with disabilities in the area were involved in self-employment activities such as poultry rearing, dairy farming, fish cultivation, agriculture, small shops and making fishing nets. Most of them lost their assets during the cyclones and were not in a position to restart their livelihood activities as they did not have the resources. Some of those most in need were identified to receive livelihood support.

The people selected had prior technical expertise in specific trades. However, most lacked adequate skills and experience in business planning and management. It was thus decided that before receiving a livelihood support grant, target beneficiaries would be trained in business skills.

First, though, the DPO's livelihood workers received training from CDD on livelihood planning and

management. They next organized this training for the persons with disabilities in their locality. A business and trade feasibility assessment was conducted prior to finalization of the trade against which the grant was provided to the recipients. They undertook follow-up of people once their livelihood was started. After one year, some people with disabilities were provided with a second grant to expand their livelihood business. Many of them are now earning and contributing to their family expenses. This has not only boosted their self-confidence but also increased their acceptance within the family and community as an equal member. The DPO's associated SHGs supported the selection process of the beneficiaries to avoid duplication and ensure that the most needy received the support. A few of the neediest members within the SHGs also received similar support.

OTHER ACTIVITIES TO PROMOTE DISABILITY INCLUSION

Education: The DPO, with the support of CDD and from its own resources, provided books to some children with disabilities who had lost their educational materials during the disasters.

Environment: In some homes, apple plums, a local tree, were planted to contribute to protection of the environment and as a source of nutrition and additional income for the family. Three years after being planted, approximately 60% of the planted trees have survived.

Drinking water: There was also a need for longer-term access to safe drinking water, but as it was a saline area and fresh water was very deep and difficult to reach, it was too costly to supply tube-wells and only a few were installed. SSDP and the SHGs gave support by cleaning up polluted ponds used for household activities.

Early warning: In 2007 many people did not receive the cyclone warnings. Making sure that people with disabilities and their families receive warning signals in adequate time for them to take evasive action is a particular challenge. To address this, in Cyclone Aila in 2009, the DPO sent SMS information to its members through a mobile phone network. After receiving this information, members supported each other in seeking safe shelters.

Getting disability needs onto various agendas: The DPO had spent a huge amount of time communicating

---

*Sharmin received an accessible house, solar panel, assistive device and livelihood support.

and coordinating with different agencies, before, during and after the disasters. It required approaching agencies, participating in different meetings and frequent follow-up in an effort to maximize coordination.

However, as the DPO leader notes:

Ensuring that persons with profound disabilities are not left out was a particular challenge, as they remain mostly indoors and are more invisible than others. Another challenge was to reach the communities of persons with disabilities living in distant areas, requiring more time and different modes of transport to reach. In some cases these areas were just not visited, even though they had a greater need.

In Barguna there is an ethnic minority group who settled in the area from neighbouring Myanmar. As these people are different, culturally, religiously, in appearance and linguistically, in times of disasters they are mostly neglected and deprived. Persons with disabilities in this group suffered doubly, because of their disability and because of their ethnicity.

'WATCH GROUPS'

Immediately after a disaster there is an unannounced race in the disaster affected region by individuals and groups based on political, social, electoral identity and capacity to take control and establish influence. Unfortunately, sometimes these people are corrupt and have an intention to exploit and profit from the context. On some occasions these local powerbrokers are so powerful that they are in complete control of the fate of the affected people. In essence, they decide who will receive support and who will not. In such circumstances it is not uncommon for disaster affected people to align themselves with these powerbrokers, or in certain cases pay them, in order to be listed as recipients for support. The DPO, however, considers that this can be tackled if a 'watch group' is formed in the locality, comprised of teachers, community leaders, SHG and DPO members, NGO representatives and religious leaders, and if this watch group is mobilized to be a part of the relief, rehabilitation, reconstruction and mitigation work of their locality.

ADVOCACY AND AWARENESS

Raising awareness was also important. It included organizing local level workshops to create awareness of the different actors of development, including disaster management. The purpose of these workshops was to increase networking among different actors and to sensitize them to the situation of people with disabilities in a disaster situation and to the possible roles these actors could play in this regard. The media was extensively involved in the sensitization process; the DPO met with national daily newspaper representatives to publish their experiences and case studies on persons with disabilities who were affected by the cyclones and then supported to face their challenges. For future reference a list of people supported was prepared and kept ready. This information can be shared with the government and other NGOs in a disaster response should a situation arise.

MOVING BEYOND CHARITY

It is not just challenges with administrations and the disaster-responding agencies that need attention. The DPO highlighted that dealing with the 'charity mentality' of many persons with disabilities, and their families, has also been a huge challenge. They invested a lot of time in counselling sessions with individuals and their family members to help them understand that charity is not sustainable; rather that they must focus on their empowerment and take collective actions on disaster preparedness instead of waiting for someone to give charity. The benefits of charity last only for a few days, but preparedness and empowerment will benefit a lifetime.

KEY LEARNING, INSIGHTS AND STRATEGIES

There are a number of important insights to emerge from CDD and the local SHGs' and DPO's experience of Cyclones Sidr and Aila that have implications for policy and practice in 'disaster and development'.

The Role of DPOs

The initiatives of the DPO have positively influenced the lives of those cyclone-affected people with disabilities that live in the DPO's area of operation. But beyond this, the majority of people with disabilities were not reached and their needs were largely left unaddressed.

The post Sidr and Aila experiences of CDD have highlighted how very valuable it is to have an established DPO and network of SHGs through which to respond to disasters; the survival, recovery and future preparedness of people with disabilities is substantially improved. They provide a critical and rapid conduit in facilitating access to relief, mobility, shelter, income, education and more, all things that are important to health, dignity and wellbeing.

What is further evident is that where these local organizations exist, and have been working for the rights and development of persons with disabilities and disability issues across all stages of 'disaster and development', there is significantly less likelihood that people with disabilities will be overlooked or ignored. Supporting the development of DPOs and SHGs can thus be viewed as a key strategy in helping people with disabilities prepare for and manage disasters.

Awareness of Disability Issues Among 'Disaster and Development' Actors

It was evident from the experiences of these disasters that the awareness of policy makers, development actors, civil society, the Government and nongovernment representatives about the imperative of addressing disability issues within disaster management was very low. On the one hand, there was an assumption that there are very few persons with disabilities, and that their needs are less than those of other vulnerable groups; on the other hand, there is little knowledge on how disability issues could be addressed within disaster management.

It is essential that sensitization and advocacy on 'disability issues in disaster management' are conducted for organizations and individuals working on disaster issues, especially those that are responsible for disaster risk reduction (DRR) and disaster response. Training and capacity building of key agencies on disability issues in DRR is a prime requirement.

People with disabilities can play significant roles to advocate that their issues are not ignored in disaster management. Together with their organizations they should be meaningfully involved in sensitization and capacity building processes. The positive influence that persons with disabilities can directly wield on people in key positions through experience sharing and interaction is much more effective and lasting than that attained through other people or through information packages.

It is important that DPOs and organizations working on disability issues maintain regular communication and network with organizations working on disaster issues, and provide technical support so that disability issues are included and addressed within their programmes. It is advisable that, if such an organization is planning to work in a disaster affected area, it partners with a local DPO, who will have more information, access and credibility of the local persons with disabilities and their families. However, it is advisable to identify a DPO that is well established in the area and has strong linkages with different stakeholders, including the local government.

Inclusion of People with Disability in Response

Following a disaster many organizations, both Government and nongovernment, initiate recovery activities. Unfortunately, people with disabilities are largely left out of these, due to the lack of availability of information and limited resources. Hence it is essential that information about persons with disabilities is made available, and that even if resources are limited and interventions inadequate, people with disabilities are not excluded. Organizations need to consider how to distribute relief and ensure the response and recovery system is appropriate for those with disabilities. Designing rehabilitation activities that consider the needs of persons with disabilities will also benefit other vulnerable groups. The disaster shelters, homes, community spaces, safe drinking water sources, sanitary latrines, etc., that are constructed after a disaster should be accessible and disability friendly.

Disaster Risk Reduction and Preparedness

More emphasis should be placed by organizations on addressing disability issues in disaster risk reduction. The vulnerability and capacity assessments conducted must include information about persons with disabilities. Community capacity development initiatives should include persons with disabilities and their families. Identification, early warning, search, rescue and evacuation processes must ensure that essential and minimum requirements are considered for persons with disabilities. Local and regional disaster management committees should also include people with disabilities.

DISASTER: AN OPPORTUNITY TO PROMOTE DISABILITY ISSUES

As CDD notes:

> Local DPOs and SHGs have created a stronger platform for addressing disability issues generally through engagement with a wide range of disaster management actors and by creating replicable examples. There have been some remarkable long term changes in the wellbeing of people with disability, as individuals and through changes in the community. However, it has to be remembered that for measurable changes to occur such DPO

initiatives need more support to continue and to strengthen. Unless more organisations, including Government and the mainstream DRR organisations show commitment and take actions, the issue of disability in DRR will never be adequately addressed. In this process the participation of persons with disabilities and their organisations needs to be ensured at all levels.

CONCLUSION

Bangladesh is moving away from a charity and relief focused approach in disaster management to a more disaster preparedness and risk reduction approach promoting empowerment of the community. This is the same for all development initiatives in the country. In this development transition and process it is essential that SHGs and DPOs are meaningfully engaged, and their experiences and contributions recognized and respected.

17

ACCESSIBILITY OUTCOMES IN DISASTER RECOVERY – A CRITICAL CONCERN, A MINIMUM REQUIREMENT OR AN AFTERTHOUGHT?

SAMANTHA WHYBROW ■ CATHERINE BRIDGE

INTRODUCTION

This chapter is based on personal reflections and observations related to my work as an occupational therapist and aid worker in Sri Lanka following the 2004 Indian Ocean tsunami (SW). My primary role with an international nongovernmental organization (NGO) was to improve accessibility during the reconstruction efforts, particularly as it pertained to people with disabilities. The aim of this chapter is twofold: (1) to illustrate how standards of accessibility can be incorporated into emergency response and resettlement efforts following disaster, and (2) to outline key considerations related to the needs of people with disabilities as a part of international response. Towards this aim the personal stories of those with disabilities following the immediate relief effort are shared.

REALITY ON THE GROUND

The tsunami resulted in wide-scale destruction with vast areas of inhabited urban and suburban space being destroyed. In Sri Lanka the influx of money and aid agencies seeking to rebuild and repair these areas was admirable; however, in many cases the idea of rebuilding to a standard of accessibility, however basic, was either unaddressed or thought to be too complicated for such a fast and furious response to a big international crisis (Whybrow et al 2010). In fact, access to relief itself for people with disabilities was

said to be marginal at best by local disability organizations. Within an international context, the situation was further complicated by the fact that the South/South-East Asian understanding and responses to disability are different from those of developed nations such as Australia, Canada, the United States and the United Kingdom (Whybrow et al 2010). Current developed nation responses to disability directed by international NGOs reflect an entitlement or rights based approach (Batavia & Schriner 2001). In contrast, the concept of a common good (Ingstad & Whyte 1995) and rights of the community underpin the quiet push for accessibility and inclusion that is in its infancy in the developing nations of South/South-East Asia (Bridge 2008, IDIRYA 2008). Appreciating this local context proved to be important to implementing any sort of 'intervention' or assistance related to accessibility following the disaster.

ACCESSIBILITY AS AN IMPORTANT CONCERN

Accessibility is important during disaster recovery and reconstruction for several reasons. First, previous work has implied that the nature of the recovery environment has important health implications, particularly as related to mental health and post-traumatic stress following disaster (Ursano et al 1995). Second, as Diamond & Precin (2004) note, lack of access to relief including food, water and sanitation, shelter and basic health care is detrimental to a person's physical and mental health and may exacerbate stress and post-traumatic symptoms. Individuals with disabilities tend to underutilize disaster-relief services because they lack access and are too often invisible in emergency response contexts. Last, timelines are critical given that immediately after the disaster there is a heroic phase, where all members of a community pull together to address immediate safety and sustenance needs. However, disillusionment often follows and solidarity wanes with potentially greater consequences for those with disabilities (Diamond & Precin 2004). If the specific needs of people with disabilities are not considered in the immediate aftermath of disaster and do not feature in risk reduction measures (e.g. early warning and preparation) people with disabilities miss opportunities for recovery and building their resilience. Furthermore, their sense of dignity and self-esteem is also greatly impacted. This is a reality that I observed shortly after arriving in Sri Lanka and meeting people like Saraswathie.

MEETING SARASWATHIE

Arriving in Sri Lanka, six months after the 2004 tsunami, I was taken to a relief camp by a worker from an international nongovernmental organization (INGO) who had a social work background. The aid worker had sought me out as she had heard of a new accessibility initiative and was personally interested in seeing what could be done for some of the disabled people that she had discovered were residing in temporary shelters in a relief camp. It was there that I met Saraswathie and her 11-year-old daughter. Together we trudged to Saraswathie's shelter, making our way across the sandy makeshift roads of the sprawling camp that was now home to hundreds of families left homeless by the tsunami. It was hot and the sun blazed down on everyone in the camp, although a few months later when the monsoons arrived this camp would be underwater. The road was higher than the shelter and we quick-stepped down a small incline to get to the front door. Saraswathie was waiting inside, sitting on a stool.

She had some trouble with mobility but in the compact and smooth-surfaced shelter she described no problems with getting about her daily activities

with one exception: her greatest concern was getting to the toilet.

SHELTERS AND ACCESSIBILITY

As in most camps of this nature the toilets (or 'latrines' as they are more commonly referred to) were situated in a separate block and were shared by everyone. The main problem for Saraswathie (and, as it turns out, many people Samantha met that day because this was a habitat inside a war zone and there were many amputees) was a combination of distance and surface: the latrines were some distance from her shelter across uneven, sandy ground (Figure 17-1). It was impossible for Saraswathie to manage independently and so she relied on her daughter to help her.

LATRINES

Once at the latrine, Saraswathie had to make it up several high steps of irregular height. Without a rail to help, she also required assistance up these steps. Using the latrine – a squat pan as is common for most rural people in this country – presented another challenge, as she could not squat. Again, this was a challenge she could not manage on her own. Nor could she manage the other elements of this activity, namely filling a bucket with water and carrying it to the latrine as everybody else did. The trouble, aside from being unable to perform a usually private task independently

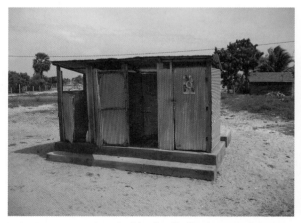

FIGURE 17-1 ■ A typical latrine facility in one of the temporary camps.

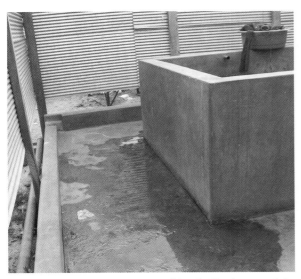

FIGURE 17-2 ▪ Community washing facility in one of the temporary camps.

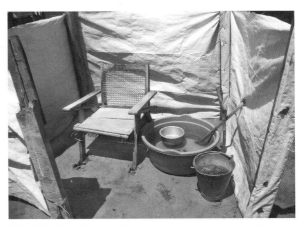

FIGURE 17-3 ▪ Parvati's solution to the access problems in the camp – a makeshift commode area.

(as she was used to in her own home), was that her daughter no longer went to school and was, instead, staying home to help her mother use this toilet and bathe as necessary (Figure 17-2).

Solving this problem meant restoring a sense of dignity to Saraswathie as well as enabling her daughter to continue her education. We ended up doing so by making a commode and bringing it to the shelter – a tip we had learned from Paravati.

Paravati was another woman with a mobility impairment living at a camp who had (entirely of her own accord) managed to rig up a makeshift washing place and commode next to her own shelter by enclosing a small rectangular space with plastic and woven fronds for privacy. Inside the washing place she placed her home-fashioned commode chair with a bucket underneath as well as a large bucket of water nearby (someone else filled that up for her) with a piece of rubber hosing attached to it. Inside this enclosure she was able to use a toilet and bathe (Figure 17-3).

INSPIRING SOLUTIONS AND RAISING CONCERNS

As we continued to work around the country in the aftermath of the tsunami, these two encounters continued to resonate with me because they illuminated the social dimension of disability and reinforced the intimate connection between space and personal dignity. I listened repeatedly to difficulties like Saraswathie's and her daughter's and endeavoured to help. Paravati's example of innovation was a constant reminder that professionals did not hold all the answers but could inspire solutions by connecting people and sharing their stories as examples and catalysts for change.

However, the stories of Saraswathie and Paravati raised further concerns about people with disabilities in response and resettlement contexts. First, what happens in the absence of an interested nongovernmental organization or government official who actively seeks out people with disabilities after disasters? What if there is no social worker to make contact? Unfortunately, this scenario is common. In my experience, many organizations appear to believe that there are no people with disabilities within the population they serve. To them, people like Saraswathie and Paravati did not even exist; they were unable to survive the disaster. This misperception made it very difficult for people with disabilities to gain access to available services, information, and facilities; when they did, it was often random.

Second, physical access barriers confined many people with disabilities to their homes, while inside their homes many relied on family members for care.

This, in turn, placed increased demands on that family member. The link between disability and poverty has clearly been established elsewhere and in Sri Lanka this was no different; for most families, extra time spent caring for a person with a disability is time taken away from wage earning, education or other duties.

Third, many NGOs were unsure of what specific assistance they could provide to people with disabilities and there was a general lack of knowledge about how to coordinate, address or meet the needs of people with disabilities in the relief and reconstruction efforts around the country.

The rest of this chapter explores these issues in greater depth through my experience with an accessibility initiative 'Access for All' – the project that brought me to Sri Lanka in the first place.

ABOUT 'ACCESS FOR ALL'

The 2004 tsunami left more than 31 000 people dead, 4000 missing, and half a million displaced in Sri Lanka (Nishikiori et al 2006). The disaster mobilized many into action, including a group of local disabled persons' organizations (DPOs), the Ministry of Health, and international (disability) nongovernmental organizations (INGOs) already in the country who formed the 'Access For All' consortium (AFA). The name of the initiative was intended to capture the basic idea of the group – to promote access for all people to both the process and outcome of relief and reconstruction efforts in order to rebuild a more accessible Sri Lanka. The two main components of the campaign were: (1) advocacy, and (2) technical advice/training/capacity building.

The theme of 'access for all' is one that disability advocates and organizations have, in their own ways, been promoting around the world for some time (Kose 2006, UNESCAP 2002). The aim of the concept is to make life easier for everyone by making products, means of communication and building environments that are more usable for more people at little or no extra cost. This means that our physical surroundings, products and services are planned and designed so that everyone can participate regardless of age and physical ability with equal opportunities to participate in modern society. In Sri Lanka local DPOs had been trying, with varying degrees of success, to promote this

message although the AFA project brought many of them together for the first time in order to do so.

The assembly of previously separate groups was itself a positive consequence of AFA as it was the coordinated efforts of DPOs through the AFA project that was a major contributing factor in bringing mandatory regulations to improve access to public buildings a year after the disaster (before the tsunami, these were 'voluntary' rather than mandatory). The idea behind AFA was that access brings opportunity; if people are prevented from or otherwise unable to access something – a service, an event, a building, for instance – then they cannot participate in decisions, activities or roles that may affect or add value to their lives, and may miss out on further opportunities. As such, the right of access was considered a basic human right.

Indeed, access or accessibility is now included in the recently ratified United Nations Convention on the Rights of Persons with Disabilities (CRPD) (United Nations 2007), the most innovative element of which, according to some authors, is Article 9, which outlines the principle of accessibility (Arnardóttir & Quinn 2009). It is this article that gives life to the principle of substantive equality. The Australian Agency for International Development (AusAID) (2008) states that taking 'measures to provide access on an equal basis with others to the physical environment … is an overarching right aimed at guaranteeing equality of access for people with disability to all facilities and services within the community' (p. 18). It benefits people at all stages of life and has other benefits such as reducing accidents.

ACCESSIBILITY AND OCCUPATIONAL THERAPY

The concept of access is also central to the work of occupational therapists who have been concerned with how valued occupations are performed and how alterations of environments might resolve them for some time (Bridge 2010). This is because it is the interaction between individuals and their environmental settings that enables the development, practice and fulfilment of personally valued activities (Schkade & McClung 2001). Thus, in terms of access, occupational therapists are concerned with the process of engagement or the act of involving oneself (participation in occupation), as well as enabling the physical artefacts (buildings, policies, equipment and the like). For occupational therapists, enabling access is not an end itself but a means to enable occupation.

This idea is highlighted nicely in our work in trying to improve physical accessibility of damaged schools after the tsunami. The destruction of these schools led to an opportunity to improve facilities for all, including those with disabilities. It meant the opportunity to build spaces that would enable students, teachers or parents with disabilities to move around and use the school's facilities. AFA worked with several NGOs building schools to ensure the facilities were physically accessible. This, we considered, was important work for it is difficult to convince people to renovate existing buildings, whereas it is relatively easy to design for accessibility when there is a 'clean slate'.

However, having a building provided in which to be educated is not the same as receiving an education. And while access to buildings was provided in many schools, until disabled students were studying in seats and playing in the playgrounds, or disabled teachers or parents were teaching in classrooms or meeting in staffrooms, there was no participation and (physical) access would not result in the desired outcome. At the time AFA did not have the time, resources or influence to address the other access barriers to education (e.g. supportive attitudes, resources, policies), and now that many schools are accessible it is important that such work takes place because even if appropriate staff, policies and resources exist, the mere fact that they exist – like the building exists – is not enough as it does not guarantee participation; the most meaningful outcome will always be the disabled person engaged in their chosen occupation of student, parent or teacher.

LESSONS LEARNT

That an advocacy arm was present in the AFA project is telling: a lot of work had to be done to convince organizations that access for people with disabilities was something that should be included as part of their routine work and carried with it benefits to all. Our idea was to conduct campaigning and promotional work to alert organizations to the need for accessibility with the expectation that they would then either start ensuring access themselves or request our assistance if

they needed it. In retrospect we were a little optimistic and underestimated how much advocacy work was required.

Early on we discovered that many organizations had not considered disabled people as part of their programme of development/relief delivery. In this regard, our team was fortunate to have a charismatic, eloquent and vivacious woman with a disability who – a lawyer by profession – made a wonderful advocate. She spent a great deal of time presenting at coordination meetings, trying to get appointments with key people in various organizations and agencies, and perhaps single-handedly changed perceptions of disabled people among many of the people she met. To us it seemed as though many people needed to meet a disabled person and see how the benefits of access to education, in particular, could impact on a disabled person's life.

While our advocate was promoting both a rights-based approach (as outlined in the UN charter), and the common good approach ('this will help everybody'), common reactions from programme workers included: (1) 'we should try to help unfortunate disabled people'; (2) 'but only two per cent of people are disabled'; and, less commonly (3) 'great, tell me how'.

The first reaction highlights the difficulty we had in breaking the charity mindset associated with disability work. The problem with charity is that it treats people as 'helpless victims' and involves waiting for people who have the time, inclination and commitment to your particular cause. While we readily acted when organizations expressed charitable intentions, it meant we relied on any time and money they had left over – of which there was not a lot. In many cases our work was seen as an optional extra.

The second reaction highlights the difficulty we had in breaking a minority mindset associated with disability work – that it does not help many people and, therefore, programmes seen to be for disabled people were not worth investing in. The idea that only 2% of people in Sri Lanka had disabilities may have come from the Sri Lankan Government census of 2002, which, for the first time, included a disability schedule and arrived at the 2% conclusion (Department of Census and Statistics – Sri Lanka 2001). However, to DPOs and by international standards this figure seems unrealistic. For instance, WHO (2008) suggests that on average, 19% of less educated people have disabilities. Disabled people themselves offer one explanation for the low official figure, with one wheelchair user who answered the door on census day pointing out: 'Even though I was in a wheelchair and had an obvious disability, the census collectors did not ask me the disability questions and I had to remind them to.'

Yet another source of the 2% mindset could be the relative invisibility of disabled people in Sri Lanka at the time. Disability in Sri Lanka is defined in the Protection of the Rights of Persons with Disabilities Act (Parliament of the Democratic Socialist Republic of Sri Lanka 1996). Under the Act, disability is defined as a condition experienced as a result of any deficiency in physical or mental capacities leading a person to be unable to ensure the necessities of life. While this definition is a reasonably broad one, encompassing both medical and socioeconomic aspects of disability, it differs from that of the World Health Organization (WHO), which views disability from a functional performance frame and considers impairments, activity limitations and participation restrictions (2008). The Sri Lankan definition, as enacted in legislation, appears to restrict concern to those requiring government assistance. One might argue that this, itself, might lead to underreporting and poor visibility of disabled persons prior to the tsunami disaster. Further, within the Sri Lankan culture there are superstitions associating persons with disability with misfortune and therefore perceiving them as harbingers or omens of bad luck (Fernando 2003). In this context, a disabled person may be perceived as someone to be supported throughout life, a burden to his or her family and community. Many disabled people, especially those who have lost their limbs in the recent civil conflict, are therefore also ashamed and depressed, as well as being impoverished (Grobar & Gnanaselvam 1993). So it is unsurprising that in nations like Sri Lanka, people with disabilities are often invisible and are not part of the decision-making that will ultimately affect their lives. Subsequently there may be a mismatch between a community that is trying to create an accessible environment and the needs of the individual trying to function in that community (Whybrow et al 2010).

This minority-thus-insignificant attitude was especially interesting to us as it came not only from local organizations (who may only have had access to the census figure) but also from INGOs who, for the most part, if working in their home countries would have been compelled by legislation and Discrimination Acts at least to address physical access concerns when building permanent structures (although probably not compelled to ensure access to information and other relief services). While we were able to demonstrate the 'common good' aspect of access to some extent, when such attitudes prevailed it was difficult to change them in a short space of time. From this perspective, an emergency/relief operation is perhaps not the best time to start an advocacy campaign if it is attitude change that is required.

In this regard, it is also important to note that the tsunami event created a new set of issues in Sri Lanka with hundreds of new agencies arriving in the country and existing agencies experiencing growth resulting from a surge of donations and aid. This situation 'resulted in challenges in coordination among the central government, the districts, and realities in the field' (Yamada et al 2006). Agencies were grappling with many new issues and it seemed a struggle for them to take on board our message.

The third reaction – 'tell me how' – though less common, was a relief to us all and we found that people who accepted the notion of 'Access for All' were the ones we mainly ended up working with. They tended to be DPOs or international organizations with an interest in health and/or disability, charities like Rotary, or those who had a worker with a personal interest in disability, like the social worker mentioned previously.

What all this meant was that access tended to be random, and, for the most part, aid organizations would report there were no disabled people among their target population when we started asking. Yet we knew this to be unrealistic in light of the country situation (Sri Lanka was still in the midst of a three-decade-long civil war at the time, although it has now ended). So why were there 'no disabled people'? One of the main problems, from our perspective, was that while most organizations may have collected a great deal of information from the people they were working with (commonly known as beneficiaries), almost none seemed to be collecting any specific information that might be relevant to disabled people, including whether or not there were people with disabilities in the families of the 'beneficiaries'. This had significant consequences since such information is used for planning purposes. It meant, for example, that some disabled people ended up leaving welfare camps because their needs were not identified or met (particularly in terms of physical accessibility, as an online discussion moderated by the World Bank on disaster and people with disabilities in 2006 found). Thus, due to environmental barriers it may, indeed, have been true that there were fewer disabled people (although unlikely that there were none).

One story told to us by the DPOs we worked with recounted the situation of Mr Chandrasekeram, a wheelchair user. Apparently Mr Chandrasekeram tried to stay at one of the temporary shelters but could find no dignified or appropriate way to use a toilet (the latrines did not accommodate him) or get around the camp so was confined to his shelter. No-one came to ask if he needed assistance or what type of assistance he needed. He quickly left for the interior of the country to stay with family. The knock-on effects of not being present in the shelters were that people who were there initially may have dropped off an NGO's list of beneficiaries and been unable to access other support services (e.g. permanent shelters and livelihood assistance).

This lack of data collection resulted in the exclusion of many disabled people from the relief process and seemed to reflect either the absence of any policy considering the needs of people with disabilities among most organizations or a lack of knowledge on how to implement them meaningfully if they did exist. This typically meant that disabled people, along with any needs of disabled people, either did not exist or were not adequately addressed. However, even if you count disabled people – as some organizations did – this does not mean their needs are addressed. Mrs Darmalingam's story highlights this.

Mrs Darmalingam was a widowed mother of three young children. She was provided with livelihood assistance and was helped to set up a small shop. The problem was that her role as breadwinner was the only one considered in the initial needs assessment; her role as sole carer for her three severely disabled children was not. While the intention of the relief organization had been to ensure that Mrs Darmalingam could earn a living – a critical need – she had an equally critical need

to be able to be a mother to her children. The problem was that the shop environment made it very difficult for her to manage both roles. Basically, she had to leave her children lying on the floor out back all day (they had no assistive devices) where she could not see them while she had to tend to the shop counter. The needs of the children were also initially missed, although the organization later referred them to a specialist disability NGO who provided additional assistance.

This failure to either include disabled people in initial assessments or adequately assess needs had yet other consequences and was observed particularly in our work in trying to influence permanent construction. By the time we contacted organizations (or by the time a request for assistance came) many organizations had already submitted, and had approved, budgets and design plans for buildings. Since the needs of people with disabilities were not on any agenda the schools or hospitals or buildings or houses they were funding likewise failed to consider them. Through this we learned the importance of the relationship between disaster and development. Trying to advocate for inclusion and accessibility in relief and early recovery contexts presented many barriers. What was needed was a longer-term focus at the centre of which lies relationship building and capacity development. We continue to work toward this aim, promoting accessibility including universal design (Goldsmith 2004) and building resilience to future disasters. Working in partnership with individuals with disabilities and DPOs and learning from their experiences is fundamental to this work.

CONCLUSION

Overall, the AFA team found that access was largely random – an afterthought or optional extra. We found it difficult to influence attitudes in the midst of a major relief operation, understandably given the massive scale of the destruction and volume of work to be undertaken. In emergency/relief operations time is scarce and chaos often prevails; asking organizations to do something unfamiliar at such times is difficult. Our experience, on the whole, was not that organizations maliciously or deliberately excluded disabled people; they simply forgot or mistakenly believed there were none.

The organizations and people we ended up working closely with were generally those who had a prior interest or were otherwise 'sympathetic' to our work. Typically we found they lacked knowledge associated with assessing needs of people with disabilities and in implementing solutions to address them and came to us for advice and training. While our work did not end up being as comprehensive or as widespread as we would have liked, through these partnerships some great work was done, including the construction of an inclusive village, accessible schools, hospitals and shelters, training of lay people and professionals, and the development of culturally appropriate access guidelines (Whybrow 2006a, 2006b).

Nowadays relief organizations routinely consider the particular needs of women and children before they even enter a disaster zone and come prepared. It is our hope that the needs of people with disabilities will also soon be an a priority consideration and not simply an afterthought.

POSTSCRIPT, MAY 2014

Yesterday I (SW) was driving around Colombo with an architect on the way to a garment factory. It was the first time we had met and I mentioned I used to work on accessibility at the tsunami time. He then relayed a story about his recent experience. It is mandatory that new public buildings be made accessible in Sri Lanka. He was the lead architect on the construction of a two-storey government building in a rural part of Sri Lanka that would provide general services/information to the public. The project was being funded by the Asian Development Bank. The architect came up with a design but the ADB rejected it and told him they would not fund a building if it did not have a lift because they needed to adhere to disability regulations. The architect informed them that such a solution was not practical in a rural area and even if they were willing to fund the lift the local government would need to pay for the ongoing maintenance and, also, that the rural people were not used to using lifts. The ADB persisted so the architect spoke to the local councillors and they came up with their own solution, which was to ensure that the ground floor was accessible and there was an accessible service counter on the ground floor that a government official could come

down to if a person was not able to access the second floor by steps. After a lot of to-ing and fro-ing this solution was eventually agreed upon. I congratulated the architect on his common sense solution, and it was both interesting and disappointing to see an example of an international development organization rigidly adhering to standards and regulations that are not appropriate for the context. This occurred a lot during the tsunami time – for some reason the big development agencies were focused on installing lifts even though the cost of installation and maintenance was, and continues to be, a barrier. Although such options were never suggested, it was and sadly still seems to be their conception of disability access.

REFERENCES

Arnardóttir, O., Quinn, G., 2009. The UN Convention on the Rights of Persons with Disabilities: European and Scandinavian perspectives. Martinus Nijhoff Publishers, Leiden.

Australian Agency for International Development (AusAID), 2008. Development for All: Towards a Disability-Inclusive Australian Aid Program 2009–2014 (November), Canberra. Retrieved from: <www.ausaid.gov.au/publications>.

Batavia, A., Schriner, K., 2001. The Americans with Disabilities Act as engine of social change: models of disability and the potential of a civil rights approach. Policy Stud. J. 29 (4), 690–702.

Bridge, C., 2008. Bringing rich dividends: enabling house environments. In: IDIRYA (Ed.), Access Ability for All: Why you?, Colombo.

Bridge, C., 2010. Home adaptations and modifications. In: Curtin, M., Molineux, M., Supyk, J. (Eds.), Occupational Therapy and Physical Dysfunction – Enabling Occupation, sixth ed. Elsevier Health Sciences, London, pp. 409–429 (Chapter 28).

Department of Census and Statistics – Sri Lanka, 2001. People with Disabilities 2001 Census of Population and Housing by District and Sex. Retrieved from: <http://www.statistics.gov.lk/PopHouSat/Des_Chra.asp>.

Diamond, H., Precin, P., 2004. Disabled and experiencing disaster. Occup. Ther. Ment. Health 19 (3), 27–41.

Fernando, W.B., 2003. National Paper – Sri Lanka. Presented at the UN ESCAP/CDPF Regional Meeting on an International Convention on Disability (4–7 November) Beijing, China, Retrieved from:<http://www.ihp.lk/publications/docs/projreports/ssi_main_report_final.pdf>.

Goldsmith, S., 2004. Universal Design: A Manual of Practical Guidance for Architects. Architectural Press, Oxford.

Grobar, L.M., Gnanaselvam, S., 1993. The economic effects of the Sri Lankan civil war. Econ. Dev. Cult. Change 41 (2), 395–405.

IDIRYA, 2008. Access Ability for All: Why You? IDIRYA, Colombo.

Ingstad, B., Whyte, S.R., 1995. Disability and Culture. University of California Press, Berkeley, CA.

Kose, S., 2006. Universal design for the aging. In: Karwowski, W. (Ed.), International Encyclopedia of Ergonomics and Human Factors, second ed. Taylor & Francis, London, pp. 227–230.

Nishikiori, N., Abe, T., Costa, G.M., Dharmaratne, G., Kuni, O., Moji, K., 2006. Who died as a result of the tsunami? Risk factors of mortality among internally displaced persons in Sri Lanka: a retrospective cohort analysis. BMC Public Health 6 (73), Retrieved from: <http://www.biomedcentral.com/1471-2458/6/73>.

Parliament of the Democratic Socialist Republic of Sri Lanka, 1996. Protection of the Rights of Persons with Disabilities Act. (No 28 of 1996). Department of Government Printing, Sri Lanka.

Schkade, J., McClung, M., 2001. Occupational Adaptation in Practice: Concepts and Cases. Slack, Thorofare, NJ.

United Nations, 2007. Convention on the Rights of Persons with Disabilities: The United Nations Programme on Disabilities.

United Nations Economic and Social Commission for Asia and the Pacific (UNESCAP), 2002. Biwako millennium framework for action towards an inclusive, barrier-free and rights-based society for persons with disabilities in Asia and the Pacific. United Nations. General E/ESCAP/APDDP/4/Rev.1, 8 November 2002.

Ursano, R., Fullerton, C., Norwood, A., 1995. Psychiatric dimensions of disaster: patient care, community consultation, and preventive medicine. Harv. Rev. Psychiatry 3, 196–209.

Whybrow, S., 2006a. Design Considerations for Accessibility. John Grooms Working with Disability, Sri Lanka.

Whybrow, S., 2006b. Improving Accessibility of Schools. John Grooms Working with Disability, Sri Lanka.

Whybrow, S., Rahim, A., Sharma, V., Gupta, S., Millikan, L., Bridge, C., 2010. Legislation, anthropometry, and education – the Southeast Asian experience. In: Steinfeld, E. (Ed.), The State of the Science: Emerging Research and Developments in Universal Design. Bentham Science Publishers Ltd, Oak Park, IL.

World Health Organization, 2008. Disabilities. From: <http://www.who.int/topics/disabilities/en/> (Retrieved 3 June 2009).

Yamada, S., Gunatilake, R.P., Roytman, T.M., Gunatilake, S., Fernando, T., Fernando, L., 2006. The Sri Lanka tsunami experience. Disaster Manag. Response 4 (2), 38–48.

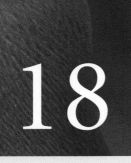

18

COMMUNITY-BASED REHABILITATION IN COLOMBIA'S ARMED CONFLICT

SOLÁNGEL GARCÍA-RUÍZ

A violent history leaving physical, emotional and cultural wounds and grieving survivors transforming despair into hope, through evolving strategies. CBR recalls its importance.

Colombia is located in northern South America. It is a country of great contrasts, ranging from the blue sea to the green mountains, including the yellow and orange colours of the tropical fruits and flowers (Figure 18-1). Colombia's cornucopia includes also the coal production of the department of La Guajira, the oil of the Llanos, the coffee of the so-called 'Zona Cafetera' region, the water of the Amazon and big river jungle areas as well as the two oceans bordering our country, the salt of Manaure, the emeralds of Boyacá department, and much more.

There are many questions about us, Colombians. What are we like? Who are we? Forty-three million people make up the country. Today's Colombians are a mix of different ethnic backgrounds: Afro-Colombian, indigenous, mulato or mestizo mixtures, and white races. We were conquered by Spaniards more than 500 years ago, and colonized by many other cultures.

OUR VIOLENT HISTORY

Armed conflict in Colombia is as old as the history of the country, and it is important to understand this through people's stories. I, for example, am a Colombian citizen who can talk about this conflict not as someone who suffers it directly in the context of

everyday life, but through the stories of others. My interpretation of the conflict is also influenced by the media's representation and by my personal history. In a broad context, the conflict is about longstanding competing interests over Colombia's natural resources. Colombia is a country that is rich in natural resources, but has many poor people. This means the wealth of the country is in the earth, but most of us who inhabit it do not benefit from this richness. The reality for Colombians is that we do not have access to good health care or social services, generally speaking, and have a low level of education. We could say this reality reflects global processes of change and a global market economy. Some foreigners have been interested in the wealth of our natural resources, but we Colombians have not been aware of the value of our resources and the interests some people weave around them.

There are several key events marking the conflict in Colombia that has spanned the past 40 years. In 1962, the Frente Nacional (an agreement by the Conservative and Liberal parties that they would take turns to govern) led to the formation of some guerrilla groups opposing this restrictive regime. There are today zones in the country controlled by guerrillas, and others controlled by paramilitary groups (opposed to the guerrillas) (Molano 2008). The country is comprised of 1 171 498 square km. The current Colombian conflict is related to land tenure, to institutional weaknesses, mainly in rural areas, and to the ineffectiveness of land reforms (CIREC Foundation 2009). As a result, armed groups have spread to areas with large economic resources or geographical advantages, and peasants

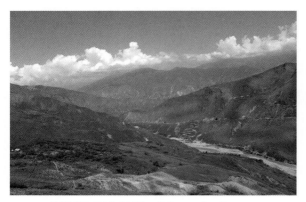

FIGURE 18-1 ▨ The Chicamocha Canyon.

have been displaced and pauperized. The decision to attack and the intensity of violence are determined by economic benefits, political power and institutional conditions (Velásquez Guijo 2008). The armed conflict stemming from these issues has caused enormous and irreparable damage to a significant part of Colombia's population.

One of the strategies in this conflict has been the planting of landmines. There are over 100 000 antipersonnel mines (APM) and unexploded ordnance (UXO) scattered across 40% of the country (Colombian National Planning Department 2009), affecting 31 of the total of 32 departments (Presidential Program for Mine Action 2009) that constitute Colombian territory. According to information published in October 2009, there have been 8081 victims of antipersonnel mines, of whom 35% are civilians; over a third of these are children. On average, three people a day become victims of landmines (CIREC Foundation 2009) – whether it is due to the explosion or by coming into contact with unexploded ordnance. It is important to understand the perversity of these weapons in that they are used to incapacitate and injure people (Lozano 2005), not to kill them. There are currently 30 553 people who are disabled or displaced (Presidential Agency for Social Action and International Cooperation 2009) by these devices.

WOUNDS, GRIEVING ...

Lesions produced by APM/UXO are classified according to the type of injury sustained by the body (upper limbs or lower face, eyes, etc.) and to the type of mine (fragmentation or explosion) used. Government organizations have defined processes for dealing with the victims of mines, including emergency care, extended care, rehabilitation help and social reintegration. I must also mention some humanitarian aid linked to education, housing and financial support.

In Colombia, most rehabilitation centres are located in major cities such as Bogotá, Cali, Barranquilla, Medellín and Bucaramanga. In order to meet the specific health care needs of the victims of landmines, the centres rely on international resources that fund projects that, in turn, promote and create specific programmes. Many of these programmes are community-based proposals looking to meet the needs of individuals and families who are direct and indirect victims of APM/UXO.

There are many stories of the Colombian conflict that could be told and have been told by journalists, anthropologists and politicians with their own interests or from their own perspectives. The stories help to understand and, perhaps, even help to resolve the conflict. All Colombians have their own stories concerning the conflict; some refer to personal experiences or those of family, friends or colleagues. What is clear is that all Colombians live with the conflict and we all experience it differently. In large cities it is easier to isolate yourself and distance yourself from stories that affect you in one way or another. I have taken a path of isolation many times, and I find I have done it because it has given me peace for a while. However, for many people this healthy temporary isolation is not possible and the conflict stays a part of their everyday life.

My mother had to leave her hometown, Caparrapí (Figure 18-2), in the department of Cundinamarca, when she was young. This was probably in the 1930s or 40s, and I do not know much about the details because it was not something she wanted to talk about. Her displacement was not spoken about at home. Those silences contributed to our version of the conflict. In the 1950s, some stories referred to my father hiding at night in the bushes because of his 'liberal' thinking, and because he feared the 'conservatives' would come for him (to make him 'disappear' or to kill him). I heard this from my grandparents and seldom from my parents. It seemed they lived full of fear and

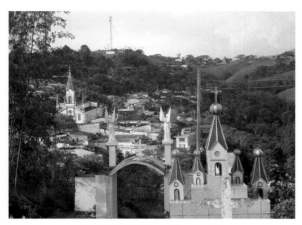

FIGURE 18-2 ■ Caparrapí.

dread, and today we have an understanding of why it was better not to speak of such things.

At home, and at work, I keep hearing stories about the conflict that make it a shadow on my everyday life. I have experienced at first hand the kidnappings of my colleagues' family members and the displacement of women who have come to my home to help me with domestic work. In all cases I have felt fear and an inability to find a solution, and I have shed tears with these victims.

STAYING OR LEAVING, THE HESITATION ...

In the 1990s and the 2000s, many Colombians of my generation left the country to find an alternative life and, perhaps, to work or educate themselves abroad to contribute to a better quality of life for our country. I have dreamt of their return one day so that we can work together; I have dreamt of them coming back to share their knowledge and experiences from other parts of the world that could contribute to the development and transformation of our country. The truth is that many of them have stayed away as I write this, and I do not feel they will be able to return. I ask myself also, what I can do for the best, to stay or leave, to get strength to manage and actively help with this national conflict.

I will continue this article, though, by relying on the story of two brave people who changed the course of their own and their families' lives. They both were

victims of landmines, and from them we can identify some lessons to contribute to Colombia's social and community development.

The stories are recorded in two projects developed in Colombia, one under the programme 'Seeds of Hope' of the CIREC Foundation, and the second within the framework of the programmes of the United Nations High Commissioner for Refugees (UNHCR).

It was Friday, March 9th, 2001. I was at home with my mum, my brother, my sister and my two cousins. My brother and cousins went to look for blackberries, and found a device that was unknown to us. When my brother returned home, he sat behind the bed, but my cousin, who was walking behind him, dropped the grenade; as he entered the house, it exploded. The impact was so strong that it propelled us all out of the house to the front yard. My cousin said to my mum, "Look at my feet Doña Martha". At that moment, I looked at my own feet and saw that my right foot was destroyed, and I noticed that all my relatives were in a bad situation. We all started to shout for help, until the other people from the town came to help us. We had to wait a few hours for the ambulance to arrive, because we were in the countryside and the nearest hospital was 2 hours away. When we reached the hospital, the pain got worse, they gave me strong medication that put me to sleep, and when I woke up I no longer had my right foot.

From **CIREC's Seeds of Hope**

In 2007, I was at the farm with my family: my wife and four children. I had some animals, crops and fruit trees. We lived off the land, and were very happy. My children went to school, I did farm work. In February, armed groups entered and planted antipersonnel mines. Unfortunately I stepped on a mine sometime afterwards, and we had to leave urgently. I lost my leg; they took me out on a stretcher; at the time, I couldn't feel anything. When I arrived to the hospital, they treated me urgently and sent me to Medellín.

From **Disability Programme of the UNHCR Reports**

Both of these incidents occurred during the 2000s, a time when accidents with landmines became prevalent throughout the country. In this war, as with all other wars, the victims and those that suffer the consequences are those that have the least to do with the interests of those that lead the conflict. They are mostly common people, citizens, whose main problem is to have found themselves in the wrong place at a given moment. It seems plausible to think that the main objective is to make them leave their lands. This way of life must change.

We survived with the help of the people in the town where we lived. The ambulance drivers told the army to let us pass, and explained that we were part of the civilian population and that we were just kids.

This situation is complex, because it is not just about the accident and what happens to a victim's body; it also affects all areas of their current life, as well as having repercussions for the future.

We survive with the help of public charity. In the municipality, they have found accommodation for us, but I can't work in the way I used to. My wife works as a domestic maid in other people's houses. With the little money she earns, we can afford to buy the necessary items for the children. They go to school, but they are teased and feel isolated, other children, ignorantly and mercilessly, call them displaced, and make fun of their clothes.

It is important to highlight the injuries that are caused to the victims' bodies by these accidents. They generally require special treatment, which is very costly for people, families and the health system. Victims sometimes suffer amputations or prolonged periods of physical rehabilitation. However, the biggest impact affects the emotions and the soul, economic production and social contact. Psychosocial support is an urgent need both for the victim and the family.

They only treated my leg, but the explosion of the mine also affected my ear and I am slightly deaf. The shrapnel got into my eyes and other internal organs, but none of that was treated.

It is common for institutions to focus on central services such as health services, rehabilitation treatment and the needs of victims with regards to grief, their feelings and fears, and all the support required at this stage. Nevertheless, the victim not only needs to receive counselling and care, but needs to be able to talk to others and to have the necessary time for anger and grief, to try to discover, understand, accept and recognize themselves in their new situation. Most often the victims are taken to the big cities to be treated, where they encounter a different world and eventually can feel completely out of place, unable to understand their current context and with limited chances to discuss their issues.

The first assistance is key to this process: 'The first treatment I received in Popayán, Cauca did not help me. They gave me a prosthetic limb which didn't have the technological features needed. At that time, I could not bend my knee. My current prosthetic limb fits my requirements: now I can even wear high heels.'

This support should be tailored to the needs of people, not to the potential supply of the institutions. It is imperative to say that this institutional lack of care does not only affect the victims of the conflict; in general, it reflects one of the main weaknesses of the Colombian health system.

… there, they gave me a prosthetic limb, but I had to learn how to use it on my own. My family nor I did fully understand what was happening. They left us alone. They took us to our accommodation, and from then on we relied on close relatives. Our relatives were scared that the armed group would seek us out, and possibly attack their family too. So, we had to find an alternative accommodation.

DESPAIR

Fear is what makes us so vulnerable, and it is what all Colombians have felt. The fear of going out, the fear of being kidnapped on the road … that kind of despair lived by everyone in the 1990s. It was in this decade that displacement began because people moved in search of security, looking for a secure place to settle down. In many cases, families became part of communities living in extreme poverty. These new inhabitants added to the so-called 'belts of misery' of the large cities.

My family does not want to return to the farm, but I would like to know what happened to the animals, the crops and our home. I am scared, though, to return because there are groups that operate outside the boundaries of the law, and we would not be very safe there. I know that one day we will return, but I fear for my wife and children. What if they were to one day step on a mine?

This situation affects the individual in a direct and indirect way. It affects whole families and communities where the conflict occurs.

Besides the collective fear, there is individual fear because of the situations experienced: 'My biggest fear was I would never walk again, and my biggest problem was to learn to accept myself. To accept the state I was in. I was so young, only 10 years old, and had lost my leg.'

Recognition of the psychological impact is critical, as well as the provision of immediate and long-term psychosocial support.

The State gave us some food only. We have not received any kind of support. Children live in fear, and have become very quiet. They do not like being here.

Of course, it is not just about getting 'things', it is also about the ongoing support that has to be provided for victims to survive in dignity and respect for themselves and others, in spite of what they are suffering.

COMMUNITY-BASED REHABILITATION

In this context, assistance, provision and support are crucial. Different circles of interaction have to work together for victims and their situation. This is where community-based rehabilitation processes become important. Consolidated action means much more than a timely response; it also entails long-term support in the rebuilding of a victim's life. This begins by addressing the immediate needs of the person. An important part of the rehabilitation process can be centred initially on the recuperation of some bodily

function, but essentially implies long-term aid for the individual, the relatives and the caregivers.

I was able to get on with my life, in Bogotá, where there was a Foundation for the rehabilitation of people with disabilities, and they helped me to learn to walk again.

Community-based processes become an opportunity to find people in the remotest corners of the country. There are many programmes throughout the country, funded by international organizations.

What helped us most was the support from my parents and the whole family. CIREC and their rehabilitation programs helped us to recover both physically and emotionally. My brother and I lost our legs in that terrible accident. We are young people, and today, we have our lives ahead of us. My brother is studying Medicine, his 5th semester, and I am in my 3rd semester of Psychology. I had an unforgettable experience with the Seeds of Hope program. It had a profound effect on my self, and produced wonderful changes in my life. I had never had the chance to interact in that way with my father. We were able to talk to each other and spend time together, and we now plan on being close the most of the time. (Barú Island, Cartagena, Bolívar department).

The Seeds of Hope programme of CIREC is supported by the strategy of community-based rehabilitation led by people who have disabilities and victims of armed conflict, who are trained as leaders. The programme leads to the consolidation of the social group that can advocate for the rights of victims of landmines. They keep records, organize local health brigades specializing in rehabilitation and form support groups where the experience of the disabled person becomes the main support for others in the same situation. The leaders form groups sharing common goals to improve living conditions and to promote access to services by people who have disabilities and need to access these services. This programme operates throughout the country (Centro Integración de Rehabilitación de Colombia, CIREC 2009).

The Colombian Constitutional Court recognizes the rise in the numbers of people who have become disabled directly as a result of the armed conflict. It recognizes the neglect that has occurred due to the individual's loss of personal independence, both before and during displacement, and the inability of some people with disabilities to flee an area if their life is in danger or if their personal integrity is at risk due to the armed conflict. The law recognizes victims of extrajudicial killings to be present, as casualties of the illegal armed groups. Their risks are magnified because of the destructive effects of forced displacement, where families' structures are put at grave risk due to the loss of social networks (Colombian Constitutional Court 2009). Victims of landmines who become disabled often become displaced because they fear returning to their homes. Displacement and disability make them doubly vulnerable.

From a systemic viewpoint, a crisis is a process that is required to experience change and to learn. It is a natural process, and it is necessary for a person's growth and development. When this point of view involves an entire country, with over 40 million people, I ask myself, what is it we Colombians have learned? What process of evolution must we experience? When will armed conflict end? Maybe then we will be able to say what we have learnt.

A reflection has to do with the differentiation of the interests that maintain or could end the conflict. As in all conflicts for power, the balance moves between individual and collective interests, between economic and social interests.

I am constantly surprised by the resilience we Colombians have. Despite the fear and pain we face, our people rebirth and recover and find ways to rebuild ourselves in time. We all reweave community and social threads. We all suffer despair, whether we are health professionals, politicians or victims. And we find strength to heal and move forward.

BUILDING HOPE

It may sound ironic, but for some people their land-mine accident has become an opportunity to strengthen personal skills. Many have become leaders who are capable of facing challenges, seeking solutions, setting goals and carrying them out. They are empowered and committed people who have rejoined their family and social life. They have also learned that organization is the way to promote and obtain results that benefit the entire population.

The process of community development, training and education of leaders is crucial. It is essential to allow for some personal growth and skills development, which contribute to the political, economic and social development of each community or communities. The leaders are able to develop better relationships at the social, group, family and community level. They obtain social recognition, as well as the consolidation of the main networks run by the participants of the programme (CIREC Foundation 2009).

Strategies such as 'Teaching lessons learned', which is based on the concept of 'Training the trainers', make a leader who has acquired all the tools and concepts to begin to lead and form another group, working at first not as a leader but as a trainer. This methodology contributes to the formation of leaders and their own development and it recognizes the family and the social network in both cases (CIREC Foundation 2009).

The processes of community development in Latin America, particularly in Colombia, are influenced by popular education proposals that encourage dialogue, debate and analysis through participatory methodologies to acquire and understand new knowledge (Freire 2007). Participation seeks to establish relationships between people based on justice, equity, solidarity and respect (Jara 2010); it entails using interactive education as a way of transforming social processes.

It is clear that the process of community-based rehabilitation that started in the 1980s and centred on the individual and his or her rehabilitation has transformed into processes that have at their core social development and collective action. This has been the case throughout Latin America and Colombia.

The opportunity to get together, associate and unite, where people share similar interests, needs and motivations, shifts the point of change from the individual to the collective. The change helps people relate to each other and overcome pain in a collective way. It contributes to the reconstruction and consolidation of community processes. In coming up with collective solutions that draw upon networks, policies and resources, change is more sustainable (Centro Integración de Rehabilitación de Colombia, CIREC 2009).

We are all citizens, regardless of how we appear. What really matters are the rights that protect us and our common humanity.

While it is necessary to identify and differentiate people with disabilities and their families, and the victims of armed conflict, their needs and problems, in general, we are the same. Disabled people have the same basic needs as people without disabilities. What I am trying to say is that sometimes the cause may be conflict, violence, accidents or illnesses. No matter what we have lived through, people have different abilities, different opportunities and different levels of autonomy in their daily lives. In terms of prevention and rehabilitation, the responsibility is enormous. It is important, as practitioners who aim to help, that we build areas and cities organized on difference and diversity.

Undoubtedly, attention to victims affected directly and indirectly by the armed conflict requires research that contributes to coming up with answers to the difficulties and problems from different perspectives. Perhaps this research can focus on the development and application of policies, the development of technologies in rehabilitation, and the development of more social and human communities.

A day is coming in which a community-based Colombia will turn out to be a place of opportunities for everyone, from one or other political perspective, with an equitable common use of natural resources, to prove that difference can make living an experience of brotherhood, respect and dignity. The only conflict would rest on agreement about the care of the land and the environment, confidentiality, and the protection and joy of integral health and evolution, as well as the joy of diversity and skills from any individual thinking collective. A day is coming where community-based rehabilitation will be a tool focused on prevention and mitigation of natural disasters.

Acknowledgements

To all the people who shared their stories.

To the Centre for Integrated Rehabilitation of Colombia, and its Seeds of Hope programme, who kindly shared information and inspiration to build this article.

To María del Carmen Botero, adviser to the Disability Programme of the UNHCR, for sharing valuable experiences and documentation.

To Kerry and Nancy, for their patience and hope in the construction of this chapter.

To Teresa Santos Rojas, for looking after intercultural accuracy in the way my ideas are written.

REFERENCES

CIREC Foundation [Colombian Integration Rehabilitation Centre] Life story. 2009. <http://www.cirec.org>.

Colombian Constitutional Court. Auto 006 2009. <http://corte-constitucional.vlex.com.co/vid/-56590397>.

Colombian National Planning Department. 2009. <http://www.dnp.gov.co/Paginas/inicio.aspx>.

Freire, P., 2007. cited by Kane, L. Community development: lessons from popular education in Latin America. Community Dev. J. 45 (3), 276–286. July, 2010.

Jara, O.H., 2010. Popular education and social change in Latin America. Community Dev. J. 45 (3), 287–296.

Lozano, María Paulina, 2005. Status of landmines in Colombia and their effects on people. In: García, S. (Ed.), Report of the Panel on Conflict and Disability at the Disability Research Colloquium. Rosario University, Bogotá.

Molano, Alfredo, 2008. Conference 'Paths to Peace'. In: Challenges, obstacles and perspectives'. III World Social Forum on Migrations. Rivas Vacía, Madrid. Maloka Collective, Spain.

Presidential Agency for Social Action and International Cooperation. Social Action. June 30, 2009.

Presidential Program for Mine Action – PAICMA. 2009. <http://www.accioncontraminas.gov.co/Paginas/AICMA.aspx>.

Velásquez Guijo, Andrea P, 2008. Formality on property rights: A determinant of the military strategy of armed actors? Development and Society Magazine. Los Andes University, Bogotá, pp. 119–164.

19

LANDMINE ACTION AND ADVOCACY: FROM LOCAL TO GLOBAL

REBECCA JORDAN

ONE WRONG STEP

My right leg was blown off by a landmine when I was 28 years old, back home in Vietnam. I was clearing a field, getting it ready for planting. I did not think there was any danger. I heard the explosion, felt myself thrown backward onto the ground, and right away knew what had happened. The pain was terrible, but I never lost consciousness. When I dared to look down at my body, I saw that one foot was completely gone. A piece of bone stuck out just below my knee, with bits of flesh hanging onto it. There was not much blood. I remember that surprised me. People came to help me. They had heard the explosion. They dragged me out of the field, even though there could have been more landmines in the same field … They saved my life.

The rest of my story is long, and each chapter was painful in its own way: the trip to the hospital, the surgery, the bandages, seeing my stump for the first time, the reactions of my family and friends … Many times I wanted to die. I thought I would be better off dead than mutilated as I was. I felt useless.

My uncle got our family out of Vietnam. The trip was horrific, but that is another story. We ended up in a refugee camp in Thailand along with tens of thousands of other refugees from Vietnam, Cambodia, and Laos. The camps were crowded, noisy, dirty, and busy, too, with schools, hospitals, offices, and huge communal living quarters packed with people squeezed together like sardines. I

marked my living space with a piece of vinyl 3 feet wide and 5 feet long. The camps were built to give us temporary shelter, while we waited to be settled somewhere else, in so-called 'third countries' like America, Canada, Australia, and France. We were all there hoping for the same thing – better lives – but the rules for Vietnamese refugees were different. We were kept in a special camp within the camp. We saw thousands of other refugees arrive, be processed and leave, while we kept waiting. We waited years.

… and a new leg

Lots of foreigners worked in the camps, teaching, working in the hospital, asking questions, filling out forms. After about three years there, two American women came through our section and made a list of people with defective bodies. Of course I was on that list. They were nice ladies, and they offered to make a fake leg, a prosthesis, for me. I agreed immediately. I was so happy to be allowed to leave the Vietnamese section of the camp for a few hours a day. The ladies really put a lot of time and effort into making the leg. They were determined to do a good job. I worked on it too, tanning the leather, and shaping some of the wooden parts with hand tools [Figure 19-1]. The knee hinge was the most difficult part to make. Some other foreigners came to give the ladies advice and someone else sent us a rubber foot in the mail. It took six months to make the leg. When it was finished, it was heavy (and ugly, to be honest) and much harder to use than my crutch. But I tried to use it, to please them.

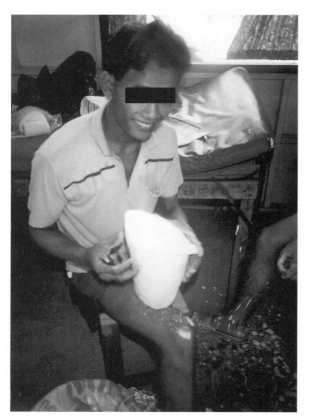

FIGURE 19-1 ■ Making a cast for my new leg.

Then, the authorities announced that all the Vietnamese people in the camp would be moved to a separate camp, with even less space and fewer services. This was supposed to convince us to go back to Vietnam, to give up on the hope of being resettled in a third country. We were told to pack our things. Each family had a weight limit. The leg the two women had made for me was a burden. My family knew I did not really use it, and they insisted I leave it behind. To be honest, they did not have to insist very much. The leg was not very useful for walking. It was just not worth its weight when it came time to move.

I hope those two ladies never found out that I left the leg behind … they would be disappointed. They had only good intentions. They were just 'off the mark' when it came to figuring out what would have been really useful to me.

WHAT'S WORTHWHILE: EARLY LESSONS

I was one of those 'two ladies' in the camp. Working with the American Refugee Committee (ARC), we ran a rehabilitation programme that targeted people with disabilities in camps for South-East Asian refugees. The story above illustrates some of what we did well: involving people in their own rehabilitation, using local materials, being creative and flexible, persevering in the face of great obstacles. But it also highlights one of the most important lessons I learned, that what a rehab professional thinks someone needs may or may not be very important or relevant or useful to that person. We did not harm the man in the story, thankfully. He did not have to pay for our services and he did benefit from being involved in the process of constructing his prosthesis. But we did not exactly help him realize his dreams. In fact, we did not even give him one jot more mobility than he already had. Maybe every therapist learns this lesson at some point, but I was only 9 months out of occupational therapy school and it was a shock to realize that even a seemingly basic therapeutic intervention – i.e. a prosthesis for an amputee – might not be literally or figuratively 'worth its weight'.

SIMPLICITY BEHIND FENCES

My colleague and I (she was a physical therapist and I am an occupational therapist) had a tremendous amount of responsibility and autonomy to manage ARC's rehabilitation programme in two refugee camps. We worked with people of all ages and all types of disabilities – amputees, children with cerebral palsy, muscular dystrophy, spina bifida, osteogenesis imperfecta, paralysis from polio, people with all kinds of sequelae from strokes, head injuries, gunshot wounds and more. We did everything – screens, assessments, direct treatment, follow-up recommendations for those leaving the camp. We trained refugees as 'rehab workers', taught sign language to deaf children, rounded up wheelchairs, had ramps built and convinced the authorities to allow extra space for those who needed it. We ran a classroom for children with mental retardation and developmental disabilities. We taught people with diabetes and Hansen's disease (leprosy) how to take care of their skin. We made adaptive equipment and therapeutic toys, wrote our own training curriculum and changed it as we needed to.

This sounds like a lot, and it was. We had the freedom to do so much, in part because the context was clear and simple: inside the fenced-in camp, we were the beginning and the end of rehabilitation services for those refugees. There were no competing organizations, no government officials looking over our shoulders, no messy political issues to limit what we did. Looking back, I am thankful that I had that kind of relative simplicity in my first position as an occupational therapist outside my own country. I gained some confidence and maturity in the camps that I would need in successive positions, where the context was anything but simple or clear.

REFUGEES BECOME RETURNEES

In 1991, some 350 000 refugees from the Thai–Cambodia border were repatriated to Cambodia under the auspices of the United Nations High Commissioner for Refugees (UNHCR). Refugees became 'returnees' (Figure 19-2) and those designated 'extremely vulnerable individuals' (EVIs) were flagged to be followed by specialist organizations. A French/Belgian organization called Handicap International (HI) was tasked with facilitating the repatriation and reinsertion of about 400 severely disabled returnees, 'severe' being defined as above-knee and double amputees, people with paraplegia and quadriplegia,

etc. I never would have applied for this job, would never have considered myself qualified, had I seen it listed somewhere. But … I was in the right place at the right time and had just enough chutzpah, sense of adventure and comfort with the unexpected to agree to take the position when it was offered. My first step was to hire a Cambodian counterpart. I wanted a co-manager, not just an assistant or an interpreter, and I wanted someone who had first-hand experience of the issues our target group would be facing. I asked HI to suggest candidates for the job and they sent me one, S.S. (Figure 19-3). Luckily, he proved to be perfect for it.

A NEW LIFE

My name is S.S. When I was a teenager, I was recruited to be a soldier. Sometimes we put

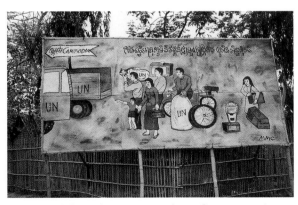

FIGURE 19-2 ■ Signage promoting refugees returning to Cambodia.

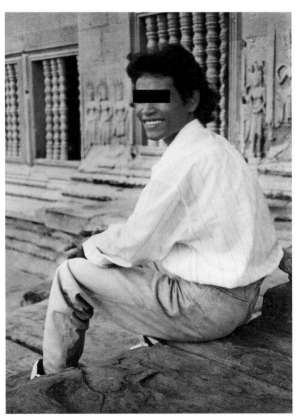

FIGURE 19-3 ■ S.S.

landmines around our compounds to protect us from enemies. Unfortunately, landmines don't discriminate among their victims, so when I stepped on one of our own landmines, it did to me what it was supposed to do to the enemy: it blew off my leg and made it impossible for me to continue being a soldier. In the Cambodian language, an amputee is called a 'neh picah' which means 'broken person'. People believe we are bad luck, that a gas seeps from the stump of the amputated limb, circles around our heads, and makes us unstable, angry, even crazy. I never believed any of those things about myself. All I knew was that I needed to find a new life, so I went back to live with my family. We fled from Cambodia, walking for weeks, me on my crutch, until we crossed the border into Thailand. In the camps in Thailand, Handicap International trained me to manage a prosthetics workshop. When the repatriation back to Cambodia was organized, HI asked if I wanted to do a different kind of job, helping other people with disabilities make the transition from camp life back to living inside Cambodia. I didn't really know how to do that, and my counterpart with HI, Miss Becky, said she didn't either, but that we would figure it out together. And we did.

THE STOP-GAP PROGRAMME

Our job as co-managers of the programme was to work with UNHCR and many other organizations to assist returnees with disabilities. It was not so difficult to know where to start. Some of the people we worked with had medical needs, but for the most part they were not sick. They were just disabled. They needed housing, food and then a way to earn a living. We called ourselves the Program of Economic and Social Rehabilitation, or PRES, in the French acronym. What we did, concretely, was to get to know the individual situation of each person on our list. We took into account each person's age, disability, strengths, skills, aspirations, family situation and the environment they lived in. We would talk with each person, sometimes for hours, and then come up with a plan for how to work towards that person's priority goals. When other resources existed, we linked people to them. For example, PRES did not do prosthetics because other

organizations were already doing that. We learned to treat pressure sores in areas where the national services for paraplegics and quadriplegics could not reach. We set up small business projects for people with disabilities because the mainstream business development programmes were not accessible to them. And so on. We were the stop-gap programme, but we eventually covered most of the country.

A TEAM OF PEERS

As PRES grew, we had to make choices about staffing. We chose to keep hiring people with disabilities who could read and write, and who showed aptitude for the work. Past affiliations or political loyalties were ignored. This meant former enemies were on the same team, working long, hard hours crammed together into the back of a Land Rover bouncing along on horrible roads for days on end. We grew into a strong team because we loved the work. It was important, and it helped people, people just like ourselves.

We saw, repeatedly, that people with disabilities gained hope and inspiration from talking through their problems and being treated with respect by a peer, by a person who was disabled, like them. Our staff benefited, too. They gained confidence in themselves as they saw their work make a difference in people's lives. We were united by the work and, oddly, by our disabilities. It's hard to explain … There was one team leader who, because his disability was a little hard to see, would roll up his pants leg to make sure that his injuries showed. He would tell people about his disability every chance he got, as a source of pride, and to prove that he belonged with the team, this big, proud, confident team of 'meneh picah'.

MORE LESSONS

S.S.'s story illustrates some further lessons that I still believe in. First, that people who have been through a trauma or extreme difficulty and who have survived or even thrived in spite of (or because of) the trauma are the best placed to inspire, motivate and accompany others who are going through the same thing. The peer to peer approach proved to be the cornerstone of PRES's success. We had an extremely hard-working and dedicated team of workers. They cared, because they identified strongly with the people they were trying to help. They also benefited themselves, becoming empowered as they empowered their peers.

Second, just about anyone can learn the basics of occupational therapy/physiotherapy/rehabilitation. It takes good training and good follow-up and support after the training. I know many professionals will disagree with this, but in countries like Cambodia and Rwanda and Mozambique, where are the professionals?

Third, that local people belong in front, and in charge. Or, as I heard someone say, foreign aid workers need to be 'on tap, not on top'. There were times when I, as an expatriate programme manager, needed to play the big boss, to sign funding proposals, or to make a speech, but the programme was always meant to be Cambodian-run, so I planned for my role and responsibilities in PRES to diminish over time, and for S.S.'s to steadily increase. As soon as he no longer needed my support, I moved on.

RWANDA'S COMPLEX EMERGENCY

In the spring of 1994, mass killings occurred in Rwanda. As the PRES programme was running well under its Cambodian management, I volunteered to join Handicap International's team, temporarily, to help with the relief efforts. I knew, intellectually, that humanitarian relief work would be different from development work, but I was not prepared for the reality of the situation on the ground in Rwanda. Kigali was mostly empty. Many buildings were still standing, but were wrecked. Any movement drew the eye. There were dogs roaming the streets in packs, and vultures flying overhead. There was no plumbing, no electricity, and no order. My job was to figure out what Handicap International and its sister organization Action Nord Sud should do regarding 'vulnerable groups' such as people with disabilities and unaccompanied minors. Everything had to be done quickly and on a large scale. I remember giving a European donor agency representative a two-page proposal for a $200 000 project to cover one district near Kigali. He glanced at it, and told me it was fine if we could triple everything: the area to be covered, the amount of money and the expected impact. This exemplifies 'emergency work' to me: big projects, implemented fast-fast-fast, some well thought out, some not.

The government of Rwanda requested that we conduct a national survey of people with disabilities. The purposes of the survey were many, some obvious and laudable, some not. After the degree of non-governmental organization (NGO) autonomy we had in Cambodia, I was surprised by the level of government intervention here. I had to let go of some of my principles in order to get something done. I could not hire disabled surveyors, could not overtly 'empower' my staff, could not do a small inexpensive sample survey, and so on. But the survey took place (Figure 19-4), as did the analysis, and the final report ended up forming one of the foundations for disability programming in the country for some years after.

In addition to the survey, we distributed clothing, provided cooking and agricultural kits, and participated in the nationwide family reunification effort. Using the ideas from a book called *Extraordinary Play with Ordinary Things* by Barbara Sher, OT, we gathered recyclable materials and then took a team of teachers on the road from orphanage to orphanage training the caregivers on how to stimulate the children with these inexpensive toys and the caregivers' imaginations and energy. That programme lasted longer than the others, probably because it morphed easily into programme activities that were still valuable long after the emergency period ended.

MORE LESSONS

Another phenomenon from that era surprised me: when I made suggestions to Rwandans to consider

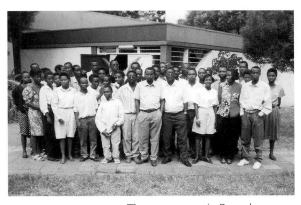

FIGURE 19-4 ■ The survey team in Rwanda.

strategies that had proved useful in Cambodia, these suggestions were not appreciated. Since then, I have heard Ethiopians reject ideas derived from Mozambique, Congolese close their eyes to strategies from Benin, and Ohioans assume they are vastly different from Kentuckians. I used to see this, a world view that pushes away or shuts out anything 'other than us', as the definition of provincialism. Maybe it is. But it seems to be a universal human trait. Widening the parameters of what is considered 'us' is perhaps the real point of international work … but it cannot be forced. I still use experiences from one place to solve problems or meet needs in another place, but I do not phrase it like that anymore. People need to believe that their situation is unique and to choose what they 'own' and care about. Those who own the problem, own the solutions.

THE YEAR-LONG COMMITTEE MEETING

Back in Cambodia, by the mid 1990s the political situation was becoming more stable and it was possible to review what was happening in the disability sector. In the early years after Cambodia reopened to the outside world, there were hundreds of NGOs swarming over the country in health, rural development, social affairs and other sectors. Because of the high prevalence of landmine victims there were lots of NGOs involved in this area. NGOs are a peculiar species of organization – full of smart, well-intentioned, hard-working, passionate people. But when each organization is free to act as it sees fit, the result can be quagmires of confusion, waste and inefficiency. For example, there were six organizations developing prosthetics programmes, each one using different technologies, referral systems and follow-up methods. As another example, wheelchairs were being produced locally, while other 'free' wheelchairs were being 'dumped' from the thrift shops of rich countries, undermining local production although the locally produced ones were much stronger and better suited for the local conditions. In short, there was a need for coordination. The Cambodian government ministry responsible for people with disabilities agreed to a study being conducted to assess the situation and make recommendations for future directions.

A task force was established with representatives from key government ministries and NGOs including persons with disabilities. The first step was to take stock of the then-current situation in each such sector: prosthetics and orthotics, wheelchair production and distribution, physical therapy services, services for blind people, services for deaf people, special education/ inclusive education, community-based rehabilitation, vocational training and more. To instil a sense of 'ownership' into the process each sub-sector was assessed by the personnel involved and the funds for the study were met by the organizations involved.

I was thrilled when Handicap International donated one year of my time to facilitating the process of stock-taking. I chaired the task force, wrote up the results of our work into a final report which was subsequently endorsed by the government, with the official Disability Action Council, a semi-autonomous national body, being established.

MY POLICY-CHANGE MENTOR

My supervisor that year was the senior international advisor to the ministry. Everything I know about national level interventions, and what shaping policy is about, I learned from this woman. The way she works is still my model for how best to achieve lasting positive changes for vulnerable groups, including people with disabilities in developing countries. From the corner of my office I saw her:

- listen to everyone involved, ask questions, listen some more, reflect, ask more questions, and slowly form a picture, using both broad-stroke and detailing brushes, of individuals, organizations, interests, challenges, conflicts, priorities and possibilities;
- work within the system that has the authority, the mandate, the long-term responsibility, but perhaps not enough capacity, for the people or issue in question;
- gently, diplomatically, respectfully nudge individuals, groups and organizations into working together, collaborating and coordinating their efforts;
- take the long view – 5 years, 10 years, 15 years – and shepherd steady, incremental progress towards lasting, positive changes.

FROM NATIONAL TO TRANSNATIONAL

I had been more or less full-time in Thailand and Cambodia for seven years. I had done short but intense stints in Rwanda, Burundi, Zaire (now the DR Congo), Vietnam and Laos. I had seen the situation of people with disabilities in all those countries, and I had my holistic, whatever-their-priorities-are-that's-what-our-priorities-should-be perspective of what should be done to help. I was inspired by my time with the Cambodian government. I could see the great things NGOs accomplished and could also see that they were drops in the ocean. The UN was engaged in issues important to people with disabilities at global and regional levels. I jumped at the opportunity to participate. I became a member of (take a deep breath) the United Nations Economic and Social Commission for Asia and the Pacific's Disability Working Group. Our main focus was to push for implementation of the UN Standard Rules on the Equalization of Opportunities for Persons with Disabilities. The Standard Rules were the best, most progressive, most comprehensive set of recommendations aimed at improving the situation of people with disabilities that existed at that time. I was energized and inspired to be a part of the process.

But then a new campaign was born, this one much narrower in scope, and fuelled by a much leaner organization than the UN. It was the International Campaign to Ban Landmines. Having seen the results of landmines on human beings and communities in Africa and South-East Asia, I was of course entirely in favour of banning the landmines, but that was not my professional interest. In fact, I agreed with people who decried the millions of dollars that went into prosthetics programmes in Cambodia (thanks to American guilt about the Vietnam War) when every other bit of funding relevant to people with disabilities had to be scraped together year after year. It did not (and still does not) seem fair that a small group – amputees, or even narrower, amputees from landmines – should receive so much more attention than everyone else put together.

But then, things happened. First, the landmine campaign was successful. In 1997, the landmine campaign won the Nobel Peace Prize and the Landmine Ban Treaty became international law. Second, that treaty broke new ground by including within its provisions the obligation that signatory countries 'provide for the care and rehabilitation and social and economic integration of landmine victims …'. In other words, this was a weapon treaty that mandated assistance for people already harmed by the weapon. When the landmine treaty became international law, governments became obliged to assist survivors of landmines. Obliged! The Standard Rules for Persons with Disabilities had no legal teeth, no formal monitoring mechanism and no obligatory provisions. The Standard Rules were suggestions; the landmine ban was a signed and sealed treaty.

I took a job with Landmine Survivors Network (LSN), an organization involved in both prongs of the landmine treaty: banning the weapon *and* assisting survivors/victims of the weapon. This organization was bold, strong and savvy in the treaty advocacy realm, but they were just beginning to figure out what to do in field-level programming. I thought I would be helping LSN develop their on-the-ground development/assistance programmes. Instead, one of the first things they asked me to do was to facilitate a global online committee. My initial role was to corral all the organizations around the world that were working with landmine survivors as their primary target or as a subgroup of people with disabilities to come up with strategies to push governments to implement the 'victim assistance' provision of the treaty. Doing 90% of the work by email, we proposed definitions for the treaty terminology, developed guidelines, presented position papers and participated in setting targets and indicators to monitor progress towards meeting the 'victim assistance' provision.

COMING FULL CIRCLE

Part of this process took place in real meetings, usually in Geneva, Switzerland. LSN made sure landmine survivors themselves were on stage at least once per meeting. The point was to insert the human face of the treaty into the proceedings by using landmine survivors' personal stories and their physical presence to emphasize the need to turn the treaty provisions into real actions. There was always a bit of resistance to putting landmine survivors on stage like that. Some felt that it was too theatrical, too undignified, too sensational. I remember one meeting in particular, when a landmine survivor from Uganda told her story to a full auditorium of diplomats. When she finished her speech, the assembly burst into applause and gave her a standing ovation. This rarely happens in diplomatic meetings. Another time, we brought a group of survivors together, scripted their stories into a dramatic reading, and had Paul McCartney and Heather Mills present the survivors with medals of appreciation. In my mind, however, having a survivor or two on stage was not enough. This was *their* issue and they deserved to be running things, not just to be showcased but to be fully involved in implementing the treaty – to be the primary advocates for victim assistance, not just the recipients of it.

So we developed a programme called 'Raising the Voices' to bring landmine survivors from all parts of the world to Geneva to learn about the treaty, to practise advocacy strategies and tactics, and to formulate plans that they could carry out back in their home countries. I felt like this programme made use of everything I had ever learned: programme recipients were at the centre of the action, and they absorbed ideas and energy from each other as much or more than they did from the 'outsiders'. They were given the opportunity to use their direct life experiences plus their new familiarity with the treaty to become advocates for their peers at home. Graduates of the programme have continued to be active leaders in Mine Ban Treaty implementation and in broader movements for social change ever since. One of the most important and successful social change movements in recent history is the development of the UN Convention on the Rights of Persons with Disabilities. Landmine survivors were involved in the Disability Convention's development from the very first meeting about it in November 2001 and they continue to be active in implementation of the Disability Convention today.

AN OCCUPATIONAL PERSPECTIVE?

It is now 21 years since I graduated as an occupational therapist, and began a journey that took me to South-East Asia, Africa, Central America, Europe and back to the US. With each move, I changed cultures, languages, climates and, sometimes, organizations. I changed my role about 10 times during those years, shifting from direct service to training to programme development to national level assessment and planning to engagement in two international treaty processes.

Looking back, I recognize three threads that ran through all those different jobs and places and organizations. One was my Peace Corps background (1981–84, Zaire). The second was my occupational therapy (OT) training. The third was personal. I do not know what to call it. I think it was my sense of wanting to do something, some work that matters.

'Promoting occupational therapy' was never in my mind. My interest has been to look for the best way to help people with disabilities, to empower them, to help them help each other. That is all. My OT training prepared me to look at disability through a number of different lenses. We examined models, theories and paradigms that underpin the practice of OT. I remember the 'biopsychosocial model' made sense to me. Then there was the model of human occupation. Nowadays, the school I attended is based on the 'science of occupation'. I do not know which of these is 'right' or which one is best for the people we serve – landmine survivors and others with disability. I still question whether I should have been consciously 'promoting occupational therapy'. I still cannot decide.

CONCLUSION

Since I started writing this chapter, earthquakes have destroyed the capital city of Haiti and thousands of people from all over the world have rushed there to help save and rebuild Haitian people's lives. I am involved from a distance, recruiting physical and occupational therapists to work there with Handicap International. I wish I could send a distilled version, a travel-sized package of all the lessons I have learned over the years, in the backpack of each therapist who goes there, especially the younger, fresher ones who might, after Haiti, go on to work in other emergency, low-income, post-conflict, developing country contexts. So, which of my lessons, if any, are worth their weight?

I guess these are the ones I have the most confidence in:

■ Being a hands-on, direct care provider is a fine way to start. Training other people to do what you know works is much better, because you multiply your effects and leave behind a permanent multiplier.

- I truly believe that just about anyone can learn the basics of OT/physiotherapy/rehabilitation, and that many people should be learning these basic principles and techniques.
- I firmly believe that people who have been through a trauma or extreme difficulty and who have survived or thrived in spite of it are the best placed to inspire, motivate and accompany others who are going through the same thing.
- I believe that local people belong in front, and in charge, that foreign aid workers need to be 'on tap, not on top', and that outsiders ought to support the system that has the authority, the mandate and the long-term responsibility (but perhaps not the capacity) for the people or issue in question.
- And finally: If you want to be present to see longlasting positive changes take hold, be prepared to stay, or to go regularly for 5, 10, or 15 years.

20

'UNITED, WE LIVE': EMPOWERING OLDER PEOPLE THROUGH DISASTER RESPONSE AND RECOVERY

KERRY THOMAS

INTRODUCTION

The world's population is ageing and social support systems are struggling to provide equitable assistance. For older people in 'developing' countries in particular, this can bring untold hardship. When disaster strikes, already difficult circumstances are exacerbated for elderly survivors, who are among the most vulnerable people in communities, and humanitarian programmes often fail to recognize the challenges and vulnerabilities faced by older people (HAI 2012). Ageing has significant ramifications for policy, planning and implementation of disaster and development programmes.

Older people are an 'invisible' population in disaster contexts (HAI 2006a). Finding ways to assist them to recover from disaster and build resilience against future emergencies is thus a pressing yet poorly appreciated global issue. Occupational therapists are potentially well placed to play a valuable role in addressing this need.

This chapter discusses a range of age-orientated strategies as implemented through the relief–recovery–development–disaster preparedness cycle, with an emphasis on recovery and ongoing development. Key insights and implications are highlighted for an occupational approach arising from participatory evaluations conducted by teams led by the author of aged-related Indian Ocean tsunami response programmes across Asia from 2006 to 2009, and related research studies. In the interests of promoting the role of programme evaluation in contributing to learning, improvement, ongoing community development and evidence-based practice, the evaluation approach is also outlined.

OLDER PEOPLE AND DISASTERS

Older people constitute a significant and growing number of those affected by humanitarian crises. Approximately 12% of the world's population is aged 60 or over, and almost 22% are aged 50 or over (UNDESA 2011). By 2050, there will be more people aged over 60 than children aged less than 15 years. Global trends show that this is not only a developed world phenomenon: by 2050, nearly 80% of the world's older people will live in emerging and developing economies, where disasters are more likely to occur and their effects are more acutely felt (UNDESA 2011). Rapid growth in the worldwide population of older people is significantly changing the demographic and epidemiological profile of disaster-affected populations (Furtade & Teklu 2012, HAI 2012). Yet there continue to be very few specific health and other interventions that target older people in disaster preparedness, response and recovery.

It is often assumed that older people's needs are met simply by implementing needs-based assistance but there is a growing body of evidence that suggests that older people are routinely neglected in humanitarian protection and assistance (HAI 2013). A study on disaster funding (HAI-HI 2012) highlighted the staggering statistics that only 0.78% of humanitarian funding proposals included at least one activity targeting older people, and that only 0.3% of these were funded. Recognizing that older people and people with disabilities may benefit from assistance designed to support the general population, the study also analysed projects to see if these groups were integrated into projects as part of a wider vulnerable group. The findings were equally stark: only 5.2% of projects analysed specifically mentioned older people and people with disabilities alongside other vulnerable groups (HAI-HI 2012, HAI 2013). These figures belie the fact that older people have specific issues, risks and needs that require particular consideration.

OLDER PEOPLE IN THE 2004 ASIAN TSUNAMI – AN INTERNATIONAL NGO RESPONSE

HelpAge International (HAI) is the primary global international nongovernmental organization (NGO) dedicated to promoting the rights and wellbeing of senior citizens in difficult circumstances. HAI designs and implements programmes in partnership with national HelpAge associations, government agencies and other local and international organizations. Through such networks unique disaster response and recovery programmes are developed that vary from country to country according to contextual needs and to the capacity of HAI partners. For example, the HAI Indian Ocean Tsunami Response Programme in Sri Lanka took a more directly operational approach, while HelpAge India was responsible for implementation in that country, and in Indonesia the HAI programme had a mainly advocacy rather than operational role. Cohesion across these countries and contexts was attained by an overarching programme design that had three main streams: enhancing social protection for older people; sustaining a livelihood in old age; and advocating for older people in disaster preparedness and response. Within these themes, activities were implemented in the health, livelihoods, social welfare and protection, and disaster risk reduction sectors.

A portfolio of activities was implemented across the region and across the disaster and development continuum, taking account of the varying places, populations and circumstances. Activities included: emergency relief actions; health camps and mobile outreach units; ophthalmic care; psychosocial wellbeing, including support for religious pilgrimages; care of the very frail and vulnerable; home/aged care; construction of new homes, villages and clinics; water and sanitation facilities including rainwater harvesting; grain banks; social pension schemes; establishment of older people's associations; livelihood assistance schemes; disaster preparedness and risk reduction; advocacy; and policy development.

PROGRAMME EVALUATION APPROACH

Monitoring and evaluation (M&E) is a requirement of international aid and development programmes. It is also a hallmark of learning organizations that seek to improve their approaches to better achieve desired outcomes and to effectively adapt to changing circumstances. From a professional perspective, M&E is a lynchpin in generating evidence-based practice.

There are many ways in which M&E can occur. Within the context of the HelpAge International Indian Ocean Tsunami Response Programme, a series of mid-term, summative and impact evaluations were undertaken of the HAI and partner programmes in three countries affected by the tsunami (Indonesia, Sri Lanka and India). While each evaluation had a specific focus, overall the purpose was to (a) assess the effectiveness and efficiency of the programme, and (b) identify lessons for future disaster response and recovery programmes. The specific objectives were to review: programme impact – how older people were affected; programme delivery – including management performance and systems; and programme legacy – for HelpAge organizations and their partners.

A multi-method, participatory approach was adopted across all of the evaluations which spanned the period 2006–9. Methods included sampling and prioritization techniques, key informant interviews, workshop discussions, focus groups (Figure 20-1), site visits, observations and document review. Particular attention was given to eliciting the lived experience of older people and service providers in tandem with quantitative evidence of activities and results. Rigour in assessing findings and compiling recommendations was enhanced by the use of triangulation and collaborative analysis techniques. There was a strong capacity-building element that included, in Sri Lanka, the

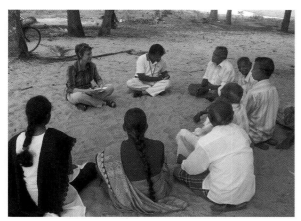

FIGURE 20-1 ■ Focus group with OPA leaders. 'It's good that HelpAge wants to know what's happened with this tsunami programme. ... A lot of good things have happened ... it's changed our lives ... now and for the future ... There are some things that still aren't so good ... can we tell you about these?'

formation and training of evaluation teams that comprised local personnel and older people representatives, and the convening of participatory 'summit' workshops whereby key stakeholder representatives critiqued findings and contributed to development of recommendations and actions arising.

WHAT DID THE EVALUATIONS REVEAL?

There were three main groups of findings that emerged from these evaluations and associated studies that have particular relevance for a socio-occupational perspective: cross-cutting issues, specific activities and the role of older people's associations (OPAs).

Cross-Cutting Issues

Humanitarian principles espouse humanity, impartiality and equal right of access to assistance. However, although there are international mandates (e.g. The Sphere Project 2011) requiring that the needs and rights of vulnerable people, including the aged, are addressed in humanitarian contexts, a wide range of age-related discrimination was evidenced across the tsunami response and recovery landscape. The following insights are summarized from the evaluation

reports (HAI-*inter*PART 2007, 2008, 2009) and other impact studies (HAI 2005, 2006b).

Lack of data on older people: Across the overall humanitarian response, lack of accurate information disaggregated by age and gender hindered assessment of the situation of older people and concealed their vulnerability. As a result they were overlooked in initial emergency relief efforts and were largely forgotten in wider recovery and rehabilitation plans. Relief workers did not think about older people or consider them as a vulnerable group with particular needs.

Accessibility: Older survivors were often unable to access relief supply distributions (including food, water and sanitation, medicines), monetary handouts, and services such as health, social welfare and livelihood programmes. Even when living with their children's families, elderly people were very often invisible. Physical, psychological, sociocultural, conflict and environmental factors hindered accessibility. Most older people wanted to return to their previous living arrangements and felt that living in camps eroded their independence; those who had lived with families wanted to stay with them, while those who lived alone wanted their own accommodation, and with the loss of documentation, some refused to leave their land.

Exclusion of older people: Because older people were poorly accounted for in situational and needs assessments, and experienced accessibility constraints, they were routinely excluded from services. In contexts where people compete for limited resources and opportunities, older people consistently lose out, even within families. Older people were rarely considered in housing reconstruction and livelihood assessments.

Furthermore, mainstream relief and recovery programmes did not recognize the positive roles and capabilities that older people can have in coping with emergencies and nurturing resilience in adapting to changed circumstances. Humanitarian workers tended to view older people as recipients of help, rather than active contributors, and made little effort to include them in camp activities.

Safety and protection: Older people experienced particular protection issues and risks, for example those arising from prevailing regional conflicts (e.g. between ethnic and political groups), while preexisting problems at individual, family or community level were exacerbated by the crisis. Lack of appreciation of contextual power relationships and understanding of such dynamics undermined recovery programmes and the achievement of expected outcomes.

Gender equality: Older women and men need to be enabled to access services equally, and to participate equally in the design, implementation, monitoring and evaluation of humanitarian and recovery programmes. Cultural and historical factors often meant that gender-specific processes were initiated. However, because women were more likely to be widowed and alone, as well as having often experienced a lifetime of gender discrimination, additional consideration was given to older females (HAI 2006b) including ensuring their equal representation in decision-making positions.

Lack of age-specific awareness, knowledge and skills: Mainstream humanitarian workers had very limited appreciation of the needs, vulnerabilities and capacities of older people. Where there was awareness, a lack of knowledge, skills and tools constrained action to engage older people, and particularly those with disabilities, and so enable their participation in programmes. Initiatives to capture and assess older people's needs and capacities, and to provide information and training for humanitarian actors helped to redress the situation.

Specific Activities

Programme design and implementation: The HelpAge tsunami programme demonstrated exemplary practice with respect to recognizing the rights, needs and capacities of older people. While specialized interventions were initiated, considerable effort was directed towards the need to substantially promote mainstreaming of aged considerations across disaster management clusters and sectors; this approach reflects the twin-track approach through which disability issues are addressed. Furthermore, in recognizing the importance of promoting post-programme capacity, resilience and sustainability, programme processes and activities were highly participatory, and where relevant gave credence to intergenerational considerations including elders' concern for the wellbeing of their children or grandchildren.

Practical strategies that made a difference: Facilitating recovery and resilience building through enabling engagement in occupations occurred through a range of activities, examples of which are illustrated here.

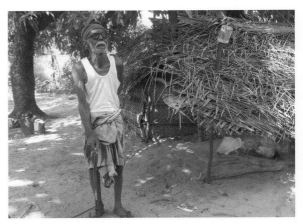

FIGURE 20-2 ■ This 84-year-old man lost his house in the tsunami but refused to move from his land for fear of losing it, preferring to live in a temporary shelter. Provision of eye glasses and a quad walking stick, to replace those he lost in the disaster, stopped falls and injuries, enhanced safety and restored independence in activities of daily living and cooking.

- *Environmental modifications and disability aids:* This included provision of aids and equipment (particularly eye glasses, walking sticks and hearing aids; Figure 20-2), making latrines accessible and safe, installing ramps and rails, and providing appropriate cooking facilities in camps and new housing clusters. These activities were provided by local programme (non-health) staff, many of whom accessed simple written guidelines to assist in providing interventions. Strengthening assessment, prescription and follow-up competencies of staff and home care volunteers and networking with other expert providers (e.g. national allied health personnel, international NGOs such as Handicap International) was an identified need – a role that lends itself to input by an occupational therapist.

- *Mobile outreach units and health camps:* These activities take services out into the community, particularly in rural and remote areas. Staffed by doctors and health professionals, clinical assessments and services are provided, referrals and home visits made, and prevention and health promotion awareness activities conducted. The camps and units were also instrumental in picking up health problems for early intervention.

■ *Home care volunteers:* In Sri Lanka 420 community-based volunteers were trained in supporting vulnerable and frail elderly people. Some of the volunteers are themselves younger elders and, unlike young people, tend to stay. They have been instrumental in helping previously hidden elders to access medical, rehabilitation and eye care services and mobile outreach units, and in getting them registered and connected with other support systems. Volunteer work is most effective when closely linked with OPAs, who may also manage and support the volunteers. Opportunities exist for occupational therapists to support such initiatives, in particular training and provision of support in managing complex psychosocial and family neglect needs and community-based rehabilitation initiatives, as well as establishing follow-up, support and supervision systems and linkages with government arrangements. Case 20-1 highlights the complexity of some situations.

■ *Psychosocial support:* This comprised a range of initiatives, the most powerful being pilgrimages in a context where religion has a strong foundation. Two day bus trips provided an opportunity for older survivors to go together to sites of significance in grieving for those lost in the disaster. This was an excellent 'entry/mobilizing point' for both

---

CASE 20-1

'Ayoma': A Case Highlighting Multiple Issues

Living in a small hut in a compound where adult, married children reside in the main house is a common occurrence among elders. Sometimes this is by choice, a way in which ageing parents provide for their children and grandchildren, and perhaps a way in which an elder can find some peace and quiet away from the busyness and closeness of family relationships. Sometimes it is the result of neglectful and even abusive behaviour by children, where elders who can no longer contribute to the material wellbeing of the family are banished to an out-place. The situation here was not clear.

We arrived to see how a recently delivered wheelchair-commode was helping Ayoma, the woman in Figure 20-3. We were all disturbed to find her half lying, half sitting in this tiny, newly constructed and very hot tin shelter. Eating a bowl of rice and vegetables, she had easy reach to a bottle of water and a ragged bag of personal effects hanging from a nail. Her reading glasses hung in a bag on another hook, and she had a long stick easily accessible to help leverage herself along and to stand up. Her very basic needs were being met, but what of her rights and wellbeing?

The two partner and programme staff were distressed at the situation, having supposedly negotiated with the family for her to be moved into the main house. When they had first visited, Ayoma had been living in a 'lean-to' shelter made of timber and fronds attached to the side of the house. The family had been seeking help in getting a wheelchair because Ayoma was affected by a hip and leg injury, deafness and increasing visual impairment. Discussions ensued with the daughter and son-in-law, the outcomes of which included the family agreeing to build a ramp up into the house, suitable for a wheelchair, and to enable access to the latrine and wash stand in the garden, and beyond. This had not been done. Also, while the chair was parked beside the new shelter, it was evident that Ayoma could not by herself get out of her shelter and into the chair. Family members were also not aware of how to transfer Ayoma safely; we later learnt that the home care volunteer was not sure of this either. Further, because of the sandy soil, the chair could not be self-propelled. Indeed, because of its narrow wheels, designed for hospital wards, it would require a good deal of strength for it to be pushed when Ayoma was in it.

Because of Ayoma's deafness it was not possible to speak with her privately at this time about what she wanted. This situation highlighted a range of issues facing personnel with respect to undertaking holistic assessment and response measures.

Case study from March 2007 Programme Evaluation, prepared by Kerry Thomas

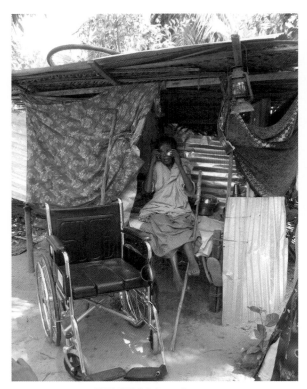

FIGURE 20-3 ■ Ayoma.

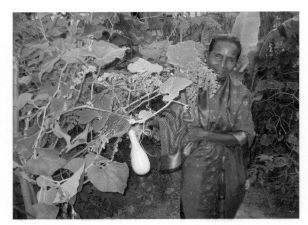

FIGURE 20-4 ■ Vegetable growing – a meaningful recovery occupation – provided improved nutrition and income through the sale of surplus quantities.

disaster response and development programmes, most particularly as a catalyst in the formation of OPAs. They were largely organized by people themselves, which itself was a normalizing occupation, and created space while travelling and on-site for mutual support. Frequently involving mixed religious groups, they also facilitated harmony in diverse community contexts, offering potential for peace-building in conflict-affected areas. Other psychosocially focused efforts in the form of spiritual, cultural, art and community activities were also noted as generating benefits for individuals, groups and community.

■ *Livelihoods:* The main livelihood activities were comprised of individual and some group enterprises and micro-credit loans and savings initiatives. These directly responded to an expressed priority of elderly people and appeared to have significantly contributed to enhancing the status and wellbeing of many tsunami-affected elders. Grants for individuals typically ranged from US$50 to US$200. Credit access and revolving loans are especially important elements in enabling successful livelihood outcomes, and have been instrumental in promoting both individual and group (OPA) savings initiatives. The opportunity to generate income and savings is a critical safety net against future shocks, as well as supporting better health, nutrition and social engagement.

Building resilience to future uncertainties and risks – including those associated with market variability, climate change and conflict – was an increasing consideration for the livelihood programme. At another very simple level, encouraging OPA members to establish home gardens was one practical strategy addressing nutrition and income needs (Figures 20-4 and 20-5), while peace-building and other more complex initiatives were developed in conflict-affected tsunami areas. While livelihood and micro-credit activities are complex in nature and management, the credit/loan programme provided many OPAs with a core role and financial function around which they may be sustained into the future.

Older People's Associations

An OPA is a community-based group of older people working together to improve the situation of older people and the community they live in (HAI 2007).

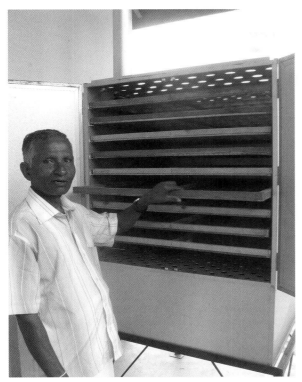

FIGURE 20-5 ■ In order to extend the benefits of vegetable growing over a longer timeframe, one OPA designed a fruit and vegetable drying process for member use.

As part of the HelpAge Indian Ocean Tsunami Response Programme, 136 Senior Citizen Committees were established in Sri Lanka, with over 16 100 members, while in India, more than 425 Elder Self-Help Groups were convened, each with 15–20 members.

Early development of OPAs has emerged as a very successful approach in supporting implementation of HelpAge response interventions as well as being an outcome in their own right, through which ongoing empowerment, resilience and development can occur. During the early phases of disaster recovery, the establishment of OPAs provided a powerful participatory mechanism through which to identify and prioritize needs and develop inclusive plans, since it built on the members' familiarity and experiences in the local area. Subsequently these associations have been the conduit for providing recovery and ongoing development assistance across a remarkable range of activities.

Figure 20.6 provides an overview of the range of activities that OPAs have gradually taken on facilitating as their capacity has developed (HAI 2007). OPAs typically implement a combination of these activities depending on the priorities identified by members. The focus and mix of activities that an individual OPA carries out depend on the context of their communities and reflect local needs and interests and member competencies.

Older people identified a significant range of benefits arising from OPA membership (HAI 2007, HAI-*inter*PART 2007, 2008, 2009). These include an opportunity to (re)gain some control over their lives – being able to make decisions about things that affect their lives, having access to funds from which to establish some income generation, and a range of psychosocial benefits that come from being part of a kindred group. In bringing these benefits, OPAs have promoted dignity and quality of life, reduced isolation, provided a mechanism to support more vulnerable members, and promoted community cohesion through organizing activities and events that involve different age groups and sections of the community. Furthermore, engagement in OPAs enhances older people's skills and confidence to plan and implement activities that benefit themselves, their families and their communities. This in turn increases older people's visibility as productive and active community members, generating respect and inclusion.

The success of OPAs is significantly dependent on the nature and quality of facilitation and support that was available and that there has been adequate time to nurture the establishment and development of these organizations (Figure 20-7). In moving forward, older people raised concerns about gaining the competencies necessary to manage OPA functions over a longer term, after the tsunami programme. These include ensuring appropriate governance arrangements, financial management associated with revolving loan and livelihood activities, and accessing technical and material support, including access to health care and other rights. Roles exist for occupational therapists to support the training and development of local facilitators and, through them, OPA management and volunteer members.

It is noteworthy that in Sri Lanka the adoption of the OPA approach cohered with and supported an

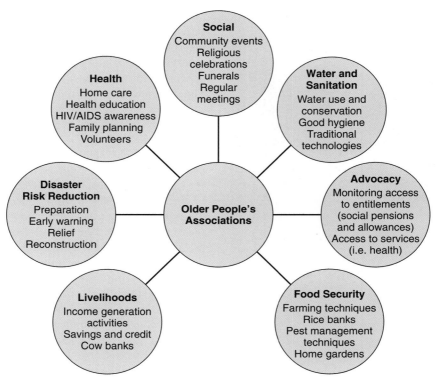

FIGURE 20-6 ▦ An overview of typical activities implemented by OPAs. *(Reproduced with permission from HAI, 2007. Older People's Associations in Community Disaster Risk Reduction. A Resource Book on Good Practice. HelpAge International, London. © HelpAge International)*

existing government policy to promote the establishment of Senior Citizen Committees (SCCs) across the country. The network of SCCs supported by the HelpAge tsunami programme was integrated into this government mechanism as the programme wound down (Figure 20-8). In India, the 'Elders for Elders' movement and federated structure that was being actively developed as a springboard from the programme led to benefits expanding beyond the end of the tsunami programme and its locale, including, for example, changes in bank loan and insurance policies for older people.

LESSONS FOR AN OCCUPATIONAL PERSPECTIVE

■ Older people have specific issues and needs that require rigorous analysis in order to understand how people of different age, gender and ability

levels are affected differently by a crisis. Systematic, aged-specific assessment and monitoring across the disaster response and recovery continuum is necessary to identify and prioritize specific and mainstream interventions. Occupation is both a subject and medium through which contextual and specific needs assessment, planning and implementation can occur.

■ Participation of older people from the outset of an emergency response through the recovery, rehabilitation, future preparedness and ongoing development phases is critical to the achievement of successful outcomes. In this sense, occupation is both programmatic and therapeutic.

■ Older people have recognized and respected roles and possess valuable experience and capacities, and yet these capabilities often remain unrecognized or underutilized during disaster situations (HAI 2006b). 'Older people play crucial roles

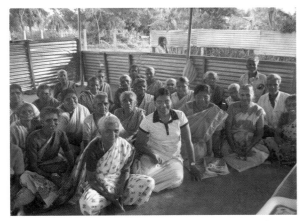

FIGURE 20-7 ■ OPA and facilitator. 'By working with us ... helping us get our Old People's group going ... you have given so much more than just things' ... 'This is something that can go on into the future' ... 'You want to know what makes it work? ... see that girl over there [group facilitator staff member] ... she listens to us ... cries with us ... makes things happen ... but does things with us ... doesn't treat us like we're old and dumb' ... 'We have a role ... we feel valued ... respected ... we've got confidence again ...'

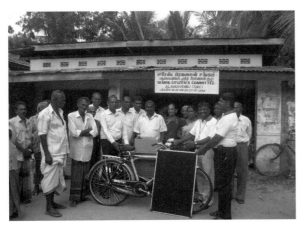

FIGURE 20-8 ■ 'United, we live.' OPAs have provided extraordinary benefits in enabling older people to unite in the face of devastation and to become even stronger and more resilient than before the tsunami.

within society, and are often pivotal in supporting response and recovery to disasters. Many care for children and make essential contributions to family income, while others hold important roles as community leaders or as holders of community knowledge and tradition. In overlooking

older people's roles and their needs, we also overlook the needs of their families and dependants, and forgo a potentially central part of community recovery' (HAI 2012, p. 1).

■ Incorporate age-friendly features into mainstream disaster and development programmes and empower older people to advocate for inclusion. Consult, communicate and coordinate across sectors in order to enable accessibility and engagement of older people to services and occupations that will enhance recovery.

■ Addressing the needs and rights of older people in disaster contexts offers a unique, practical and highly relevant role for both experienced and entry level occupational therapists in disaster management. However, it requires critical consideration, preparation and willingness to work in different ways.

SUMMARY

Awareness of aged-specific special needs and human rights remains poor among governments and humanitarian organizations. Where these are acknowledged, there is a substantial lack of knowledge and skills to implement appropriate actions. The situation is exacerbated because older people are not widely considered as legitimate stakeholders in disaster rehabilitation and development. Changes are required in how relief and development programmes are designed and implemented: specialized interventions for older people are needed, as well as mainstreamed age-friendly strategies. In the context of ageing communities and an increasing prevalence of disasters, overlaid with global resource constraints, the need to build 'self-help' systems is both paramount and possible. Central to enabling this is an 'occupational' perspective that nurtures the roles, capacities and resilience of elderly survivors and the aged community. Occupation characterizes effective relief and recovery programmes with and for older people and has potential to promote inclusion and empowerment through which elders' rights and wellbeing are achieved. With care, consideration, participation and capacity building, there is a myriad of practical ways in which occupational therapists can make an immediate and long-lasting impact with communities.

REFERENCES

Furtade, C., Teklu, M. 2012 The Sphere Project Handbook: Standards for Humanitarian Response Address Growing Problem of Chronic Diseases. Presentation to the Geneva Health Forum.

HAI, 2005. The Impact of the Indian Ocean Tsunami on Older People. Issues and Recommendations. HelpAge International, London.

HAI, 2006a. Rebuilding Lives in Longer-Term Emergencies. Older People's Experience in Darfur. HelpAge International, London.

HAI, 2006b. Older People in Aceh, Indonesia. 18 Months after the Tsunami. Issues and Recommendations. HelpAge International, London.

HAI, 2007. Older People's Associations in Community Disaster Risk Reduction. A Resource Book on Good Practice. HelpAge International, London.

HAI, 2012. Protecting Older People in Emergencies: Good Practice Guide. HelpAge International, London.

HAI, 2013. Protection Interventions for Older People in Emergencies. HelpAge International, London.

HAI-HI, 2012. A Study of Humanitarian Financing for Older People and Persons with Disabilities, 2010–2011. HelpAge International and Handicap International.

HAI-interPART, 2007. 'United, We are Living Again' – An Evaluation of the Sri Lanka Tsunami Response Programme. Kerry Thomas interPART, HelpAge Sri Lanka and HelpAge International, Colombo and London.

HAI-interPART, 2008. Fostering Pioneers – An Evaluation of the Sri Lanka Tsunami Extended Response Programme (ERP). Kerry Thomas interPART, HelpAge Sri Lanka and HelpAge International, Colombo and London.

HAI-interPART, 2009. HelpAge Tsunami Programme Evaluation. Kerry Thomas, John Myers, Mano Kumarasuriyar, interPART & Associates, Australia, and HelpAge International, London.

The Sphere Project, 2011. Humanitarian Charter and Minimum Standards in Humanitarian Response. The Sphere Project, UK.

UNDESA, 2011. World Population Prospects: The 2010 Revision, Highlights and Advance Tables, Working Paper No. ESA/P/WP.220. Department of Economic and Social Affairs, Population Division, United Nations, New York.

21

DROUGHT: SLOW-ONSET DISASTER AND ITS BURDEN UPON FAMILIES

JENNY BIVEN

SURVIVING DROUGHT IN THE MURRAY MALLEE: GETTING THROUGH THE TOUGH TIMES TO FACE ANOTHER YEAR

Carol's* Story

I live on a broad acre farm, located 40 km from a small rural town in the heart of the Mallee country of SA. My husband Doug and I were together on this farm for 22 years. Sometimes I wonder why we stayed but something about the mallee bush gets under your skin and we just didn't think of leaving despite several years of drought and little money coming in. Our three sons would help Doug on the farm when they could although all were still in school, the youngest in primary school. Doug always seemed happy when they were out on the farm with him. I know for both of us we got through the hard times because we dreamed of those illusive rains coming at last, getting rid of the debts piling up and making improvements to the farm so we had a viable place to pass onto our sons. There was an unstated assumption, I guess, that one of our sons would want to take over the farm eventually. I helped Doug when he needed me, but much of my time was occupied with just keeping the house running, getting the boys to school and their sports commitments. Our neighbours lived several kilometres away ... we knew them but didn't see them much. Doug used to be involved in the football club when he was younger but when he left and

times got tough with the drought, Doug didn't go out that much. Doug had always assumed responsibility for overseeing the farm's ongoing viability and, like many farmers, shared few of his concerns with me or anyone else. I thought ... Doug was just 'getting on with things'. But one evening I woke up when I heard the sound of a gunshot. Oh ... that awful feeling you get in the pit of your stomach when you hear that sound. Doug had gone outside to the shed ... and ... shot himself. It was such a shock. I hadn't suspected anything. I felt so numb ... and so angry ... all at the same time.

To get help I had to reach out to people ... to my neighbours. Gee, so much has changed since then. Everyone was so good to us and when the crops were due to be harvested a number of local men came to help and they got the boys involved which seemed to help with their grief in losing their dad. I never thought about leaving, I was determined to hang on to the farm for the boys' sake and for Doug's sake but it was hard accepting the help, really hard, after years of just getting on with things by ourselves. I was never inclined to get involved with local activities, just helped with some school events occasionally so this stuff of getting help was all new for me. I was given names of counselors and initially I thought 'no I don't need this', but eventually I was convinced to attend an 8 week emotional strength building program being run by a local woman who is a community health worker. I'm so glad I did this. There were about 9 other women and there was this warm welcoming atmosphere ... very soon I found myself crying,

*Name changed to protect identity.

sharing how I felt and making friends. It was such a relief. Through this program I found out what assistance was available and other options of support and this experience gave me the strength to do what I needed to so that keeping the farm was a more viable proposition. I now work part-time in town, after updating my work skills from pre-farm days, and the other days do what I can to help my eldest son who is working full-time on the farm. He and I have attended farm management workshops and tapped into financial counseling assistance. I sing regularly with a local choir and this keeps me going when I feel down about what happened. I don't know whether my sons will stay on the farm but I want to keep the option open for them so perhaps Doug's dream and his hard work may not have been in vain.

J. Schroeder, personal communication 2009

THE MURRAY MALLEE – WHAT'S IT LIKE?

Driving through the Murray Mallee region of South Australia, it can appear a harsh and tough landscape to the first time visitor. However, as with Carol and Doug's experience, there is a certain 'mallee magic' in this landscape that allows people to see past its tough exterior to appreciate the flora, the fauna and subtle features this environment can offer. The vista of grain crops and pasture paddocks is occasionally broken by clumps of the distinctive mallee trees where they have survived the rampant clearing of earlier years. The mallee tree is not your classic upright, majestic or handsome tree. It is a small, multi-stemmed tree with gnarled, tough roots highly sought after for firewood. Its understorey is dotted with clumps of spinifex, an equally tough grasslike plant but a haven for native birds, reptiles and insects. This is the understated but very unique ecosystem that many locals appreciate despite the rigorous environment (Figure 21-1).

Both the mallee tree and spinifex have adapted well to the progressively drier climatic conditions of this region (Nickolls & Angel 2002), where rainfall, even in what is classed as a 'good' year, is low, droughts are common and can extend over a number of years, mice plagues come and go, and dust storms are a regular

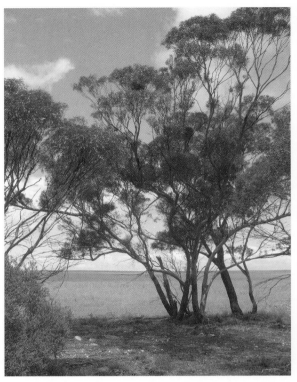

FIGURE 21-1 ■ 'Beneath the dappled olive canopy of the mallee is a myriad of small surprises and wonderful adaptations to an extreme environment.' Local resident. *(Quote from Nickolls & Angel 2002.)*

feature. Temperatures can drop as low as 0°C in winter and reach 44°C plus in summer. Altogether these conditions have proved to be a challenging environment for those seeking a productive and viable income.

When I first started working in the Mallee a mouse plague was in full swing and I remember vividly sitting in a farmhouse with one couple as they calmly emptied and reset mouse traps every couple of minutes during the time I was there. It was done in a matter of fact fashion, without fuss, and as I left I passed by the front door a 44 gallon drum two-thirds full with dead mice. This acceptance, persistence, down to earth attitude and resilience in the face of adversity I have come across again and again and also the deep attachment people have to their land despite its challenges. Maybe it is the 'magic' of the Mallee but it is also 'the intimate connection between the farm as a place of work, residence, family tradition and identity' (Drought Policy

Review Expert Social Panel 2008, p.12) that keeps them going.

Carol's family is just one of about 1432 farming families located in the Murray Mallee region, which covers approximately 23 000 sq km, taking in the plains spreading eastward from the ranges that separate it from the state capital, Adelaide. Half of the area's approximate 37 000 people live in the major business centre, Murray Bridge. The remaining population live in the small towns dotted across the region and on farms growing crops, grazing sheep and cattle and some that have diversified into stud farming, grassland and horticulture irrigation on the floodplains of the Murray river, piggeries and, recently, potato growing (Repper 2009).

LIVING IN THE MALLEE – PAST AND PRESENT

The opening of a railway line during the early 1900s and parcels of land given to soldiers returning from World Wars I and II eventually led to an increase of settlers into the region. However, much of this area is marginal farming land, and land clearance plus dryland salinity and wind resulted in widespread soil degradation, making farming extremely challenging. Many of the women who accompanied their husbands were unfamiliar with such a harsh climate, the isolation, few or no local services and having makeshift houses made of tin and wooden slabs. These days the slab huts have gone but you can find many families living in very rundown houses unchanged since they were built in the early 1950s because 'if it doesn't make a profit it doesn't get fixed' (J Schroeder, personal communication 2009).

Despite these drawbacks, fourth-generation farming families can still be found living on the original land settled by their forebears as well as the relative newcomers such as Doug and Carol, eager to carve out a future for themselves in the business of farming.

In years past, people in these small rural communities would meet each other regularly at church on Sundays, community service groups, local Saturday dances and movies shown in the local halls. Children went to the local schools and people shopped locally where possible. The loss of farming families in a district can have the domino effect of closing schools and local businesses, which in turn can affect the cultural and social fabric of the local town and its meaning within that rural environment. Now local sports clubs or going to the local 'pub' for a drink provide the few opportunities to meet up with others on a regular basis and only one or two community service groups are still in existence.

My parents' generation all went to church on Sundays. Now no-one would know where you are or what you are doing. Many tend to travel to the city for the weekend.

J Schroeder, personal communication 2009

THE 'TOUGH TIMES' AND THEIR EFFECTS ON LIVELIHOOD, HEALTH AND WELLBEING

Mark's Story

'Why come to this area?' I asked.

'Here overall expense of land was affordable, less yielding but better and … I was drawn to the place … then one of the first families I met … chappy said his father worked with man of the same name … found out Dad worked here as a young lad clearing paddocks and stuff.'

'How has the drought affected you?' I enquired.

'Been here for 15 years … first 5 years were good then first encounter with drought, had one good year since but price of grain plummeted so that wasn't environmental drought but financial drought carrying over from other years when I lost money. That was the last year I sowed a crop. We owned the place when we came here … now it's bank owned and just pay the interest! My house is falling down around me but rather be here and penniless than be forced off to go and live in Adelaide.'

'Wife left 6 years ago with our daughter … love of my life … came out here together … she was working in the local school, found it too cliquey and took things personally … but put in the money she earned so since then have tried to make ends meet. … she went to Adelaide to live for a while and then said she didn't want to come back, sort of lifestyle she didn't want … she couldn't understand my reasoning for not joining her.'

'... and last couple of years had to put in for drought relief because earning capacity less than what I had to maintain the farm ... just cost of diesel to check sheep and fences. And 18 months ago went through one of those black dog stages I s'pose ... went to the doctor ... said ... nothin' wrong with me but feel like shit ... he put me on pills but they didn't agree with me. I still have twinges and that is where Bronte [drought counsel/or] comes in ... something triggers it. Farming different to factory work ... 24/7 things on my mind ... thinking there is something you should be doing but then that's what I like about it ... no boredom, have to be multiskilled. Need to talk to other people ... I was going out and picking up dead lambs every day in that long hot weather ... but talking to my physio ... she said previous client had lost 200 sheep in one day ... you can think you are the only one but when you talk to others ... realize others in same boat or worse off.'

M. Challan, personal communication 2009

The Murray Mallee region has experienced its latest drought conditions for the past six years and has been classified as an Exceptional Circumstances district due to ongoing drought. Some farmers are selling up, relieved not to have the ongoing burden of debt and constant need to speculate on financial returns during the next season. Farms may be bought by neighbours keen to increase their income potential but in return adding to their workload and their stress. Other farms go to large corporations bringing in managers who can be more detached from historical and obligatory ties to the land on which they work. However, as with Mark, 'although it is difficult many want to stay because they want to be there ... the risks can happen ... you choose ... try to reduce the risks but have to accept the consequences'.

Unfortunately these consequences can be devastating and unexpected, as with Doug's suicide, and the effects of ongoing drought on men and women, sons and daughters, impact not only on family relationships but on communities as a whole.

'Blokes see themselves as the ones to fix things ... so they don't know what to do – it is out of their hands – lots of depression around.'

'Newer farmers are affected ... don't have the background or reserves in stock or concepts of being able to diversify. Older farmers have their reserves and say "what drought? ... this is just a natural part of life ... what are you worried about, she'll be right it's just another year that we'll get through eventually".'

B. Warneke, personal communication 2009

Men can be silent battlers, often taking on the full responsibility for the farm's success or feeling the burden of a poor season and all the while trying to keep their pride in place.

The men think 'I am useless, all my fault it's going wrong' ... don't seek help ... like the men in my family ... and when they talk at the footy or golf club it is more about how the team went, they don't get to the other layer ... shut off from the farm that is not working ... then the alcohol comes into it.

J. Schroeder, personal communication 2009

This sense of loss of status, the burden of debt or lack of income, and perception of their poor farm management can contribute, as Mark found, to poor mental, emotional and physical health and also affect their social and spiritual wellbeing. 'The hardest part is for men to step back and look at the big picture ... men find that intimidating ... not masculine or manly to do these things' (B. Warneke, personal communication 2009). Depression, anxiety, eating and sleeping disorders, alcohol abuse and in some cases domestic violence, in its various forms, can be the result. Children can be affected, such as one case in which an 11-year-old boy regressed to bedwetting due to the stress at home.

Often the use of alcohol and drugs is huge ... that is what they are turning to trying to relieve the pain.

J. Schroeder, personal communication 2009

Binge drinking among younger men is a common occurrence and the drugs 'ecstasy' and 'speed' are becoming more culturally accepted by both men and women. Risky behaviour in vehicles can accompany the high alcohol consumption, often with dire consequences.

Although I originally started work in the Mallee as a senior occupational therapist, my position as a lifestyle advisor supporting people to modify risky lifestyle behaviours brought me in contact with men and women living in the Mallee who have experienced the effects of drought on income, family relationships and their own health. Poor mental health from adversity can lead to a lifestyle of health-damaging behaviours of alcohol abuse, poor diet, smoking, social withdrawal and anger as a survival strategy (Friedli 2009).

In comparing experiences with other service providers in the Mallee, lack of trust, feeling vulnerable and a negative perception of self is a common factor encountered with clients and it is not uncommon to hear 'this is the first time I have told anybody about this'. I have heard men tearfully unburdening themselves of lost relationships and past traumas. Bronte, a drought counsellor, told of 'the stress of the moment now bringing up stress of the past and complicates it all … in these worrying times post traumatic stress disorder is coming out as flashbacks from times in the past' (B. Warneke, personal communication 2009).

A farmer did one lap on his header and then jumped off and shot himself. If you can't see a way out you can see this as a ray of hope.
J. Schroeder, personal communication 2009

South Australian rural suicide rates for men up to 44 years of age are among the highest in Australia (Suicide Facts and Statistics 2009). Specific numbers are difficult to determine due to the nature of how it is reported. If farmers are not sharing their feelings of despair and frustration with others in their community, suicide can be the way out when they cannot see how to improve their situation. As Judy related, it is usually after the event that people start to talk … there is the grief and the guilt: 'oh god, I was only talking to him the other day' or 'he wasn't looking good in the pub but he said he was alright so I backed off' (J. Schroeder, personal communication 2009). If other men are going through their own stuff they may not be able to offer help at the time and, if it rains, this can be the 'bandaid' that keeps them going.

A recent commentary on climate change and how it could impact dramatically on health highlighted the negative effects on people's mental wellbeing experienced when there is disturbance of the healthy links between themselves and their home or environment. These effects have been related to psychoterratic illnesses. A disturbance such as the experience of drought can be seen to have the effect of limiting meaningful occupational engagement. 'Solastalgia', a specific psychoterratic illness, causes distress and lack of solace in response to this resulting occupational deprivation and the negative perception of one's home environment (Pereira 2009). Discussions I have had with those working in the Mallee have described people affected by drought who perceive farming not just as a business but as their lifestyle and who have few or no other interests. Drought therefore affects their sense of who they are, their purpose and the meaning of what they do. Grief and loss reactions can result from the sadness of losing yet another year to poor seasons and the personal and community repercussions this entails.

The grief and loss when kids go away … like half of you is missing. You're left with a partner you hardly ever see.
J. Schroeder, personal communication 2009

Doug and Carol's sons attended the local schools but there is a tendency for families who are prepared to make the sacrifice, and who can afford it, to send their children to the city for their high school years to give them an added advantage for the future. However, this means exposure to a different way of life and opportunities that can make it difficult for young people to accept a life back on the farm when they leave school, particularly when they have watched their parents struggling to make a decent living through years of unpredictable seasons and drought. Judy, who has lived in the Mallee for 30 years, told of her son who came back to the farm saying 'is it worth it all when you average 16 hours a day?', having also had his partner leave because 'there was nothing there for her and she was not going to endure that sort of workload' (J. Schroeder, personal communication 2009).

Blokes don't have it (the need for others) as much, seem to be able to manage alone … my husband is lucky he has got his son there and before that his father.
J. Schroeder, personal communication 2009

Prolonged drought can mean that women like Carol work off the farm to supplement the farm's income. It can provide much needed socialization and support for them but means leaving men for longer stretches working alone on the farm. Some men juggle another job off the farm to keep debtors from the door. Other families find they are unable to provide a wage to sons or daughters who want to stay and help.

> I see a lot of … neglect … not looking after their teeth, unopened envelopes they can't face.
>
> **J. Schroeder, personal communication 2009**

Some women have enough of the hardship and leave altogether, with devastating results when they claim a share of the farm and plunge their ex-partner into often insurmountable debt.

Farm properties are usually handed on to a son, daughters missing out in the succession process. A son who wishes to get off the land and not battle continuing hardships can find this is unacceptable to older parents who may not have relinquished their decision-making powers. This can cause increased frustration and resentment with the son and projected expectations onto a grandson.

PROMOTING RECOVERY AND STRENGTHENING RESILIENCE

Mark's Story Continued

> 'What has helped you get through' I asked. 'Lots of things out there if you know where to look … I saw an ad in the paper … from Anglicare … got some financial help … needed money to pay council rates and needed dental care so they helped with that. Also Country Women's Association were giving out food vouchers … then I got this call from this bloke who said he wanted to have a chat – that was Bronte from Centacare. He's prepared to listen to the complexity of what is happening to you, can bounce things off … when I feel alone in the way I am thinking … he can tell me how it is with others … so I get a bit of feedback. When Bronte goes away … I am on a high.'

I have become acutely aware of the number of men and women, like Mark and Carol, who, despite the harsh

environment and prolonged drought conditions, have a deep attachment to their land that keeps them hanging on in the face of emotional and financial hardship. The question is how to provide support to these often isolated, proud farmers who expect to manage a successful farming enterprise without assistance and find discussing problems, financial or otherwise, difficult even with family members. One local worker described how 'the first crash brings them into the system but then … longstanding relationship issues come to the fore that had not been addressed until the drought situation brought them into services'. And not to forget … how to support the women and children affected as well.

> One farmer copes by building fences but he is going to run out of fences to build.
>
> **B. Warneke, personal communication 2009**

Gaining a person's trust has been a consistent factor mentioned by both workers and those who receive services. Services, activities and events that engage, connect and provide support, either individually or as a group, foster communication and sharing, and provide information about help that is available, have had positive results in strengthening resilience and promoting recovery (Box 21-1; Figure 21-2).

Free education and training is encouraged through up-skilling in areas of environmental and business management, realistic succession planning and consideration of the concept of accepting dryness as an ongoing occurrence that needs to be managed differently. Exploring other areas of personal interest can connect and de-stress, and provide another avenue of expression. Supporting people to adapt and adjust to changing circumstances and continuing dryness is essential in strengthening resilience in the face of what the future holds. Resilience is not just about surviving disasters or hardship but being positive, having the ability to act and problem solve and being able to manage the numerous stresses that inevitably come and go in our lives (Repper 2009). Enabling the process of adaptation through a variety of opportunities promotes resilience and assists people to regain health and wellbeing, moderate psychological distress, broaden their safety net of support and provide them with alternative means of consolation when the going gets tough (Greenhill et al 2009).

BOX 21-1
ACTIVITIES AND EVENTS
THAT HAVE OCCURRED IN THE MALLEE AREA

- Free barbecues held in a local park by a group of local service providers with 80 men attending.
- Free boat cruise organized through the local drought support service attracting 60 people.
- Lunch or dinner provided with a programme of speakers who can discuss their services and engage with locals over a meal.
- Information sessions about rural grants, new farming methods, support networks and one-to-one programmes available.
- Forums, seminars or workshops offering training in property management and succession planning.
- Annual sheep fairs and local agricultural shows providing further opportunities for information dissemination by service providers, and locals being available for a supportive chat.
- Encouraging involvement in local sporting clubs. This has proved to be an important social avenue for men to keep in touch and look out for each other.
- A dedicated group in one township made the decision to counteract what was a dying commercial centre by rallying community support to purchase four closed shops. This process not only improved services to those

shopping in the town but made a statement that the community had found a resilience to not give in and to try and turn a negative into a positive outcome. The businesses are making a profit that now goes back into funding projects in the local community.
- Drumming groups have been conducted with participants making their own drums and learning to play them. Some groups have continued to meet.
- Eight-week emotional strength building programmes for women living with anxiety and depression use different activities to assist people to understand their depression, work through grief and loss issues, and enhance mental wellness. Activities include guest speakers, massage and manicures, singing, dancing, tai chi, yoga, creative arts, claywork and collage. Feedback is always very positive.
- Groups bringing women and men together on a regular basis through picnics have sprung up in a number of districts throughout the Mallee, initiated by a proactive local, health worker or church minister.
- In one community a Lutheran minister organized farmers to meet in each other's sheds, have a fire, provide food and have a topic to discuss. It has been very successful.

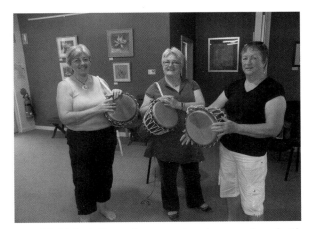

FIGURE 21-2 ■ Drumming groups have been conducted with participants making their own drums and learning to play them.

Initially there needs to be an avenue to disseminate information about events and services such as local newspapers, doctors, town noticeboards, letter drops and cold calling farmers (unannounced phone calls).

KEY LEARNINGS AND IMPLICATIONS FOR PRACTICE

Mark's Story Continued

I could do something else but I don't want to ... it comes from there [pointing to his chest] ... it just does. We do live in one of the driest states ... there is always someone out there who does it tougher ... here if you try and bring things to a seasonal thing ... it just doesn't work.

From a worker perspective the informal events described above are avenues for initial engagement, building trust and to show commitment and interest. Understanding the strong connections to the land, knowledge of the local farming history and the positives people associate with living in that area, and contacting key referral sources such as local doctors are crucially important. Get to know the communities by travelling and exploring the area, engaging in chats with locals over a coffee, being mindful of the role of small businesses within farming communities and the social capital available, and reading local newspapers. All these provide insights and knowledge that can contribute towards gaining the trust and confidence of people so they can be open and frank, not feel self-conscious or judged, speak of their sadness or suicidal thoughts and feel there is genuine interest in their situation.

Farmers and their families want you to take the time to find out what they really need. There will be resistance, but persistence can pay off. I have been told that cold calling farmers has been appreciated when trialled in drought areas. For some, being sensitive to the 'need to disassociate personal problems from the individual, inquiring about the health of the business … gets a better response than discussing the mental and physical health of the person separate to business' (Repper 2009, p. 11).

Post-traumatic stress and issues unrelated to the drought may be expressed, and listening and empathizing are vital in affirming their needs. In these situations knowing who to refer onto is helpful; however, having your own 'toolkit' is also beneficial. For example, I have found acceptance commitment therapy (ACT) and relaxation and mindfulness techniques helpful. Another worker has used interactive drawing therapy with good effect, particularly with men.

Bringing different sectors of the community together to work with the issues, particularly the concept of prolonged dryness, using local knowledge and word of mouth, and providing up-to-date information on grants and financial assistance are what farmers are finding helpful, as is being able to assist farmers to explore alternatives if deciding to leave the farm. Be mindful of supporting local workers as they can be experiencing drought hardship themselves.

From an occupational perspective, I have come to realize that for people who have experienced ongoing natural disaster that has impacted on their health, wellbeing, livelihood and relationships, supporting the person to find what motivates them towards caring for themselves is often the starting point. Encouraging an individual to explore how they can strengthen their sense of self-worth can be the initial step towards regaining 'a balance of physical, mental and social wellbeing attained through socially valued and individually meaningful occupation' (Wilcock 1998, p. 110). Engagement can be a step towards gaining insight into their capacities that contribute to surviving the tough times and strengthening resilience.

In the Mallee, when it rains, there is quick recovery, like the mallee tree which is so resilient – this 'mallee magic' – people take that on too.
J. Schroeder, personal communication 2009

Promoting and strengthening resilience could be further improved through: (1) taking the focus away from 'drought' services, therefore reducing stigma and reflecting a more holistic, inclusive and responsive support service hub for farming and small businesses and their communities within a business and economic framework – 'the stigma associated with a possible mental illness, however temporary, continues to be a barrier to open conversation on the topic and help-seeking behaviour' (Repper 2009, p. 11); (2) workers having contracts long enough to enable them to connect and make a difference; (3) mentoring by experienced farmers for new or younger farmers; (4) supporting women to have greater recognition within the farming culture as viable successors; and (5) utilizing community capacity assessment to assist a community to determine strengths and weaknesses and enhance their resilience (Repper 2009).

In summary, surviving ongoing drought is difficult but many find their sense of place is intricately tied to their land; leaving is not an option. People can lose sight of their personal resilience when there does not seem to be an end to tough times. Finding appropriate and acceptable ways for engaging and connecting in which information is disseminated and support made available can strengthen resilience. This in turn can lead to surviving prolonged drought on a more sustainable level that can focus on being prepared for future dryness through adaptation and adjustment, adoption of self-reliant approaches and being more aware of the health risks and where to find help (Box 21-2).

Acknowledgements

I want to acknowledge the contributions of Judy Schroeder and Bronte Warneke in sharing their experiences, knowledge and stories through working and living within the Murray Mallee region. Also Mark Challans, a Mallee farmer, for sharing his story.

BOX 21-2
INDIVIDUAL CAPACITIES THAT CONTRIBUTE TO SURVIVING THE TOUGH TIMES

- Being able to communicate and be open with others.
- Trusting in others who can provide support.
- Having the history on the land: to be able to say 'what drought?' – this is just the 'natural part of life', the way of things.
- Looking after one's own mental health and wellbeing.
- Connecting to a club or friendship group – e.g. service club, sports club or going to the pub on a regular basis – so that one is missed when not there and blokes look out for one other.
- Good business skills and being open to learning new ways of property and business management.
- Not confusing the business of farming with lifestyle and wellbeing.
- Being able to look longer term than just the immediate situation.
- Sense of belonging and 'place' in the community.
- Having skills or qualifications to find off-farm work.
- Having off-farm investments/savings.
- Discussing health and wellbeing with local doctor.
- Being prepared for prolonged dryness.
- Preexisting viability of business.
- Access to internet/information on health issues, etc.
- Off-farm interests and maintaining friendships.
- 'If it doesn't make a profit it doesn't get fixed.' Only spend money on essentials in time of drought – fixing the header comes ahead of house renovation.
- Prenuptial agreements to decrease risk of farms going into debt or being sold after a marriage breakup.

REFERENCES

Drought Policy Review Expert Social Panel, 2008. It's about people: changing perspective. A Report to Government by an Expert Social Panel on Dryness, Report to the Minister for Agriculture, Fisheries and Forestry, September, Canberra. <http://www.agriculture.gov.au/SiteCollectionDocuments/ag-food/drought/publications/dryness_report.pdf> (viewed 21 August 2009).

Friedli, L., 2009. Don't worry, be happy. Ment. Health Today, 10–13. 2009.

Greenhill, J., King, D., Lane, A., MacDougall, C., 2009. Understanding Resilience in South Australian Farm Families. Rural Society 19 (4), 318–325.

Nickolls, J., Angel, A., 2002. Mallee Tracks: A Wanderer's Guide to the South Australian and Victorian Mallee. Pinnaroo, S Australia.

Pereira, R.B., 2009. The climate change debate: ageing and the impacts on participating in meaningful occupations. Aust. Occup. Ther. J. 56 (Commentary), 365–366.

Repper, J., 2009. 'Enhancing the resilience of Murray Mallee communities.' A report to the Department of Health and Ageing (DOHA) for enhancing the capacity of communities within the South Australian Murray Mallee region to better manage the psychological impact of drought, on behalf of Murray Mallee General Practice Network.

Suicide Facts and Statistics, 2009. Mindframe National Media Initiative. <http://www.mindframe-media.info/for_media/reporting-suicide/Downloads/?a=6011> (viewed 21 August 2009).

Wilcock, A., 1998. An Occupational Perspective of Health. Slack, Thorofare, NJ.

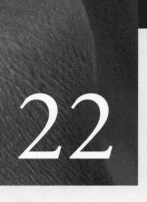

22

SUPPORTING COMMUNITY RECOVERY THROUGH INDIGENOUS ENGAGEMENT AND THE NATURAL ENVIRONMENT

TANIA SIMMONS ■ PENNY SCOTT ■ CHANTAL RODER

On 3 February 2011, vast areas of Australia's Far North Queensland were devastated by Severe Tropical Cyclone Yasi – the largest, most powerful cyclone to hit Queensland in living memory. While many may have considered this a once in a lifetime event, it followed a remarkably similar course to Severe Tropical Cyclone Larry, which wreaked major havoc only five years earlier. The close timing of these two cyclones provided the community with the opportunity to actively apply relatively recent experience in preparing for, and recovering from, such an event.

Terrain NRM is a not-for-profit organization supporting natural resource management (NRM) in the Wet Tropics region of Australia. With climate change scenarios indicating greater severity in weather systems impacting the tropics, a key goal of Terrain is to build long-term community and environmental resilience in the face of natural disasters. Terrain was able to tailor its response to Cyclone Yasi to achieve multiple outcomes across the environmental, social, cultural and economic spheres.

One key lesson Terrain learnt from Cyclone Larry was the strong link between community recovery and the recovery of the natural environment. Despite this, response efforts tend to focus on 'cleaning up' vegetation debris, often impeding the environment's natural recovery processes. There was a clear role for Terrain to play post Yasi to minimize the negative impact of the well-meant recovery effort on the region's environmental assets.

Terrain became involved in one of the early recovery programmes, which funded work teams to assist local landholders to 'clean up'. Employing 50 workers through this programme, Terrain focused its efforts on ensuring the 'clean-up' of key environmental assets was as sensitive as possible. Terrain developed and delivered comprehensive environmental awareness training to its own teams, as well as many of the other teams employed through other non-environmental organizations.

Although the protection of the environment was Terrain's main driver behind participating in the work team programme, there were clear economic and social outcomes of this project. The 50 workers recruited were either unemployed as a result of the cyclone or classified as long-term unemployed, and as well as ensuring the work teams had sufficient environmental training, Terrain tailored the programme to emphasize the wellbeing and motivation of the teams, and to ensure that socioeconomically disadvantaged participants gained as much as possible. Motivational initiatives included:

- running additional wellbeing training, such as nutritional and budget management;
- a worker of the week award, with the prize – a supermarket voucher – decided by the teams;
- a 'brag book' to profile the feedback from appreciative landholders, many of which reflected the level of personal engagement that the teams had with landholders – printed copies were provided to each relevant team member;
- a large photographic display in the Terrain reception area, publicly showcasing the highly valued work they were doing;

- collective lunchtime cooking providing higher quality nutrition, cost savings and enhanced social cohesion.

Unlike many other labour market programmes, attendance was excellent, drop-out rates were exceptionally low, and in most cases people leaving the teams were going to longer-term employment – often in the environmental sector.

Many team members have been traditionally on the receiving end of assistance. To be on the giving end was a source of tremendous pride, particularly during a period of great community need. This enhanced sense of self-worth contributed positively to their own ability to recover. The accolades for their work are testament to the contribution they made:

> *I would to thank and praise the crew that came to clean up the waterways at Dundee Park … they have left Dundee looking better than it has ever done … When the crew returns I will be serving them morning tea because just saying thank you does not seem to be enough.*

Traditional Owner group Girringun Aboriginal Corporation (GAC) through this programme also recruited 60 additional rangers, to complement their existing Girringun Ranger Team (Figure 22-1). During and immediately after Cyclone Yasi, many within the Traditional Owner community felt disempowered and excluded from the broader community response. Despite this, Girringun were determined to ensure their post-cyclone project was an integral part of the response programme and a community-building tool. Not only did this programme provide Traditional Owners with employment after the cyclone, it gave them a strong sense of pride to be helping people in the community. Employment also meant the rangers spent money within the local community, with much needed flow-on benefits to the local economy and businesses. The critical role the rangers played had a very positive impact on the reputation of the Girringun Rangers within the wider community.

> *From a public image perspective our guys were out there helping no matter who they were, black, white or brindle, and in the hour of need they were there*

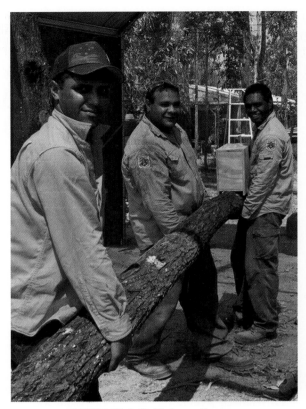

FIGURE 22-1 ■ Girringun Rangers.

> *in force helping the broader community recover. There's been a lot of really positive feedback from the broader community … if we were to do a social analysis of the experience I think the contribution would be enormous.*

> ### *Phil Rist, Girringun Aboriginal Corporation*

The disaster recovery process provided a conduit for previously unrealized local partnerships. Terrain work teams were given the task of 'cleaning up' the Cardwell Country Club golf course – a highly valued community recreational asset that also provides critical shelter and food resources for the endangered mahogany glider. The entire habitat footprint of this species was heavily impacted by Yasi, and through Terrain's post-cyclone work the value of the local golf course as a vital habitat corridor was identified.

During the clean-up activities, a Terrain team felled a damaged tree that contained an active den for a resident mahogany glider. Due to the training the team had received, the glider was recognized and saved, but the incident led to a major rethink about the 'clean-up' of the site and mobilized enormous community support for ensuring the newly recognized habitat values of the golf course were not only preserved but enhanced.

With support from Terrain and local environmental groups, a landscape enhancement plan was developed for the golf course, aimed at closing the gaps between trees, increasing the understorey with native flowering shrubs – providing increased amenity values as well as food for the gliders – and the installation of interpretive signage. The Cardwell Country Club is planning to rebrand its facility as the only one in the world to provide habitat to the endangered mahogany glider.

Girringun were already working with the Queensland Government in post-cyclone mahogany glider recovery, including installing and monitoring feed stations and den boxes. A natural partnership between Terrain, Girringun, community groups and the Cardwell Country Club blossomed, with joint work team days held for tree planting and the installation of 40 den boxes. Importantly, this project brought together all the players around a collective asset – a place of environmental, social and cultural value.

Although the cyclone has inflicted enormous pain on the community and environment of the Wet Tropics, the response presents a range of sustainable partnership opportunities to explore and build on. The foundation established through the Cardwell Country Club project is now evolving into a longer-term arrangement which may see commercial opportunities for the Girringun Rangers in guiding night spotlighting tours, new indigenous 'artscapes' across the golf course as part of the new landscaping plan, and a greater level of engagement between the Traditional Owners, environment groups and general community of Cardwell.

Importantly for Terrain, community perception of the endangered mahogany glider has moved from conservation nuisance to community asset. The Yasi recovery effort has been the driver for a monumental shift in community attitude in a range of areas. For Terrain, engaging in a major labour market programme required a major shift from core business in order to achieve its desired environmental outcomes. However, it enabled Terrain to deliver a triple bottom line outcome. Both Terrain and Girringun have provided many individuals with not only a job during difficult times, more skills and a sound knowledge of environmental management, but also a tremendous sense of satisfaction and an enhanced feeling of self-worth – critical to personal recovery and long-term resilience.

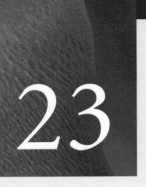

23

CLIMATE CHANGE AND CHILDREN: THE NEED FOR INNOVATIVE RESPONSES

KERRY THOMAS

This chapter discusses the impact of disasters on children and offers a perspective on how human-induced climate change is affecting children. It outlines strategies related to community-based adaptation (CBA), disaster risk reduction (DRR) and child-centred approaches in disaster management, highlights key programmatic areas and child protection considerations, and identifies lessons and directions for ongoing future attention.

A YOUNG PERSON'S STORY

I felt numb. It was like something very big was on me. I felt I could not survive. When the second wave hit, I got loose and was able to go on to the surface. Then, I just went unconscious. When I was in the water, it was like being in a washing machine. Everything was spinning. I felt the sunshine as I woke up on a hillside. I found myself buried under the mud with my head sticking out from the ground. I struggled to pull myself out of the mud and started to run up the hill. My lips were cut through and I was bleeding here and there. I found a couple of farmers on the hill and they told me to keep walking to the village. I walked until I met my mom. I was crying while my mom was washing my face with fresh water. Then she went down to look for my younger brother. It took her several hours to find his body. He did not survive.

Ismael, a 17-year-old boy from Ranong Province, Thailand, elaborating how he and his family were affected by the tsunami in 2004

THE IMPACT OF DISASTERS ON CHILDREN

Millions of people are acutely affected by disasters every year; around 50% of these are children. Children under the age of 5 years, and particularly those who are poor, are most at risk.

Children are one of the most vulnerable groups during disasters because of their age and dependency on others. In the event of a sudden-onset natural disaster, children can become separated from their families. Their carers may be killed or seriously injured, and forced rapid displacement can result in children or parents being left behind. In addition to family separation, emergencies result in children facing heightened risks including psychological distress, physical harm and gender-based violence (ISCA 2008a). The vulnerability of children, especially those who have been separated from their parents and carers, makes them an easy target for exploitation. This is particularly true where local support and protection structures at community level may have been impaired or broken down following a disaster. Boys and girls are at greater risk of being recruited to work in hazardous conditions, such as agricultural labour, factory work or prostitution. In countries affected by both natural disasters and armed conflict, children face the additional risk of being recruited into armed forces or militia groups.

It is for these reasons that children are formally recognized as a 'vulnerable group' in disaster and development policy and practice. As stipulated in the Sphere Project's Humanitarian Charter and Minimum

181

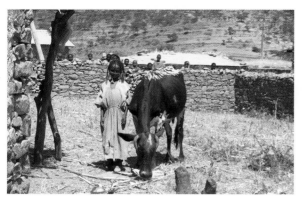

FIGURE 23-1 ■ Girls are particularly vulnerable. Ensuring they have equitable access to disaster response and resilience building initiatives, including livelihoods, is important.

Standards in Humanitarian Response, children are entitled to protection and rights in critical circumstances. This and related instruments demand that special measures be taken to protect children from harm and ensure their equitable access to basic services. Among children, girls and children with disabilities are especially vulnerable, and as such additional attention is required in addressing their protection and needs (Figure 23-1).

Disaster response strategies thus have provision for child-focused action, led by international agencies such as UNICEF, governments, and nongovernmental organizations, most notably the International Save the Children Alliance, Plan International and World Vision. This being said, challenges remain in adequately addressing children's needs across the myriad of actors involved along the disaster management continuum.

DISASTER, CLIMATE CHANGE AND CHILDREN

As Part I of this book elaborates, there is a very evident increase in the frequency, distribution and intensity of disasters across the world, a trend that will continue to escalate with the impact of now undeniable human-induced climate change. The effects of climate change will impact on children directly and indirectly, and will be felt unevenly, hitting children and other at-risk groups including people with disabilities, in developing countries, hardest of all.

Climate change is already beginning to compound existing threats to children's health, food security, livelihoods, protection and education, and escalate degradation of the natural resources upon which human life and wellbeing is completely dependent. Decreasing rain and crop yield, reduced livelihood options and rising food prices all increase the possibility that competition for scarce resources may lead to increasing tensions and violent conflict (ISCA 2008a), migration and poverty (Baker 2009). The combination of the overwhelming nature of disasters and the massive losses they engender gives rise to a complex clinical and social picture with long-term physical, psychological and social effects on children, families and communities (Laor et al 2003). As the frequency of hazards and disasters continues to rise, some families will be facing extremely stressful, almost perpetual dislocation, losing their assets including land and material items, finances, physical and mental health; every time having to start from scratch … and turning to ever more desperate means of survival. All affect child survival, health and wellbeing.

Despite children having no role in causing it, Save the Children (2007) estimate that in this current decade up to 175 million children every year are likely to be affected by the kinds of natural disasters brought about by climate change. An estimated third of the entire global childhood disease burden is attributable to changeable factors in food, soil, water and air (McMichael et al 2008) – diseases and conditions that are predicted to worsen with climate change. As Box 23-1 shows, the resulting impacts are staggering.

While children can show great bravery in the face of adversity, they can also be easily frightened, in large part because they cannot yet fathom big issues like climate change. Children and young people, even in more affluent countries, are especially susceptible to a sense of impending and unavoidable doom: one 2007 survey of Australian children's fears and aspirations for the future revealed that as many as one in four believe that the world will end in their lifetimes (Tucci et al 2007). These feelings may be aggravated by the sense that adults are not responding to the risk appropriately – that, in effect, grown-ups are not protecting their future or, worse, are potentially abandoning their children (The Climate Institute 2011).

So, while climate change is a global phenomenon, adapting to its impacts is very much a local process. In this respect, it is important to remember that *people do not adapt to global trends; they adapt to the changes they experience in their day-to-day lives.* These are in part caused by global climate change, but they are also interwoven with a lot of other factors, including social, cultural, environmental and economic dynamics. Climate change is therefore just one of many things people have to manage simultaneously with other problems, risks and vulnerabilities (Raihan et al 2010). The uncertainty created by natural disasters interplays with other factors, such as unemployment, lack of protection, poverty and unequal distribution of power (Baker 2009, UNICEF 2006, UNICEF n.d.).

In order to understand how climate change affects everyday life, we have to start by asking local people – including children – living with the changes. The effects of climate change are highly contextual; they can intensify existing problems and create new problems, but always within an existing local reality (Raihan et al 2010).

CLIMATE CHANGE: APPROACHES IN ADDRESSING CHILDREN'S NEEDS

While the effects of human-induced climate change are already being experienced, approaches to climate change are largely grounded in 'adaptation' and 'risk reduction'. Climate change 'mitigation', namely efforts to reduce the rate at which the climate is changing by managing the causes of that change, such as reducing greenhouse gas emissions, is noted but not explored in this chapter. Within climate change adaptation and risk reduction, family- and child-centred approaches provide specific guidance on ways to ensure that the perspectives of children and youth are heard through their voices.

Community-Based Adaptation (CBA)

'Adaptation' is about adjusting to current climate realities or expected climate changes and their effects, so that harm is reduced and people can make the most of any benefits that may arise from the changes.

'Good' community-based adaptation, like other forms of participatory development, is community driven, empowering, and strengthens local capacity. Much CBA draws on participatory approaches and methods developed in both disaster risk reduction (DRR) and community development work, as well as sector-specific approaches such as farmer participatory research and participatory primary health care. While DRR approaches are designed to build the resilience of communities to disasters such as floods and drought, CBA incorporates longer-term climate change and its predicted impacts into community-based planning (IIED 2009). Broader participatory community development and livelihood approaches should also be taking into account the effects of climate change, if development gains are to be sustained. It is through these participatory, often cross-cutting processes that the lived experience and views of all

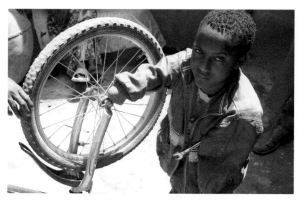

FIGURE 23-2 ▪ Children with disabilities have special perspectives. This young fellow, living rough and ostracized by many in his community, exemplifies the extraordinary tenacity and resilience that exists among many marginalized people. Even without hands, he can change and repair bicycle tyres in minutes, providing himself with a livelihood and respect. He has clear ideas about what will help him in the face of adversity.

community members – including families and children – can be ascertained and built on (Figure 23-2).

Communities have a wealth of knowledge about the local environment, and have been adapting to and coping with change for years (Box 23-2). Although this knowledge and traditional coping mechanisms may become less effective as climate change leads to greater unpredictability in weather patterns (e.g. rain coming at any time rather than at predictable times) and more extreme events (e.g. droughts and floods), they remain an invaluable resource and the platform for local action.

Initiatives directed towards directly engaging children and youth in CBA are emerging. These can be seen through the growth and utilization of youth environmental groups and representatives in broader community planning, action and advocacy activities (e.g. interPART 2006). Across the globe, education curricula are expanding to include consideration of climate change, sustainability, and social and environmental development issues; school kitchen gardens are blossoming and environmental monitoring and action is being nurtured.

Supporting such initiatives are resources such as *Climate Extreme*, a youth-friendly summary of a publication produced by the Intergovernmental Panel on

Climate Change (IPCC 2012), the *Special Report on Managing the Risks of Extreme Events and Disasters to Advance Climate Change Adaptation* (IPCC 2012), which looks at how climate change affects disasters, how people are being impacted now and will be in the future and how we can support people to become more resilient. *Climate Extreme* (Fawcett 2012) describes how young people around the world are contributing and stimulates thinking about what else can be done by children, youth and the wider community to adapt to the risk of climate change related disasters.

Disaster Risk Reduction (DRR)

Disaster risk reduction is a process of improving people's preparation for future disasters as well as the response to, and recovery from, disasters when they happen. This can take place at local, national and international levels.

Child-centred DRR (CCDRR) recognizes that children can play an important role in helping their families, villages and communities to reduce the risks associated with natural disasters.

As the case study in Case 23-1 illuminates, children can and should be involved in all aspects of DRR work in their communities, from assessment to implementation.

Child-Centred Approaches

Despite an emphasis on 'vulnerability', it is important not to presume that children are incapable of coping during disaster. They are not helpless victims. While children are in a particularly susceptible developmental stage in their lives without the benefit of the life experience of adults, many of us have witnessed the impressive ability that many children have to stay resilient during calamities, and that their high energy and participation efforts during emergencies can be of crucial value.

As the case study in Case 23-1 highlights, empowering children through their participation is also an important protection strategy; it prevents them being alienated from their rights and reduces their vulnerability in critical circumstances. Very often it is an organization's or adult's lack of knowledge and awareness that can inadvertently exacerbate children's vulnerability, in both normal and critical circumstances. In fact most children have remarkable

BOX 23-2
CBA: UNDERSTANDING AND ACTION AT THE LOCAL LEVEL – SOME KEY CONSIDERATIONS IN FACILITATING COMMUNITY-BASED ADAPTATION PROCESSES

- *Local people know local conditions.* These conditions include weather patterns, changes in ecological systems, what grows where, when and under what conditions, the effects of environmental changes – all are dynamic factors that underpin environmental health and productivity, including food and water security.
- *Livelihood is the number one concern.* Ability to access basic needs (food, water, shelter, safety) and to achieve health and wellbeing is a fundamental concern for all people, particularly families and children, and especially for the majority world who are poor and have limited access to social welfare safety nets.
- *Climate change as one factor among many: people don't just live in a climate, but in a world shaped by social, cultural, environmental and economic factors.* Integrated, holistic approaches based on local scenarios assist people to manage climate change challenges simultaneously with other problems, risks and vulnerabilities.
- *Adaptation must build on local experience: it is difficult to distinguish between climate change impacts and other problems that people experience in their relationship with nature and their efforts to make a living from it.* Adapting to climate change is thus not something that requires an entirely new approach. It is essentially about community development and sustainability.

- *Three types of knowledge are important: local knowledge, scientific knowledge and knowledge about rights.* Local knowledge enables people to analyse their situation and helps them gain a practical understanding of their context. Adaptation must also draw on scientific knowledge to ensure an understanding of climate change and its causes. Adaptation initiatives must provide people with knowledge about their rights and how to demand them. Together, these types of knowledge can empower people to take collective action.
- *Protecting people and assets from disaster.* Development of adaptive strategies takes time and, given climate change unpredictability, may not be fully effective in mitigating the impact of disastrous events. There remains a simultaneous need to strengthen actions to better protect people and assets, especially in high-risk and vulnerable communities.
- *Fostering capacity for collective action.* While the needs of individuals cannot be overlooked, the scale and complexity of climate change impacts demand collective action – at local and regional levels, up through national and international forums – if resilience, transformation and rights-based approaches are to have the impact necessary to transition successfully into the emerging new world.

Adapted from Raihan, M.S., Huq, M.J., Alsted, N.G., Andreasen, M.H., 2010. Understanding climate change from below, addressing barriers from above. Practical experience and learning from a community-based adaptation project in Bangladesh. ActionAid Bangladesh, Dhaka.

coping capacities and can play an active role in recovery and development activities aimed at reducing their risk and building resilience, provided their abilities are recognized and their issues and concerns are mainstreamed in all stages of programme interventions.

This being noted, there are nevertheless important ethical and protection considerations in working with children across the disaster management arena. In disasters, children are particularly vulnerable due to a range of risks: family separation, sexual exploitation and gender-based violence including rape. Box 23-3 summarizes key programming priorities that international organizations have identified as deserving highest consideration when designing protection efforts for children in emergency situations. It is interesting to consider these also from a climate change adaptation perspective.

As part of disaster response, recovery and preparedness programmes, child-centred strategies are continually being piloted and refined for wider implementation by international NGOs in partnership with local organizations and government departments. They lend themselves to application in climate change CBA and DRR initiatives, and can intersect with family-based and community-based approaches, particularly where families and communities are risk. Indicative examples include:

- *Child friendly spaces (CFS),* which are now a feature of emergency and longer-term recovery programmes. They can be constructed in any available space, such as under trees, in a tent or in a courtyard (Figure 23-3). With support from families and community members who volunteer to lead the activities, children have the

CASE 23-1

Children and Disaster Risk Reduction (DRR)

In 2004, six provinces in southern Thailand were severely affected by the Indian Ocean tsunami. More than 50 000 children and families lost their lives and livelihoods. International nongovernmental organizations (INGOs) responded to the needs of children and families through livelihoods and psychosocial support in the first phase of the disaster response. One INGO initiated a 'Child-Led Disaster Risk Reduction' (CLDRR) programme with school children in four of the worst affected provinces in the second phase of recovery. This 'bottom-up', participatory approach to DRR was a new approach in Thailand.

Participation is among the basic principles of children's rights, as stated in the UN Convention on the Rights of Children, and is also a fundamental community development principle. With these in mind, the goals of the DRR initiative were to: (1) build children's knowledge of DRR; (2) build the capacity of children for DRR actions within their communities through an educational campaign; and (3) sensitize adults and civil society (schools, communities, government officials, partner organizations) to the importance of involving children in DRR.

The programme was implemented through local partner organizations with an emphasis on advocacy, children's rights, and capacity-building towards empowering children to have a meaningful role in DRR activity. The CLDRR project targeted children in 40 schools in Phuket, Ranong, Phang Nga and Krabi, and as an entry point to also reach children in the community. The age range of children participating in the project was 10–18 years old. The children engaged in DRR activities related to building knowledge of DRR concepts and definitions, conducting community surveys, producing community risk and resource maps, and providing an educational campaign in schools and communities.

Together, local partners used participatory methodologies to engage children in learning about the relationships between disaster, hazards, vulnerability and capacity in order to provide a foundation to analyse disaster risk in their local community. Children prepared interview questions for community members and observed community activities. Based on these data they analysed the community's risk and developed a resource map identifying the disaster/hazard risk area, capacity and vulnerability of the community. In the final step, children implemented a DRR educational campaign involving drama, a puppet show and poster to educate and change attitudes and behaviours of community members. The ultimate goal was to build a safer culture in their community.

Through the CLDRR project the children gained knowledge, skills and self-confidence, and revealed their inherent capacities to play a key role in DRR and in building their futures. This experience demonstrated that children can act as positive agents of change, protecting themselves as well as their families and communities in the face of disaster. In addition to several significant successes, there were a number of challenges that illuminated the need for adult support at a higher level (e.g. provincial and national) to support the engagement of children in DRR. Although adults at the community level showed extensive support for children, those at provincial and national level were yet to recognize the children's capacities. In order to receive recognition and strategic support from central government, it may be argued that programmes such as CLDRR need to provide evidence at the national level that children can play an active and genuine role in reducing disaster risk in the community. This requires further development of children's technical knowledge and skill in DRR and cultivating opportunities for children to work alongside INGOs to advocate for their role in DRR.

Case study developed from Save the Children experience, ISCA, 2008a. In the Face of Disaster: Children and Climate Change. International Save the Children Alliance, London; ISCA, 2009. Reducing Risks, Saving Lives. International Save the Children Alliance, London; Save the Children Sweden, 2010. Living with disasters and changing climate. Children in Southeast Asia telling their stories about disaster and climate change. Including W. Chaimontree interview note; Vanaspongse, C., 2007. Towards a Culture of Prevention: Disaster Risk Reduction Begins at School. UNISDR, Geneva.

BOX 23-3
CHILD PROTECTION: SOME KEY CONSIDERATIONS IN DISASTER MANAGEMENT

- *Protect children from physical harm, exploitation and gender-based violence:* design programmes and establish systems to prevent the occurrence of abuse; provide activities that care for survivors and reintegrate them back into their families and communities where appropriate; provide special protection for especially vulnerable children (e.g. children with disabilities); establish child friendly spaces; implement strong monitoring systems.
- *Protect children from psychosocial distress:* prioritize programming that enhances families' protective behaviours in crises and encourages the development of pro-social behaviours for children including enhanced self-esteem, hope and a sense of self-efficacy; strengthen children's resilience through humanitarian action; establish child friendly spaces; provide careful, culturally appropriate therapy.
- *Protect children from family separation:* prioritize family-based programming and preparedness activities and connect with coordination systems; facilitate the reunification of families when it is in the best interest of the child; provide support and occupational engagement opportunities for unaccompanied minors.
- *Protect children from risks related to displacement:* prioritize programmes designed to address risks (e.g. trafficking, prostitution, militias, as well as disease risks) through increased access to meaningful occupational activities, education, livelihoods and health services; avoid inadvertently exposing children to further harm; establish strong monitoring systems.
- *Protect children's access to rights:* ensure access to impartial assistance; facilitate access to health and education; build children's capacity to claim their rights.

CPWG, 2013. Minimum Standards for Child Protection in Humanitarian Action. Child Protection Working Group, Global Protection Cluster: Save the Children, Terre des Hommes, UNICEF; Save the Children UK, 2006. Watermarks: Child Protection During Floods in Bangladesh. Save the Children, London.

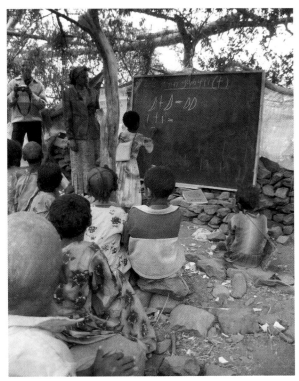

FIGURE 23-3 ■ Access to education is a fundamental right and facilitating it is a child-centred disaster and development activity.

opportunity to play, sing and socialize with their peers – and to regain a sense of normalcy in difficult times. CFS provide places where therapeutic activities can also be provided. They also help keep children safe during the day, giving parents/carers an opportunity to focus on finding support and services and to rebuild their lives. Experience of CFS is widely available through, for example, published case studies and various manuals (e.g. *Child Friendly Spaces in Emergencies: A Handbook for Save the Children Staff*, ISCA 2008b).

- *'Pictures for Life'*, where children consulted communities in undertaking a social equity audit (SEA) to assess whether relief and reconstruction had been distributed efficiently and equitably. Children attended training and then conducted surveys, backing up their findings by taking photos of the people they interviewed. The children gained a sense of responsibility through their meaningful endeavours, as well as the respect of their home communities (Plan International 2008, India).

Video methods have also been successfully used. In 'Amplifying Children's Voices on Climate Change', Tamara Plush (2009) describes how the process of participatory film-making proved more effective than traditional methods, such as workshops and lectures, in helping children understand climate change impacts, identify coping strategies, prioritize their adaptation needs and advocate for change, and through the process of 'doing' built skills and resilience and was a catalyst for change (Change with Children in a Changing Climate, the Institute of Development Studies and ActionAid Nepal).

■ *Reducing risks and enhancing safety* by mainstreaming child-centred DRR into schools and conducting sessions to teach essential survival skills and ways that children can prepare themselves for natural catastrophes (Plan International 2008, Philippines). In applying the knowledge they acquire, children can keep themselves safer and can also pass this knowledge on to adults, who may not be as well versed in disaster preparedness. Incorporating DRR into education and after-school activities is an important way of increasing the skills base, confidence and capacity of local communities (ISCA 2008a).

■ *Concern and contribution trees*, where children (and adults) write or draw their concerns or problems either directly onto a poster, or on coloured 'leaves' which are pasted or hung on a 'tree'; using another coloured 'leaf' they are also encouraged to identify things they could do or contribute to address issues. This can be done over time to allow people to contribute as and when they feel comfortable, and anonymously if needed, but as a public tree the results can be read, discussed and actioned together. Actions can be documented in the tree's root zone, reflecting the nutrients that can build the tree's strength and resilience. Activities such as this use a problem–assets based approach that empowers through building common understanding and confidence and capacity through collective action.

Variations of this technique include *happy-sad boxes* where children can post notes or pictures in secure boxes where designated counsellors, teachers or centre staff read and can then offer advice and support. In contexts where young people are shy, diffident or wary of speaking out about their troubles, such processes help to build trust. It also promotes greater openness

about the challenges children face (Plan International 2008, Sri Lanka).

Children should thus be considered as key stakeholders in disaster management and climate change action – they can be excellent advocates, communicators of good practice and active agents of change. Experience shows that enabling the participation of children and young people in preparedness, emergency response, rehabilitation and reconstruction initiatives not only generates more effective programmes but is also therapeutic and healing for young people who may have experienced trauma.

Use of peer approaches can be particularly effective and is readily adapted to CBA, DRR and disaster response and preparedness activities, while appropriate youth representation and engagement in mainstream planning and decision-making forums can bring multiple awareness-raising and outcome benefits if adequately supported or facilitated. Age, gender and cultural factors influence perspectives and need to be considered in successfully enabling such participatory processes.

Child-centred approaches are more commonly applied within those programmatic domains that have particular child-focused disaster management concerns. These include health and rehabilitation, water and sanitation, shelter, food security and nutrition, livelihoods, education, child protection, disability and development. However, given the nature and experiential perspectives of climate change, more cross-sectoral, holistic child-centred initiatives are emerging and evolving. These aim to access a range of views, knowledge and experience to generate actions that can be effective now but also have a positive influence on the future (Figure 23-4).

Lessons Learnt and Future Challenges

■ *Rights:* Across the disaster continuum and climate change approaches, it is crucial to include children's views in assessing the situation and their needs. Plans and responses should be built on children's specific needs as reflected in local contexts and occupational interests and experience; these should not be based on general assumptions. In doing so, the real needs and issues experienced by children are addressed, and children's rights will be upheld.

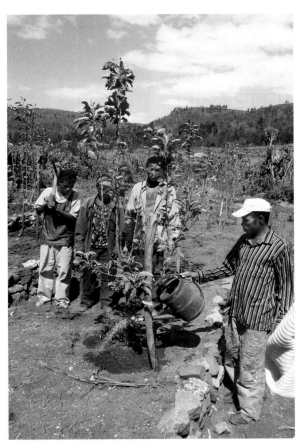

FIGURE 23-4 ■ Children and adults working together, in cultivating mixed, drought-tolerant crops, generates multiple benefits that strengthen capacity to respond successfully to climate change impacts.

- *Protection:* Children have a right and expectation to be protected from harm. Climate change, and the myriad type of disasters that may result, brings significant and particular risks for children. Standards and guidelines exist to protect children in emergencies and need to be followed. Supporting organizations and personnel to understand, implement and monitor these obligations requires ongoing work.
- *Participation:* Children's participation is equally as important as child protection. Children's participation in designing, carrying out and evaluating DRR and other strategies is key to achieving a sustainable approach to building resilience among children and families. Involving children in understanding the root cause of the problem through DRR activities helps survivors regain their lives, supports capacity building and provides empowerment in the face of climate change. However, children's participation as a concept and approach requires careful and ethical facilitation to ensure it is meaningful, informed and genuinely respected. Furthermore, it should be inclusive of all groups of children, boys and girls, including those with disabilities and from different cultural, socioeconomic backgrounds.
- *Adult facilitation:* The involvement of adults to support children's capacity in CBA, DRR and child-centred approaches is a key area to be strengthened. Children's participation and capacity in CBA and DRR cannot solely rely on their own agency; adults at different levels, from community to national, must take a role in supporting children. Sensitizing and enabling strategies directed towards enhancing adult understanding of the importance and value of children's participation and a positive attitude towards children's capacity are an ongoing need.
- *Roles:* Research (IIED 2009) and experience show that children and young people can participate in climate change and DRR activities in a number of different ways:
  - as *analysers* of risk and risk reduction activities;
  - as *designers* and *implementers* of projects;
  - as *communicators* of risks and risk management options (especially communications to parents, other adults, or those outside the community);
  - as *mobilizers* of resources and people; and
  - as *constructors* of social networks and capital.
- *Advocacy:* Advocacy activities are required to promote appreciation for children's capacity and their outputs from participating in CBA and DRR activities, such as risk and resource maps and child-designed and implemented education. Advocacy should emphasize and support the active involvement of children across the disaster continuum, including during disaster responses. Where agencies listen to children's needs and opinions, accountability for children is improved;

not only does it enact children's rights but it contributes to ongoing community building, resilience and transformation.

■ *Policy and institutional arrangements:* In tandem with 'bottom-up' strategies, effective CBA and DRR depend on policy action and services that support community initiatives. This includes action to curtail carbon emissions as well as establishment of cross-sectoral programming arrangements to integrate climate risk information and address adaptation as it is lived. To manage climate impacts adequately, specific strategies are also required to strengthen health systems, food security and nutrition, livelihoods and social protection programmes, as well as ongoing investment in community- and child-centred DRR and CBA. At national levels, commitment to implement the Hyogo Framework for Action, particularly building local capacity, is also required.

■ *Research and evaluation:* In support of programming and policy development, and the promotion of 'best practice' approaches to address and engage children in disaster management and climate change adaptation, further research and evidence is required. At another level, there is a need to better understand and manage the relationship between the human mind, the socioeconomic fabric and climate change, including addressing fear, despair and a sense of powerlessness that can paralyse action. Opportunities also exist to strengthen mechanisms for sharing results and learning, and utilizing these to improve performance.

■ *Personal action and role modelling:* As disaster practitioners, educators and policy makers, we are also citizens in global and local communities, with mutual concerns for health, wellbeing, sustainability and intergenerational equity. In addition to facilitating personal, family and local emergency preparedness actions as appropriate, we can each take responsibility to actively 'think globally and act locally' in relation to climate change by embracing sustainability and adaptive management practices. If each and every one of us took mindful action to reduce our own greenhouse gas emissions, and adopt reduce–recycle–reuse and renew and replenish practices, we would be contributing to a more viable future for our own children and grandchildren as well as those who are most at risk of climate change impacts.

■ *Occupation:* Across the challenges of climate change and disaster, and responses that address immediate needs while promoting resilience and transformation into the future, it is occupation that provides the conduit for engagement and achievement of desired outcomes. Occupation is both a process and a product in these initiatives, serving children and the wider community.

Considering that children comprise around 50% of those affected by disasters, strategies to address their needs and to actively engage them in disaster response programmes and in climate change DRR and CBA are an imperative.

Children are the future, and are capable of co-creating their own destinies.

Young people have a unique perspective both about the risks they face themselves and about those present in their communities for others. Young people also have unique abilities to lend to climate change adaptation and mitigation. They are a strength, both for the present and the future.
Climate Extreme (Fawcett 2012)

Acknowledgements

Development of this chapter was supported by contributions from Sophapan Ratanachena and Chitraporn Vanaspongse, who previously worked with Save the Children in Thailand.

REFERENCES

Baker, L., 2009. Feeling the heat. Child Survival in a Changing Climate. International Save the Children Alliance, London.

CPWG, 2013. Minimum Standards for Child Protection in Humanitarian Action. Child Protection Working Group, Global Protection Cluster: Save the Children, Terre des Hommes, UNICEF.

Fawcett, A., 2012. Climate extreme: how young people can respond to disasters in a changing world. Produced by Plan International on behalf of the Children in a Changing Climate coalition (UNICEF, World Vision, Plan International and Save the Children); Australian Aid. <http://plan-international.org/about-plan/resources/publications/emergencies/climate-extreme-how-young-people-can-respond-to-disasters-in-a-changing-world/>.

IIED, 2009. Community-based adaptation to climate change. Participatory Learning and Action 60. International Institute for Environment and Development, London.

interPART, 2006. 'We Make a Difference': An Evaluation of the Catchment Care and MurrayCare Programs. For the South Australian Murray-Darling Basin Natural Resources Management Board. interPART and SAMDB-NRM.

IPCC, 2012. Managing the Risks of Extreme Events and Disasters to Advance Climate Change Adaptation. A Special Report of Working Groups I and II of the Intergovernmental Panel on Climate Change. Cambridge University Press, Cambridge.

ISCA, 2008a. In the Face of Disaster: Children and Climate Change. International Save the Children Alliance, London.

ISCA, 2008b. Child Friendly Spaces in Emergencies: A Handbook for Save the Children Staff. International Save the Children Alliance, London.

ISCA, 2009. Reducing Risks, Saving Lives. International Save the Children Alliance, London.

Laor, N., Wolmer, L., Spirman, S., Wiener, Z., 2003. Facing war, terrorism, and disaster: toward a child-orientated comprehensive emergency care system. Child Adolesc. Psychiatr. Clin. N. Am. 12 (2), 343–361.

McMichael, M., Friel, S., Nyong, A., Corvalan, C., 2008. Global environmental change and health: impacts, inequalities and the health sector. Br. Med. J. 336, 191–194.

Plan International, 2008. From Catastrophe to Opportunity: Children in Asia Creating Positive Social Changes after Disasters. Plan International Asia Regional Office, Bangkok.

Plush, T., 2009. Amplifying children's voices on climate change: the role of participatory video. In: IIED 2009 Community-based Adaptation to Climate Change. Participatory Learning and Action 60. International Institute for Environment and Development, London, pp. 119–128.

Raihan, M.S., Huq, M.J., Alsted, N.G., Andreasen, M.H., 2010. Understanding climate change from below, addressing barriers from above. Practical experience and learning from a community-based adaptation project in Bangladesh. ActionAid Bangladesh, Dhaka.

Save the Children Sweden, 2010. Living with disasters and changing climate. Children in Southeast Asia telling their stories about disaster and climate change. Save the Children Sweden, Bangkok.

Save the Children UK, 2006. Watermarks: Child Protection during Floods in Bangladesh. Save the Children, London.

Save the Children UK, 2007. Legacy of Disaster: The Impact of Climate Change on Children. Save the Children, London.

The Climate Institute, 2011. A Climate of Suffering: The Real Costs of Living with Inaction on Climate Change. The Climate Institute, Melbourne.

Tucci, J., Mitchell, J., Goddard, C., 2007. Children's Fears, Hopes and Heroes: Modern Childhood in Australia. Australian Childhood Association, Melbourne.

UNICEF, 2006. Child Protection Information Sheet: Trafficking. UNICEF, Geneva.

UNICEF. n.d. Child Trafficking. Available at: <http://www.unicef.org/eapro/activities_3603.html>.

Vanaspongse, C., 2007. Towards a Culture of Prevention: Disaster Risk Reduction Begins at School. UNISDR, Geneva.

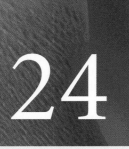

24

MEDICAL ASSISTANCE TEAMS: REFLECTIONS ON EMERGENCY RESPONSE EXPERIENCE

VALERIE RZEPKA ■ NATHAN KELLY

In this chapter, two practitioners reflect upon their involvement with Canadian Medical Assistance Teams (CMAT) and the paths they forged into the field. Both practitioners speak of human resilience in their efforts to respond to the medical and public health needs of people affected by disaster. Their stories are interconnected yet offer unique perspectives on the challenges and triumphs of volunteering in the field.

'HOMELESS, ROOFLESS, BUT NOT HOPELESS'

VALERIE RZEPKA

Resilience. Of all the experiences a relief worker has when working in a disaster zone, the most profound observation is resilience. Whether it is children who are playing soccer in a field next to their collapsed school, or local merchants setting up their fruits and vegetables on top of the rubble that was once the walls of their shop, strength of character and the resilient nature of the human race is something I find incredibly awe-inspiring.

My first experience responding to a disaster happened by chance. I had booked a vacation to Thailand to depart on 2 January, 2005. Little did anyone know that on Boxing Day a week prior to my scheduled departure, a 9.8 magnitude earthquake would spawn a tsunami that would sweep the Indian Ocean, taking over 250 000 lives in its wake. Having spent several years working as a registered nurse (RN) in paediatric critical care, I was not sure if my skills would be of use, but I decided to try anyway.

On a visit to the island of Koh Phi Phi Don, off the coast of Phuket, Thailand, I came upon a volunteer-run clinic being managed by ex-pats. They heartily accepted me as a volunteer, and I proceeded to treat both local and foreign patients with what limited resources we had. The 'clinic', which was housed in the washed out remains of a hotel lobby, provided basic health care services. We had some medications, basic first aid supplies, and our own skills and knowledge – a far cry from the highly technical, complex critical care I was used to providing in a downtown Toronto hospital, with resources and assistance at my fingertips.

As I would come to learn, after a tsunami there are generally not very many injuries; one either lived or died. It was communicable diseases such as dengue fever and acute watery diarrhoea that our patients were dealing with in the aftermath. Any physical injuries that we treated were generally related to the clean-up and recovery effort, such as puncture wounds from nails, or lacerations from glass or metal.

Aid work is not without risk, as I too caught dengue fever while in Thailand, resulting in my early departure from Asia, a short hospitalization and prolonged recovery at home. But I did not let illness weaken my resolve. I had discovered in myself a sense of satisfaction, and a new passion that compelled me to redirect my career trajectory and become a humanitarian aid worker.

While many people desire to travel to far-off places and help the world's poor and suffering, being a humanitarian aid worker is not for everyone. The work is exhausting, the hours are long, and the conditions are extremely difficult. The experiences are also emotionally taxing, and there is a high level of post-traumatic stress experienced by humanitarian aid workers. Anyone considering becoming an aid worker needs to be confident enough in their own skills to be able to think critically and respond creatively when unusual or unexpected situations arise. They must be self-directed enough to find tasks and duties that need to be done, and yet able to take direction when needed. Most importantly, an aid worker needs to be self-aware and realize their limitations. While delivering aid is a noble gesture, especially from those who volunteer their time, recognizing physical and emotional exhaustion and burnout in oneself is the key to remaining a resilient aid worker.

Not long after I had recovered fully from my illness, a 7.6 magnitude earthquake struck northern Pakistan, centred near the city of Muzaffarabad, Kashmir. Within a few hours I was in contact with an informal Canadian relief group and agreed to travel to Pakistan as their Field Medical Officer. Over the course of the ensuing three months, I oversaw several rotations of teams who treated hundreds of patients in this remote region of the Himalayan lowlands.

In this theatre in particular, we found that the provision of postoperative nursing care and rehabilitative services was severely lacking. This was attributed to the fact that many local nurses and allied health care staff perished in the earthquake when hospital buildings collapsed. Those who did survive had their own families and homes to attend to, and were unable to return to work in the immediate aftermath. We collaborated with local and federal authorities, coordinated by the United Nations 'Health Cluster', and set up our clinic inside a local hospital, which was the only one of the three that remained standing. In the early days we delivered the front-line care for patients who were clustered in tents in the grounds of the hospital. As the weeks of recovery wore on, and people began to return to work, we felt it was important to make the transition as smooth as possible, and so we developed a training programme for the local staff, to teach them proper aseptic wound care techniques. After a few weeks the transition was complete and the local workers took over full responsibility for providing health care for their community.

Our team rotations of Canadian nurses, nurse practitioners, doctors and paramedics found that although there were a significant number of ex-pat volunteer surgeons who came from around the world to the region to provide medical and surgical care, there was little or no concern for the medium to long-term postoperative follow-up, which was either sorely lacking or completely absent.

We found that we were treating patients who had been operated on several weeks before who had never once had a dressing change done, the majority of whom had significant wound infections and occasionally bone infections. We saw children whose broken bones had healed using external fixation rods, but without anyone to surgically remove the rods the children were running around on their healed legs with rods sticking out of them.

Most importantly, we treated pain. The postoperative patients who were seen in our clinics had very poor pain management and control, but did not voice complaints. Their stoicism and resilience were evident and we were able to treat their pain successfully with basic acetaminophen or ibuprofen. However much they had lost in this disaster, the relief and gratitude on their faces was immeasurable.

By the time our project in Pakistan wrapped up, I knew that disaster response and humanitarian aid had become my primary area of interest and passion. While I pursued a Master's degree on a related subject, several colleagues and I came together to formally incorporate Canadian Medical Assistance Teams (CMAT), a grassroots disaster relief organization. Funded solely by private donors at present, CMAT's volunteer roster is made up of health professionals and nonhealth-related volunteers who give their time and resources to provide medical aid to the victims of natural and complex disasters around the world.

Since its inception, CMAT has responded to earthquakes in Pakistan, China, Haiti, Chile and Japan. We also sent volunteers to provide primary health care services in flood-affected regions of Bangladesh and Pakistan. More recently, our teams responded to the typhoon that struck the Philippines in November 2013. In all, CMAT's health volunteers have treated over 25 000 patients, delivered dozens of babies, and made huge impacts on countless lives around the globe.

As we approach the tenth anniversary of CMAT's inception, we are looking to expand our mandate. At present, due to limited resources, CMAT responds solely to major global natural disasters, and has a presence in the field of 60–90 days. The purpose of our deployments is to help fortify the surge capacity of the local communities and their first responders, allowing them the opportunity to recover. By helping the community in their transition from recipients of relief to active participants in recovery, CMAT helps to foster the development of higher quality health care delivery. We encourage the involvement and employment of local staff in all our deployments, and typically utilize local nursing and allied health students as our translators, allowing them to gain useful and relevant work experience to help them enter the workforce.

Through all our work we endeavour to promote a culture of resilience, starting with our volunteers. One of our CMAT volunteers, a registered psychologist, has helped CMAT to develop a member wellness programme that allows our team members the opportunity to address their own emotional response to the events they have experienced. CMAT is also now in the process of developing a system of online training modules and skills workshops for our volunteers, many of whom have already received training in the Sphere Minimum Standards in Humanitarian Response.

In the greatest of hardships, it is the resilience of the human spirit that always seems to shine through and guides us in our efforts to provide humanitarian assistance. In November 2013, following the third largest tropical cyclone in recorded history that struck the central Visayas region of the Philippines, I was reminded of the resilience of the human spirit. The devastation left in its wake was immense, and together with the rest of the humanitarian world, CMAT's assessment team was mobilized immediately. On arrival in the province of Leyte, the scene was one of total destruction: fields of palm trees toppled over like a box of toothpicks; roofs of major buildings like hospitals and shopping malls blown clean off. It was believed that electricity would not be restored to the area for at least 6–8 weeks. In the early evenings, smoke from cooking fires made our eyes burn. The streets of Ormoc were littered with debris, broken tree limbs and

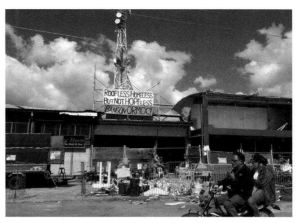

FIGURE 24-1 ■ Homeless, roofless, but not hopeless.

shattered glass. Amidst this loss and devastation, we saw neighbours helping neighbours clean up the mess. And in the centre of town on one of the main buildings there was a hand-painted banner (Figure 24-1) that read:

'Roofless, Homeless, but not Hopeless. Bangon Ormoc! ['Rise up!']

HAITI: A RETROSPECTIVE FROM A CMAT VOLUNTEER
NATHAN KELLY

The 6.9 magnitude earthquake that struck Haiti in January 2010 caused widespread destruction and loss of life, and affected the health and wellbeing of males and females of all ages. This, in a country that is already experiencing longstanding chronic disaster as related to the social determinants of health, political instability and corruption, corporate exploitation, lack of employment and gender inequality, allowed for a further decline into calamity. Hundreds of thousands of Haitians lost their homes or shelters, became internally displaced persons (IDP) and were forced to move into large camps where space was available. The camps housed thousands of persons and families in small shelters made of sticks and plastic tarps. Most camps did not have access to fresh water and sanitary outlets. These cramped, hastily built shanty towns quickly became a destructive and unsafe environment for the vulnerable, especially females. These were my preliminary observations in the first few days of my humanitarian pursuits in Haiti.

The earthquake struck just as I had graduated with my Bachelor of Science in Nursing from Brock University in St Catharines, Ontario, Canada. Writing the provincial licensing exam could not come soon enough, as my thoughts were with friends and colleagues who were volunteering and had boots on the ground in the devastated country. Once I was confirmed as a living, breathing RN, it was not long after that I received a call from a good friend, Valerie, the executive director of the NGO, Canadian Medical Assistance Teams (CMAT). Valerie invited me to join a team going to Haiti that comprised a doctor, nurse practitioners, registered nurses and paramedics. I was humbled by the opportunity and accepted. A couple of weeks later I found myself on an Air Canada flight out of Montreal bound for Haiti. It was not until we were taxiing on the tarmac for takeoff that I came to a realization that this would probably influence my perspective on life, the world, and the moments that define relationships both with family, friends and colleagues. Indeed it has, and it has tempered me into a more well-rounded person and registered nurse.

I will always remember when the crew cracked open the cabin door after we landed. The heat and humidity were overwhelming and would continue to be so throughout the two weeks ahead. Clearing through customs took some time but we gathered as a team and proceeded through the chaos of people who greeted us as we stepped through the gates into Haiti. Our driver found us amidst the sea of people and we loaded into a Toyota pickup truck and travelled onwards to Petionville, a more affluent area of Port-au-Prince.

You see, CMAT had partnered with another NGO to provide health care services from basic primary care to triage to trauma (Figure 24-2). They had set up camp on the only nine-hole golf course in Haiti, which now housed (for lack of a better term) 60 000 internally displaced persons. Our partner organization was responsible for the building up of the IDP camp including roads, trenches, fresh water, latrines and showers. This was not done alone but with the assistance and collaboration of many other NGOs. CMAT provided the medical personnel of various backgrounds to assist Haitian medical personnel to treat and respond to the diverse needs of the sick, injured

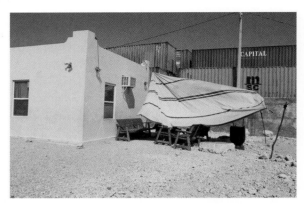

FIGURE 24-2 ■ Triage and waiting area.

and infirm. As a recent graduate my critical thinking and theoretical knowledge would be put to the test. Never did I think that my first practice setting as an RN would be a disaster zone. Luckily, I was deployed with an amazing team of health professionals who would guide my thinking and practice and help me to manage the situations and environments that I had otherwise not seen in a structured health care setting in Canada. Our partner organization had set up a large military-style field hospital tent. It housed 14 stretchers for general treatment, a trauma area, a maternal/child birthing area and a small pharmaceutical and supply area. Every working day would start at 08.30 and end at 16.30. Each day I would observe a lineup of approximately 500 people looking for medical service, of whom our team would see half. Most would start lining up in the early hours to ensure they would be seen, as by midday it was too hot to wait any more.

At the age of 36 and as a new graduate RN, I had a lot of life experience mixed with new knowledge base from a medical perspective. Much of what I noted from the people I triaged was high blood pressure, dehydration, undernourishment, wounds, follow-up wound care, sexually transmitted infections (STIs), gender-based violence (GBV), urinary tract infections (UTIs), yeast infections, birthing, febrile seizure, and post-traumatic stress disorder (PTSD) across the lifespan. Although we were one of the better equipped NGOs we were still limited in what we could deliver, especially regarding mental health care. Luckily, other NGOs had set up in a building within the IDP camp with mental health professionals to assist those in need. I found myself to be wearing many caps as I put together clinical interventions for each individual that presented themselves in front of me. To this day I take the knowledge and experiences learned and apply them to my day to day practice, whether in the hospital or community setting.

Although not nearly all of my experience is captured here in these words, I am offering a mere glimpse and my perspective of the challenges faced in an austere environment within one of the largest IDP camps in Haiti. This experience has sparked a larger interest in disaster response and I am currently pursuing my Masters of Science with specialization in Disaster Healthcare from the University of South Wales, Wales. As we grow as a global village, and disasters grow in frequency and magnitude, as doctors, RNs and allied health professionals, we need to be prepared to work collaboratively and offer our skills and resources as needed.

In June of 2011, I made a second trip to Haiti as a volunteer with another NGO that was involved in long-term recovery and development. The focus of this NGO was maternal and child health, gender-based violence, well-woman/well-baby checks, sexual health and community development projects. A small clinic and teaching facility was built in Wharf Jeremy, a small neighbourhood within Cité Soleil, the most impoverished, violent and neglected community of Port-au-Prince. I took a four-week leave of absence from my hospital job in Canada to return to Haiti to continue the hard work of recovery from the earthquake in 2010. The government had just been reinstated, with Michel Joseph Martelly having been voted by the Haitian populus as their president. As I travelled throughout the Port-au-Prince area in the coming weeks I observed a sense of optimism from the Haitian people I met, of all ages. President Martelly was extremely popular and seen as the president to bring truth to the government and the rebuilding of the economy to bring jobs and address the chronic systemic abject poverty that affects most of society there.

I arrived in Haiti with my friend and colleague Rebecca, and met with Mark from an NGO founded in the United States. Mark brought us to the compound where we would be staying for the next few weeks. The home was owned by a wealthy Haitian who owned motels in the Port-au-Prince area and lived in Montreal as well. He and his family were kind enough to house various micro-NGOs in the short term as well as the longer-term volunteers in a spacious home surrounded by tall cement-built walls with barbed wire on top. Access to the inside was only possible by a locked thick steel gate. We paid US$25 daily to stay in the compound which provided us with a shared bedroom, three meals daily, access to washrooms and water as well as electricity, wifi and security. This daily fee also provided jobs for local people to clean the home and prepare meals, giving all a sense of inclusiveness and belonging. During our stay the evenings were often enhanced by songs in chorus, mostly church related, underscoring their strong Catholic faith and the commitment to moving forwards with their lives.

Upon our arrival we met with Maeve, a young, fiercely dedicated Irish RN who was the medical director of the clinic in which we would be practising. We instantly got along, which made our experiences richer and our ability to bring about health care service easier and more successful. To this day we all remain friends and continue to talk about further collaborations in the future. Maeve explained that the clinic had just been up and running for a few weeks and she was grateful for the professional help. A schedule provided consisted of a commute with a hired Haitian driver across Port-au-Prince to Wharf Jeremy that would take 35 minutes to an hour depending on the traffic and other incidents such as flooding, broken-down vehicles, human traffic, accidents or rallies. It was estimated we would arrive at the clinic at 09.00, set up and begin seeing women and children who would have been arriving hours beforehand. On Tuesdays there would be a Haitian doctor available for assessments; on Thursdays a Haitian obstetrician–gynaecologist would be present as well as an ultrasound technician who had moved to Haiti from the Midwest United States (with functioning equipment!). Mondays, Wednesdays and Fridays, the clinic would only be occupied by us volunteer RNs, two hired Haitian nurses, and our two hired Haitian translators. When we were presented with patients whose conditions were beyond our capabilities, we would have them transported by our Haitian driver, RN and translator to the nearest appropriate hospital for treatment. As you can imagine, our translators were our lifeline and as I only knew enough French to get by on the street, and no creole, I relied heavily on them and grew to appreciate their friendship beyond measure. Our days would conclude by 15.00 or 16.00 when people would stop coming as they would be getting on with their days and responsibilities (as well as the sweltering heat). On an average day we would have 60–70 people waiting for us when we arrived, with the Haitian nurses triaging, taking vital signs and interviewing for presenting complaints.

Much of what we saw was undernutrition, dehydration, headache, febrile illness, UTIs, yeast infections, STIs, GBV (Figure 24-3) and sexual abuse. We struggled as a team to help as there were few or no resources to refer to or supplies to treat effectively. We had a small pharmacy supplied with donations of various medicines, rehydration salts and vitamins. As I happen to be a male RN it became evident over time that word was spreading throughout the neighbourhood that I was there, because more and more males would come to the clinic to see me. Many had STIs that they were afraid to bring to the attention of a female nurse. Most were assessed and treated by me and the Haitian doctor on Tuesdays. Reflecting on the weeks spent in this clinic I can now say that we provided gold standard care to an impoverished neighbourhood overlooked by the international NGO response in the acute and longer-term phases of the Haitian disaster.

After a week or so we noticed that the numbers of people coming to the clinic sharply decreased. This perplexed all of us and so we decided to walk about the neighbourhood with our translator and the hired

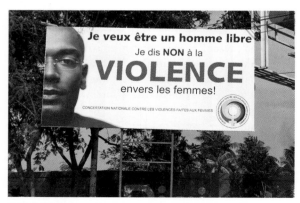

FIGURE 24-3 ■ Government awareness campaign in 2011 addressing gender-based violence.

security guard that lived in a tent behind the clinic. Garcon was a popular person within this established community of around 3000 and brought us to all areas including his destroyed and crumbled home that he shared with his wife and children. He recalled the earthquake and how they escaped injury and how the community came together to assist one another during the time of crisis. As we continued on, we walked along a deep ravine with a slow trickle of water making its way to the wharf nearby. As there were no services for garbage collection pre and post disaster, people would just throw their refuse along the ravine and into the water. As the plastics and other garbage broke down, the land and water would become toxic and contaminated. These toxins would enter the water system in the wharf where the fish were caught and entered the food chain. Also, free range pigs and goats would meander through the ravine eating the refuse, including the plastics, and would be used as a food source by the locals. This highlighted the need for education linking environmental health to human health but seemed to be a daunting task as this neighbourhood was representative of all the IDP camps and neighbourhoods and presented a systemic problem wherever I travelled.

Through further dialogue with Garcon we were able to uncover the reason why our clinic numbers were declining. It seemed that a local gang had been coming to the clinic after hours and intimidating Garcon and his family. As a result, Garcon had agreed to charge an upfront fee for those seeking health care from the clinic to give back to the gang in exchange for protection. This had been happening for a few days, explaining our decline in numbers. We asked Garcon to ask the gang members the next time they met if we could meet with them and negotiate some terms. Garcon agreed and the following day when we arrived he stated that they would meet with us the next day at the clinic. When we arrived the next day in the morning there were four young men at the clinic doors. All were friendly and shook our hands. We decided as a group to walk over to a small scantily built structure that passed as a bar on the main road leading to the neighbourhood. It was one room with a few chairs. There was an electric freezer in disrepair at the back and a small bar with a selection of beers and liquors. We purchased a round of beers for them and began a dialogue with our translators. Soon after, it was identified by these young men that they were unemployed and did not have any hope for employment. They spoke of their families and neighbours living in poverty and the struggles to survive from day to day. As an offer of good faith in the spirit of negotiation, we offered to assist in resuming building as well as to offer education in English in the small two-room school next to the clinic in exchange for people to have free access to our clinic services. To the advantage of all they agreed and would come to the clinic and the school in the coming days and weeks. By partnering with these young men and focusing on building capacity, we were able to foster tangible self-efficacy and as a result supported the resilience and rebuilding of community ties from within.

A few days later, after a walk about through Wharf Jeremy, we returned to the clinic and were met by a well-dressed older man. He introduced himself and stated he was a teacher at the local school. I asked where the school was and the grades involved. He stated the school was for younger children from 6 to 12 years. I made plans with him to meet the following day at the clinic and to have a tour of the school. He was quite excited and proud to have us express interest in what he did and the school at which he taught.

We met with him and two younger male teachers the following morning. He brought us to a small cinder block building with a partial corrugated metal roof, the rest being covered with tarp and pieces of plywood. The school was near the bar where we had met with the young men whom we were now assisting. The dirt floor was uneven and susceptible to flooding due to the large exposed areas of the roof. Inside were partitioned areas with hardwood benches three deep. The areas were separated by large plywood boards used as chalkboards. The teacher explained that each separated area was a different grade and that school was not currently in session. Much discussion was had regarding school attendance and the struggles for funding to provide a quality education. During our conversation I did suggest that the nurses and other staff at the clinic could provide, from time to time, some public health education appropriate to each grade. I suggested that the younger children could be taught to identify potable, safe water for drinking and personal use as well as proper handwashing and hygiene. I had also suggested educating the older children regarding sexual health, gender-based violence and proper nutrition. All the teachers this day were happy to hear of this collaboration with the clinic and the potential it had to positively influence young minds and hearts. Myself, I was feeling a sense of joy as this was a terrific opportunity to provide a foundation of lifelong knowledge supporting the notion of health and safety. Most of the follow-through was completed by other clinic volunteers weeks and months after my departure back to my life in Canada.

Disaster can strike anywhere, at any time; for others, particularly in poor regions of the world, it is a part of everyday life. As an aid worker, whatever your background, you cannot remain detached from the communities you become committed to, and it is important to acknowledge and monitor stress levels. I have learned much from my experiences in my trips to Haiti and can speak to the power of resilience, not only within the individuals and communities we serve, but within ourselves as humanitarian aid workers. Witnessing calamity and hardship from day to day may cause an unacknowledged decline in coping, but continuing forwards in fostering resilience in individuals and communities will bring positive influences to the hearts and minds of humanitarian aid workers with boots on the ground.

25

DRINK A DOZEN CUPS OF TEA: LESSONS ABOUT LISTENING AND LEARNING

ADELE PERRY

SNAPSHOT OF TODAY

I sit writing this in a guest house in Islamabad, listening to the sound of afternoon prayers and conversations in Urdu drift in the window. I am here for a short time working as an inclusion advisor for the international nongovernmental organization, Handicap International. The conflict that continues in the northwest of the country and natural disasters that have occurred in the last 10 years leave an increasing number of vulnerable and poverty stricken people, including persons with disabilities. My one-month mission here is focused on assisting Handicap International develop a new strategy that will support all vulnerable people, particularly persons with disabilities, to participate fully in society and benefit equally from humanitarian aid and development programmes.

THE SEED IS PLANTED

My journey to this point began nine years ago, at the end of my first year at university while studying occupational therapy. Not understanding occupational therapy at this point, and disillusioned with the prospect of working in a hospital for the rest of my career, I attended a lunchtime presentation on 'Operation India'. I heard about the experiences of occupational therapists (OTs) who had completed their fourth-year clinical placement in India. The terms 'community-based rehabilitation' (CBR) and 'community development' were coupled with words such as 'challenging', 'creativity' and 'initiative', and phrases like 'think outside the box', and 'make a difference'. By the end of

the presentation I was intrigued and excited and, for the first time since beginning my course, felt like maybe there was some part of this profession that was for me. Three years later, as a result of the mentorship and encouragement of those members of faculty with a passion for CBR and community development, I boarded a plane bound for India.

THE FIRST STEP

Operation India was my first step into the world of 'development' and despite all the briefings, cultural awareness and theory of CBR that occupied my mind, as soon as I stepped off the plane into the humid, sweet yet putrid smell of the Bangalore night, I realized that all the theory in the world was not enough to prepare me for the reality of life in a developing country.

Over the next seven weeks my fieldwork partner and I struggled to apply the theory of CBR to our situation, floating from confusion to frustration, from enthusiasm to exhaustion, but all the while learning by trying, learning through doing and questioning why? how? what for? for whom? By the end of our placement, with the help of my supervisors and local colleagues, I felt that I had connected the theory with my experiences and gained a clearer understanding of CBR and its place in development.

However, on a personal level I realized that more important than the professional learning was what I had learnt about myself – about how I cope in challenging environments and also about culture and cross-cultural relationships. I kept a reflective journal throughout the experience through which I gained valuable insights into my communication style and the profound impact my Anglo-Australian, upper middle class upbringing had on my communication with, and view of, people of other religions, cultures and classes. It is hard to come to terms with the realization that you are, to put it bluntly, an ignorant snob. I had good intentions to help and lots of enthusiasm, but lacked understanding and appreciation of the local context and experience. It was a significant first step in a long journey of self-realization and learning that continues today. Operation India had given me a glimpse into the world of development and, despite still feeling confused about what I had learnt professionally and personally, I felt that I had found my direction as an OT.

MAKING THE LEAP

Six months later, urged by my always encouraging mentor, I headed to the Solomon Islands as an Australian Youth Ambassador for Development (AYAD) to teach at the Solomon Islands Community Based Rehabilitation Unit. Apprehensive and feeling completely unqualified for the position, I embarked on a journey that took me on sheer cliff learning curves, everything from managing a project, to teaching and supervising students, into deep valleys of exhaustion and frustration at the laidback culture and conflicted situation in the Solomon Islands, and into sleepy villages on remote islands. Through these experiences, I learnt that development is a long, slow process that can only be achieved by drinking numerous cups of tea and chewing kilos of betel nut in order to understand the situation and build trust with the community.

By the end of the 12 months, my understanding of how to work effectively in another culture had deepened thanks to a lot of practice in cross-cultural communication, support from my mentors, and simply time spent in the field. I had gained valuable new project management skills and had contributed to the development of CBR in the Solomon Islands. Importantly, I had seen that my background as an OT was useful for working in development.

THE NEXT STEPS

International development is a tough business to break into and with only one year of experience in the field and an OT degree, my chances of getting a 'decent' job were very slim. After half a dozen applications and a reminder from my mentor that I needed to 'do the time' and get more experience, I relented and began searching for volunteer and internship positions. My first stop was the Australian Volunteers International (AVI) website, and it was not long before I sat staring at the description of my next job: OT with the United Nations Relief and Works Agency (UNRWA) for Palestinian refugees in Syria. It seemed like my OT skills were again the thing that would get me into the field.

My 18 months as an AVI volunteer with UNRWA provided me with an opportunity to learn more about the complexity of the Israeli-Palestinian conflict, the impact of conflicts in Lebanon and Iraq, the Arabic language, and the beauty of Arab culture and Syrian hospitality (Figures 25-1 and 25-2). I was exposed to the frustrations and joys of working for the United Nations (UN), juxtaposed with the lives of refugees, and the reality of development and humanitarian aid within Middle Eastern politics. My time in Syria again challenged my ability to cope and forced me to wrangle with my own beliefs, prejudices and weaknesses.

My role with UNRWA was supposed to be focused on building OT capacity within the physical rehabilitation section of the disability programme, but as it turned out my OT skills were used for more than just training professionals and helping people recover from illness and disease. After several months of not really knowing what I was supposed to be doing, but seeing

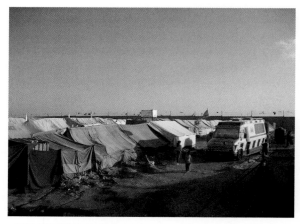

FIGURE 25-1 ■ Refugee camp on the Syria–Iraq border.

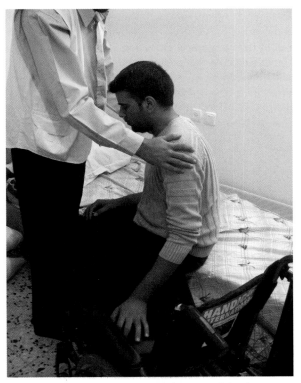

FIGURE 25-2 ■ Occupational therapy training in Gaza.

the potential of OT beyond individual rehabilitation, I knew I had to convince my UNRWA colleagues that OT was a profession whose core business was to promote participation in occupation. I needed to show that my skills could be used to assist people with disabilities participate actively in their lives and communities through more than just therapy.

Having my colleagues recognize my potential to contribute as an OT was only part of my successful integration into UNRWA. I realized that after five frustrating months of feeling like I had achieved nothing of significance, I had actually achieved the most important things of all by sitting in people's offices asking questions, drinking tea and attending endless meetings in Arabic. I had built positive relationships, rapport and trust, the very foundation of any real development work. Although my results-driven head told me I had achieved nothing, I had laid the foundation for effective work of true value.

For the remainder of my time with UNRWA I worked on promoting participation of refugees with disabilities in occupation and further developing my skills in project cycle management. This involved: writing a situational analysis of the disability programme; mainstreaming disability issues in the UNRWA Syria strategic plan; making recommendations on the Agency's disability policy; and starting rehabilitation services for Iraqi Palestinian refugees with disabilities in Al Tanf refugee camp – all of which was possible because of my OT perspective on enabling participation through occupation.

WALKING THE LINE BETWEEN DEVELOPMENT AND HUMANITARIAN AID

After two and half years of volunteering and gaining varied knowledge and skills, I felt qualified and up to the incredible challenge of working in an emergency context. In the wake of Operation Cast Lead in Gaza, I was offered a job with Handicap International as part of their emergency team. My role was to work with the UN Cluster system as the lead of the disability sub-cluster. Through my work, I continued on from what I had done with UNRWA in Syria, and mainstreamed disability issues in the work of other clusters. The other part of my role was to promote coordination among organizations providing humanitarian assistance to persons with disabilities.

Unlike development work, I learnt that emergency humanitarian work requires a quick response: rapid needs assessments, decisions made on information available at the time to preserve life, and not necessarily the level of input from the community that you require for development. However, despite the need for a quick response, the one lesson that I took away from my time in an emergency team is that you still need to make the time to drink those cups of tea. You need to truly listen to the people you are endeavouring to help as the starting point of all intervention. At some point the emergency will end and what you have done must still contribute to long-term development.

Following the conclusion of HI's emergency response, I stayed with HI in the role of Gaza programme manager. After 12 months in Gaza – 4 months in an emergency role and 8 months in the transition back to development – I left Gaza feeling physically and emotionally exhausted and frustrated by the complex and dire situation. Despite this, it was rewarding to know that I had contributed to changing the lives of a few people with disability.

I returned to Australia, where I began working for CBM Australia as an International Programmes Officer, managing projects that empowered people with disability to participate in their communities and live meaningful and purposeful lives. I continued to use my core OT skills in some way or another, all the while developing new, complementary skills. I was also reminded daily of the need to stop and listen, to hear what my colleagues and the beneficiaries were saying, and then act. This was especially important when I visited projects in China, Indonesia or the Philippines. With only a short amount of time to visit each project, it was important not to make assumptions but to listen, observe and ask hundreds of questions. With the information gathered, I could better assist project partners to empower people with disability and work for their inclusion in society.

After 18 months I took a job with the CBM-Nossal Partnership for Disability Inclusive Development, building the capacity of humanitarian and development organizations to include people with disability. I again had the opportunity to learn new skills, but I was also able to use my knowledge and experiences to guide disability inclusion work. More recently, I have taken some time out to complete a Masters of International Development. This provided me with a theoretical basis for all I have seen and done and an opportunity to do research which has better equipped me to support the inclusion of people with disability in humanitarian and development work.

So as I sit here in Pakistan, reflecting on my journey, I can tell you that whenever I start a new piece of work I still have to remind myself to stop and listen, to drink those cups of tea and hear what people are saying rather than making assumptions. I often have to fight the feeling that the situation is too hopeless and that what I am doing is not making a difference. But whenever I meet a project beneficiary who has been empowered to participate in their community, I am reminded that by using my core OT skills and accumulated knowledge I have the ability to support change in the lives of at least a few people with disability and the communities in which they live.

MOVING FORWARD

Working in development and humanitarian aid is not easy. There are plenty of challenges, but also many opportunities to learn and to have a positive impact. To survive the challenges and work effectively in emergency and development contexts, I have learned to:

- Believe in the strength and resilience of the people you are trying to help and believe that you are making a difference.
- Drink a dozen cups of tea and listen before acting.
- Get yourself a good mentor and network with others who share a vision.
- Trust your ability to problem solve and use your core OT skills in any environment.
- Remember that the lives of those you are assisting will go on after you have left; all you can do is strive to empower people.

My advice to others – do not be scared to take that first step or even that leap into the world of development, but be prepared to listen, learn and be challenged, both personally and professionally.

26

CHANGING FIELDS OF PRACTICE: TRAINING IN THE FRONTIER PROVINCE, PAKISTAN

MIRIAM KOLKER

The car is surrounded by people, including a young boy selling lollies. It is mid-morning and we are inching our way through a town in North West Frontier Province so slowly that the boy is literally leaning on the car while giving imploring looks for a sale. The main street is also the market and is lined with stalls selling everything from fruit and vegetables, to goat carcasses to clothes, fabric and toys. Dust fills the air and people are going in every direction. I look out for women and count about four. For once, I am grateful for the dubatta over my head, as I can hide under it from the stares as men brush past the car.

I am in Pakistan, working for an international NGO (nongovernmental organization) that has been here since the earthquake that devastated this region in 2005. It is 2008 and there is still much 'rebuilding' to happen. We are working alongside the government to address issues affecting people with disabilities, who in these mountainous northern areas have had little or no access to services. The number of people disabled by the earthquake is now realized to be small when compared with the numbers of previously unidentified people with disabilities living in these remote earthquake-affected areas. I am on my way to run a training workshop on 'access and home modifications', and this is only about the second time I have felt really productive since arriving in Pakistan some three months ago.

The project I have come to work on is constantly changing under conflicting pressures from the government authority we are working with and the funding body. The team is somewhat inexperienced and organizational support seems far away. Or maybe headquarters have not been made aware of the issues being faced; I am not in a position to know. My role is the intermediary between the office in Islamabad and the four regional offices/resource centres. So far I have not travelled out to these centres as much as I had expected, due to a combination of security issues, being required to 'hold the fort' in the absence of other staff in Islamabad, and my line manager wanting me to remain in the office to learn as much about the project as possible before venturing into the field. I feel it is taking too long to get out there and be 'doing' something but bury my frustration. I know from experience and the few trips I have made so far that actually being in the field is more productive (and rewarding) and you learn more than being stuck in the office.

I am also the voice for the field staff, their link with the multitude of changes coming out of the Islamabad office and the key support in helping them deal with resulting difficulties in working with their government counterparts. The government also has centres in the same towns as us and while the working relationship on the ground is reasonable in most places, it is tricky at the intermediate level, which impacts on our staff at times.

So there I was on my way to do the second lot of accessibility training. It was a great opportunity to use my occupational therapy (OT) skills and broaden my role within the project. I think about the planning behind these training sessions and how at the outset I wondered how I would squeeze four years of study into a three-day session. How can you impart

205

professional knowledge and clinical reasoning in three days? Who do you train? One person on the project expected I would train everyone including the community-based workers (who have the least amount of education). I queried the ethics of this and whether it would lead to unsound recommendations, so it was decided I would train our staff and others from partner organizations who are physiotherapists or have already received training around disability.

I felt the first workshop was great. The group (which included one female) thrived in the interactive setting; they loved the small group work, and the community visit to practise assessing public building accessibility and to measure for a ramp. They were hungry for knowledge and ideas and absorbed everything I could share with them! And I was pushed to unearth my most creative training skills (with no electricity most of the day, we put butcher's paper and participatory techniques to good use). Throughout the process, I learnt more about their skills and knowledge and identified gaps that may impact on successfully putting the training into action. It felt productive and rewarding!

REFLECTIONS ONE YEAR ON

Now, a little over a year later, I am back in Australia, browsing photos and reflecting on the whole experience. I think as OTs we are taught to reflect very well, and it usually generates valuable insights.

I guess if someone had asked me in the beginning why I went to Pakistan, I would tell them I went to Pakistan for a change. After several years working with remote and Aboriginal communities in the Northern Territory (in Australia), I left hoping to work in an environment where I could make some real difference and could see that difference in a timeframe of a year or so. I also wanted to get experience working in overseas development, to gain skills so I could continue in this line of work. My goal was to learn as much as possible. I wanted to learn about project management, about planning, monitoring and evaluation, and proposal writing, and have the opportunity to practise these skills. Finally, I was also going for some adventure and to work within a country and culture that intrigued me many years ago when travelling through that part of the world.

When I first returned from Pakistan, my thoughts and concerns were about the fact I had left pre-

maturely and that it felt as if I had not gained the skills and experience I had hoped to gain. I guess I was thinking about getting another job and writing up the curriculum vitae. But over time I relaxed about that and started to reflect on what an amazing and challenging encounter I had just had. I realized that through it all I had learnt a lot – just much of it not what I expected to learn. Thinking about the whole experience – why I was there, what I was hoping to achieve and whether I did actually make a difference in any way – made me realize the really important thing was not about what I was there for, it was not about building my own capacity but about building the capacity of the local people, so they could carry on when I left. This awareness has, in particular, made me rethink some of the initial concerns I had around the training in accessibility and home modifications.

I found myself thinking about the first training session in remote Azad Kashmir and in particular the young man I met, made paraplegic by the earthquake. Aqeel was one of the lucky ones; his house had been modified and he was independent within the house. He did, however, need the assistance of two or more strong people to negotiate the ramp to the street, a short steep ramp constrained by the lack of space all around within a crowded town on the side of a very steep hill (Figures 26-1, 26-2, 26-3 and 26-4). What I remember most about this meeting is his mother's tears and how, with little English, she conveyed her despair for her son's future, particularly in securing a wife or another job in

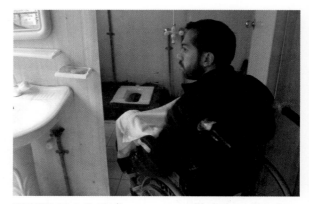

FIGURE 26-1 ■ Finding ways to enable independent functioning in activities of daily living is part of the training for survivors and disability workers.

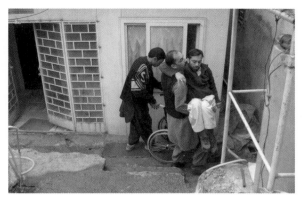

FIGURE 26-2 ■ Aqeel requires assistance to access the street from his home (the space is too steep and small for a suitable ramp).

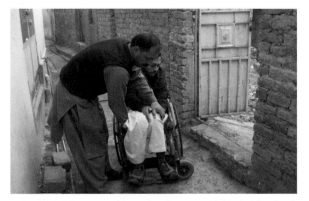

FIGURE 26-3 ■ Aqeel is assisted to re-position in his wheelchair after being carried up to the street.

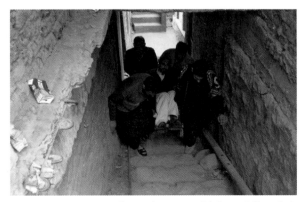

FIGURE 26-4 ■ Aqeel experiences multiple mobility challenges in getting out into the community.

his profession of engineering. I guess this emphasizes the limits of the training … access to life and occupation might well begin with physical accessibility, but there was just not the space there to build a 1 : 14 gradient ramp … and so the environment mocks my original concern about community-based workers making 'unsound recommendations'.

Regardless of how good my training might be, all those I train will be forced to make modifications that will not meet any standards due to the physical setting – the natural barrier to accessibility that so many people face in these mountains. But I do believe the training will help them to make the best modifications possible, to make informed decisions based on knowledge. So I hope those I trained, and those they go on to train, pick up most on the message that accessibility is far more than just having a ramp that meets standards, and can employ their best problem-solving skills to make it easier for people like Aqeel to get out and achieve those other goals in life. I also hope the training contributes to raising awareness around the issues facing people with disabilities.

LETTING GO

In reflecting on these hopes and the extent to which I may or may not have been successful in encouraging them, I now realize that it was right to 'let go' and not let 'professional ownership' get in the way of providing this training, that the ethical thing to do was to train locally based people. My initial unease with trying to pass on all my education and experience disappeared soon after I started preparing the sessions. I realized I was dealing with needs and issues that go way beyond anything I was taught at university and now see that the crux of this training was the 'teaching' of problem-solving skills. My learning curve was probably as steep as that of my students; I had never been taught to modify a house made from stacked stones or a squat toilet! We were working in remote areas that would require a lot of creative, locally sourced solutions. There are so few OTs in Pakistan and the need for this sort of knowledge and skill is too great. I can see now that if I did not empower local people to make recommendations for home modifications or equipment, then how else would things change for people with disabilities? Their need far outweighs my 'professional' dilemma, and with ongoing support and extra training to address identified gaps in knowledge, I felt our staff could make a real difference for people with disabilities and their families. In these remote, under-resourced areas they were already working to raise awareness and encourage other community-based organizations to include people with disabilities in their programmes, so now they could help people with disabilities to 'get out' and access all that is on offer, such as education, livelihood training and participation in community life.

LEAVINGS AND LESSONS

Unfortunately I ended up leaving Pakistan earlier than intended and did not get a chance to address the gaps identified or see the modified homes. Amidst increasing security and changing programme management, I was not able to properly wrap up, or even to say goodbye to some colleagues. This feeling of 'unfinished business' has been difficult, even though it can be rationalized as a factor to contend with when working in disaster and development contexts.

Reflecting on the experience – and even the writing of this story – has helped put the whole experience into context. I did not get to practise all the project management skills I thought were so important, and I may not have achieved what I thought I would, but together with the local communities we did achieve many things and the experience taught me some important lessons.

We made a difference at many levels, starting with the local staff. They are the key to this; even when our project ends, they will go on to work on another project or somewhere else and will take their learning and experience with them … and so the ball will roll on. They will make the difference, not me, and that's the way it should be if impact is to be sustained and extended.

My personal achievement is a lot simpler. I worked in Pakistan for a year, survived and had my eyes opened to development work. The emphasis shifted – the desire to meet my personal and professional needs faded and the focus became the people and communities I worked with, which is really what this sort of work should be about and is what I would really like to do more of. With this has come insight and learning that will continue to inspire and impact on my life and practice as an OT, wherever I travel and work. In addition, the experience motivated me to enrol in a Master of Public Health (MPH) qualification and through that I have gained many of the desired skills and a more thorough understanding of the principles underpinning work in development contexts.

For those wanting to work in disaster and development contexts, here are a few pointers that may help you be prepared, survive and be successful:

- Countries like Pakistan, where conflict and security issues infiltrate development work, are not easy places within which to work; there are significant religious, cultural and language differences to manage. Consider leaving your comfort zone locally before jumping head first into somewhere really tough overseas.
- Learn as much about the employing organization and programme as you can before you leave, and insist on an orientation even in 'emergency' situations.
- Identify and access all the resources and supports (human and technical) available to you, before leaving and on arrival; network.
- Once you are there, especially in a country with security issues, be flexible and attentive. Seek and listen to the knowledge and experience of the local people. Do not leave for tomorrow what you could do today.
- Look after yourself: try to keep a work/life balance, have supports and keep a sense of humour. Make sure you know your own stress signs and have strategies to deal with stressful situations. Do not always rely on your organization to do this for you and do not hesitate to ask for support if you feel you need it.
- Record your journey along the way (e.g. a diary, journal, emails to friends, photos). Do not forget the amazing experiences and people you meet that offset the challenges. This will help you to process/reflect upon the experience.

27

MOBILIZING A THERAPEUTIC RESPONSE IN A DISASTER ZONE, CHILE 2010

CECILIA FARIAS BASADRE

BACKGROUND

On 27 February 2010 an earthquake with a recorded intensity of 8.8 on the Richter scale (the fifth most violent ever registered) and tsunami struck Chile. Chilean territory lies where two geological faults converge. Our country is not only used to enduring earthquakes but it is also well prepared to resist them from an engineering and architectural point of view. People who live in the coastal zones know how to evacuate their homes in case of a tsunami. This is evidenced by the fact that there were only just over 300 casualties from the 27 February earthquake and tsunami, in an affected region of 7700 inhabitants. The destruction of infrastructure and high-rise buildings was not of an apocalyptic nature as in other countries that experience an earthquake of that magnitude. However, many people's lives were affected that day. Not only did they lose their homes and belongings (Figure 27-1) but many also lost their job sources, particularly those involved with fishing, farming and forestry.

The earthquake struck 450 kilometres south west of Santiago where I live and work as an occupational therapist. I am from Chile and so I was able to see the need and respond immediately, mobilizing what I call a 'therapeutic operation' to go to the most affected zones of the country, assess the situation and help the victims in dealing with the tragedy. Drawing upon my personal, professional and institutional networks I summoned people to assist on a voluntary basis through personal invitations, emails and phone calls. I requested assistance in the form of team members

willing to collaborate, offer their skills and provide a sustained commitment of time, or donations of money or items to support 'leisure' and 'wellbeing.' The response was immediate, numerous and enthusiastic.

THERAPEUTIC OPERATIONS

We targeted the district of Pelluhue, located in the Maule region along the coast. The chosen locations were Pelluhue, Curanipe, Chovellén and Salto de Agua. We partnered with the health department of Pelluhue and together we defined the human groups and spaces for intervention and our project aims:

Groups/Spaces for Intervention

- Staff at the health department engaged in response activities.
- A primary health care station located in Curanipe.
- Two emergency camps for displaced persons.
- The rural community of Salto de Agua.

Project Aims

Over the course of one year, the project aimed to:

- Establish 'wellbeing spaces' where people could go to rest, reflect, access peer support or engage in leisure or relaxation activities.
- Reintegrate people affected by the earthquake into their usual occupations.
- Build the foundations to support 'occupational performance'.
- Promote 'occupational redesign' in order to improve quality of life.

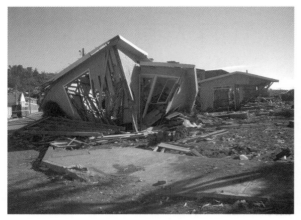

FIGURE 27-1 ■ Destruction of a home in the Terapeutica Pelluhue Curanipe area, March 2010.

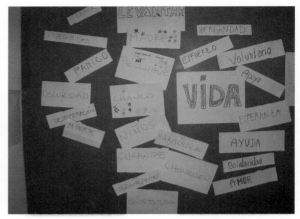

FIGURE 27-3 ■ Therapeutic activity with the local health team. During the process, team members were invited to express in a few words the different emotions they had lived through and experienced:
- *Past:* during the earthquake and tsunami: darkness, fear, panic, desperation, etc.
- *Present:* at that time of the intervention: wake up, mother, kids, the names of locations.
- *Future:* what they envisage after this: life, effort, hope, volunteer, support, love, brotherhood, solidarity, help.

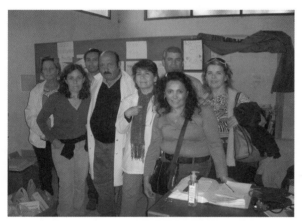

FIGURE 27-2 ■ Members of the combined health and therapeutic team.

- Strengthen mental health and wellbeing.
- Increase disaster preparedness.

Several operations were planned over the one-year duration involving teams of skilled volunteers from diverse backgrounds (Figure 27-2). Our first operation occurred three weeks after the earthquake and included seven professionals (one medical doctor, two psychologists, two occupational therapists, one sanitary civil engineer and one administrative worker). The second operation occurred about a month later and included six team members (four occupational therapists, two assistants). The third operation followed the next month and consisted of eight people (one psychiatrist,

one psychologist, three occupational therapists, two agronomy engineers and one driver). The next operation, four months after the earthquake, involved six people (four occupational therapists, one business administrator with an MBA in Public Health, one driver).

ACTIONS AND RESULTS

Staff at the Health Department

Staff from the health department had been working non-stop to provide aid to survivors for 21 days since the earthquake. They worked at a local church facility which had been adapted as a medical first aid post. Many of the staff presented with symptoms of post-traumatic stress. Our intervention involved 19 employees and centred upon grief support and stress relief to help them manage the challenges of their roles. They received donations to support leisure (guitars, radios, books, games, etc.) and stress relief. We helped them to set up 'wellbeing spaces' in the adapted work space where they could engage in stress-relieving activities and access support (Figure 27-3). The staff began to show positive improvement in their mental health and so the intervention quickly evolved to focus on improving their relationships within the workplace and supporting occupational performance. The staff started then a reviewing process of their performance, specially focused on their own dependency and autonomy levels, within the institutional bureaucracy.

Primary Health Care Station of Curanipe

At the primary health care station of Curanipe we created a 'children's wellbeing corner' (Figure 27-4) for public use, which was later identified as a 'play zone'. Individual and family psychiatric support was also provided to the users of this space as needed.

Difficulties encountered included:

- During reconstruction within the building the 'wellbeing spaces' that had been defined by the staff had not been considered by officials; this caused discontent among staff and users of the space.
- Staff felt overwhelmed regarding their demanding work routine, that they faced impossible challenges and that they lacked a supportive work environment.

In response to these challenges our intervention extended to staff and focused on psycho-education

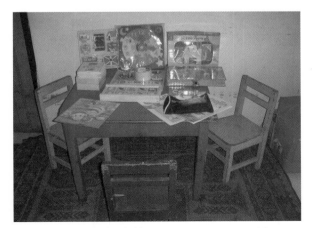

FIGURE 27-4 ▪ The children's corner: we set up this space for children's use at the improvised health service.

related to achieving 'occupational balance' in difficult and demanding environments.

Emergency Camps – 'La Trilla', Pelluhue (20 Families) and 'Fuerza Curanipe' (16 Families)

In the emergency camps we focused on building informal support networks and strengthening bonds within and between families. There was no community meeting space in the camps so we proposed that a common area be built in each camp in order to support wellbeing.

Through this initiative we created a space for women to connect and support one another as well as play and recreation spaces for children. We guided women in self-knowledge, skill development, empowerment, catharsis, sharing and mutual support. With children, by means of games, we worked on the mourning of their lost loved ones and pets. Psychiatric support was provided in situ. Seeds were donated for families to grow vegetable gardens and various other donated items supported recovery (books, games, musical instruments, bed linen and clothes, etc.).

The Community of Salto de Agua

Our intervention in the rural community of Salto de Agua focused on restoring the livelihoods of 12 farming families. A paramedic from the staff of the primary health care station of Chovellén was of great help due to knowledge of people in that village. Activities were developed on site including sowing broad beans and green peas. We provided instruction on the care and sanitary aspects of handling the crops and distributed seeds so that each farmer could sow them on their land. Farmers showed high interest in this activity, which resulted in good communication and participation. We also worked with a group of older women, re-engaging them in knitting and the production of fruit marmalades. However, with no formal route for commercialization established, the sustainability of these activities as a source of livelihood is limited.

Simultaneously the therapeutic team made individual and collective assessments related to the families' health and wellbeing. Elderly farmers were

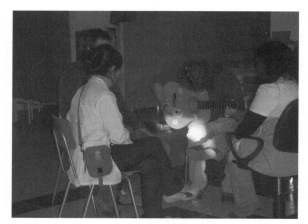

FIGURE 27-5 ■ Learning to relax. Some of the younger local health team members enjoying leisure, playing guitar and singing, after our therapeutic activity; a way to come together, ease stress, and energize themselves for continuing work.

identified as particularly vulnerable due to isolation and lack of economic, social and legal resources.

CONCLUSION

The therapeutic operations involving these diverse groups of people – staff members, women, children, the elderly, farmers – helped them to cope with the disaster and conditions of poverty. Through the creation of 'wellbeing' spaces', which essentially enabled occupation, a process of personal and social transformation occurred. The groups discovered their own strengths and inner resources and tapped into their potential not only to heal but to influence their environments without relying on formal support and institutions (Figure 27-5). Not only did this have a positive impact on individual and community health and wellbeing but it increased their resilience, better preparing them for future disasters.

28

REFLECTIONS FROM EXPERIENCE ACROSS THE ASIA-PACIFIC REGION

KERRY THOMAS, WITH CONTRIBUTIONS FROM
VARIOUS COLLEAGUES*

INTRODUCTION

The Asia-Pacific region has been hit by several disasters in recent times: earthquakes in China, Indonesia, Japan and New Zealand, hurricanes in the Philippines and Australia, tsunamis, volcanic eruptions, wildfires, floods and droughts, not to mention the devastation caused by nuclear radiation in Fukushima, Japan.

Increasingly, occupational therapists have become involved, as both survivors and responders. Experience arising from these encounters was shared and discussed in a symposium I was invited to convene during the November 2011 Asia-Pacific Occupational Therapy Congress in Chiang Mai, Thailand. This chapter summarizes key elements from selected forum presentations and group discussions from a symposium titled 'Learning from the Unexpected: Disaster Response, Recovery and Preparedness'. Insights are further supplemented with information arising from other conference papers, and disaster-related presentations at the 2012 Occupational Therapy Congress in Japan. Overviews of evolving concepts including the relationship of occupation with disaster and development contexts, and the disaster and development occupational perspective (DDOP) framework were also presented and discussed at these conferences; these are elaborated in Parts I and III, respectively, in this book.

Experience, ideas and practical innovation related to occupation in relation to six aspects of disaster response, recovery and preparedness are presented in this chapter. For each of these areas, a pithy illustrative focus is provided, drawn from the experience of the contributing presenter. Reflections and insights gained through sharing of experience and group discussion among symposium participants are then summarized and presented at the end of the chapter. These are informative in providing additional comment as well as an indication of current perspectives and understandings. Collectively, these in turn can contribute to implications for policy, practice, education and future research (discussed in Chapter 32).

GETTING STARTED: PERSONAL – PROFESSIONAL PREPAREDNESS – NEW ZEALAND

ADAPTED FROM A PRESENTATION BY RITA ROBINSON, NEW ZEALAND

On 22 February 2011, an earthquake severely damaged New Zealand's second most populous city of Christchurch. In total, 185 people were killed, making it the second most deadly natural disaster in the country's history. Strong aftershocks continued to hit the region for more than a year after the initial event.

During the emergency phase, the New Zealand Association of Occupational Therapists (NZAOT) responded in differing ways. The response was affected by three interconnected factors: people, place and processes. Arising from this experience were insights for personal and professional preparedness.

- *People.* Association members in Christchurch included those directly affected by the earthquake, those who were present but not in harm's

---

*Symposium presenters: Rita Robinson, Noriko Tomioka, Suchada Sakornsatian, Buwana Cahya, Masayuki Watanabe, Miho Yoshida and Kit Sinclair.

way, and those out of Christchurch but worried for others in the quake zone.

- *Place.* The needs of people were defined by the status of their physical place as well as their place on Maslow's hierarchy of needs. For those directly affected by the earthquake, the lower levels of Maslow's hierarchy of needs defined what they needed – that is, the more basic requirements for survival and living. For those watching and wishing to help, Maslow's higher levels were a better fit. The Association tried to cater to all the members' needs. Those members in the earthquake were receivers of assistance while those outside the quake zone became the givers. Each group of people had a different need, a different occupational requirement and differing roles.
- *Processes.* The processes arising from this situation thus reflected two primary influences: those directed to assisting people in the quake zone, and those to people outside the disaster zone. Processes that were put in place reflected that different members had differing priorities. These priorities were influenced by the status of members' physical place and the place along the time continuum from the quake, and the needs associated with these, as well as the needs expressed by people themselves.

Process activities included things such as: exchanging 'update' emails with members, be they service 'receivers' or 'providers'; communication with government agencies to extend timelines around differing accreditation tasks established during this time; setting up support including free supervision processes for those providing assistance; and facilitating access to accommodation outside Christchurch for a break away.

Processes subsequently extended to establishing disaster preparedness arrangements in the NZAOT office to support staff and strengthen office functioning should disaster strike in the future. Documenting the NZAOT response in the journal Occupational Therapy International, and ongoing workshops at professional events were important for both debriefing and improvement. These in turn influenced the opportunities created for occupational therapy students to complete community projects among the earthquake

affected community. A translation project of civil defence advice was also established with Auckland University of Technology.

GETTING STARTED: PERSONAL–PROFESSIONAL PREPAREDNESS – JAPAN
ADAPTED FROM A PRESENTATION BY NORIKO TOMIOKA, JAPAN

This part of the chapter conveys experience about personal–professional preparedness arising from the Japanese Occupational Therapy Association's engagement with the 2011 Great East Japan Earthquake (Fukushima) disaster (Figure 28-1).

General and traditional preparedness as a community:

- Disaster happens when you forget to be prepared.
- There are different types and levels of disaster to be considered: the most dreadful ones include earthquake, wildfire and typhoon; you need to visualize what the effects might be so you can prepare appropriately – as an individual and family, professional and community.

Personal preparedness depends on your and your family's past encounters with varieties of natural and/or man-made disaster:

- Have a minimum survival kit prepared: water, food, radio, medication, light, etc.

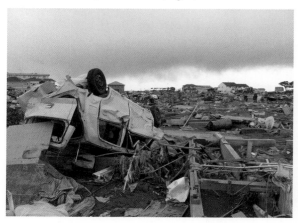

FIGURE 28-1 ■ Fukushima devastation 2011 (Courtesy of Masayuki Watanabe).

- Have agreed communication strategies in place: for safety inquiries, how will people know where you are?
- As a volunteer, do whatever your heart tells you: e.g. information networking, donating, collecting things that are needed, etc.

Professional preparedness depends on the following:

- Does your professional organization have a disaster manual?
- Do you belong to and/or have a connection with NGOs, institutions, and/or volunteer groups that recruit professional volunteers? They provide training and resource materials.

Author note: As citizens and professionals, preparedness and survival guidelines can increasingly be accessed from your local government and disaster management organizations.

GETTING CONNECTED WITH DISASTER MANAGEMENT SYSTEMS – THAILAND
SUMMARIZED FROM A PRESENTATION BY
SUCHADA SAKORNSATIAN, THAILAND

I am currently displaced myself due to the widespread flooding impacting on Bangkok, but this presentation summarizes the importance of being connected with formal disaster preparedness, response and recovery systems and organizations. Following the 2004 Indian Ocean tsunami, and through my national position with the Department of Mental Health, I became a member of the national committee and the Mental Health Centre for the Thailand Tsunami Disaster (MHCT). MHCT was based in Bangkok and worked through the Suan Saranom psychiatric hospital in the disaster-affected area.

Being connected at a national level enabled occupational therapy and therapists to be immediately engaged with the tsunami response through the psychiatric departmental response system. It could equally have been another department or response programme. Being actively attached at the national level provided a pathway to facilitating occupational therapy staff in the affected area to be mobilized and networked with other service providers, both government and NGOs (non-governmental organizations). When we established the Recovery Centre, occupational therapists connected in with the existing public health system and the educational system as well as community.

In summary, because I was a member in the Central Operational Centre, occupational therapy was represented at the national department level. In the operational area, occupational therapists and others were mobilized as staff in the Psychiatric Mobile Team, while at the Recovery Centre, my role was as supervisor in recovery services. Senior occupational therapists can thus play an active role in coordinating the engagement of the profession in disaster preparedness, response and recovery (DPRR).

Throughout the response and recovery phases, the importance of being aware of and linking in with the overarching Disaster Coordination System was critical to coordination, networking, providing data for planning, facilitating referrals, mobilizing and managing both local and international volunteers, and so on. Through this active involvement, awareness of occupational therapy and the role we can play in DPRR is promoted.

MOBILIZING OCCUPATIONAL THERAPISTS TO ENGAGE IN DISASTER MANAGEMENT – INDONESIA
SUMMARIZED FROM A PRESENTATION BY BUWANA
CAHYA, INDONESIA

Occupational therapists in Indonesia first became formally involved in disaster management (i.e. DPRR) at the time of the 2004 Indian Ocean tsunami. Since then there have been the Yogyakarta and Pangandaran earthquakes in Java in 2006, and subsequently other, less widespread but nevertheless locally devastating natural disasters, including the Sidoarjo mud flow, many more earthquakes, volcanic eruptions and floods, all causing significant loss of life, injuries and internal displacement and resettlement. Occupational therapists have been both survivors and responders.

As a profession, mobilizing a response is like building and working a beehive. There are many factors to be considered and interconnected. Three of these include what we do, the resources we have internally as a profession, and mixing and matching these to the needs and situation of local contexts.

- Occupational therapy work includes: orthopaedic, psychosocial and community-based rehabilitation, technology and assistive devices for older people, children and adults.
- Occupational therapy resources include: occupational therapists who are survivors, service providers and students, national and local occupational therapy associations, WFOT (World Federation of Occupational Therapists), and occupational therapists' links to community, government, nongovernmental and other organizations.
- Occupational therapy within community contexts includes: an understanding of local sociocultural, religious and political dynamics, infrastructure and governance arrangements, and an assessment of needs using local personnel and resources.

A description of our response to the Yogyakarta earthquake is provided in Chapter 29.

EMERGENCY RESPONSE STRATEGIES – JAPAN

SUMMARIZED FROM PRESENTATIONS BY MASAYUKI WATANABE, JAPAN, INCLUDING A SEPARATE PRESENTATION OF A STUDY CONDUCTED INTO THE EXPERIENCE OF OCCUPATIONAL THERAPISTS AS VOLUNTEER RESPONDERS (WATANABE ET AL 2011)

On 11 March 2011 the East Japan Great Earthquake occurred (commonly referred to as the Fukushima disaster in the global community). With a magnitude of 9.0 on the Richter scale, it triggered an extremely destructive tsunami in the Tohoku region of the country. The authorities confirmed 14 616 deaths, 5278 injured, and 11 111 people missing across 20 prefectures, as well as 77 336 totally collapsed and 29 899 partially collapsed houses as of 29 April 2011.

While occupational and physiotherapists were not commonly included in disaster medical assistance teams (DMAT), occupational therapists were involved in rendering assistance to disaster sufferers both at home and in evacuation centres.

We undertook a study to identify issues and explore ways to improve occupational therapy involvement in disaster relief activities within the context of rehabilitation for survivors from an early stage of the disaster.

The following findings come from this study and our own experience.

We found that volunteer work in relief varied according to the time and the sites of the affected areas:

- First, emergency supplies including water, food, clothes, batteries and radios were delivered in the areas where various lifelines were dysfunctional.
- Some survivors needed gloves, boots and materials to fix their houses and so have safe shelter.
- We helped with access by clearing paths in the city area (Figures 28-2, 28-3 and 28-4) and constructing accessible water taps, toilets and shower corners in appropriate locations.

We attended daily meetings among non-profit organizations and volunteers to report our activities and exchange information, and provided cluster reports.

The challenges we faced included:

- The law governing physical and occupational therapists which restricts our medical care services to doctors' prescription.

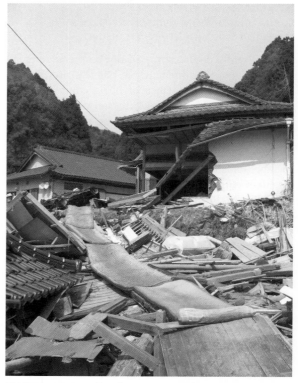

FIGURE 28-2 ■ Creating access to houses (Courtesy of Masayuki Watanabe).

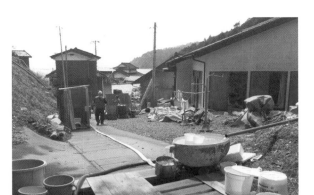

FIGURE 28-3 ▪ Facilitating access to basic needs and services (Courtesy of Masayuki Watanabe).

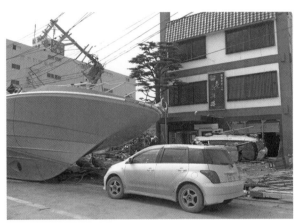

FIGURE 28-4 ▪ Ongoing reminders of nature's power extend into the recovery phase (Courtesy of Masayuki Watanabe).

- Obtaining the necessities of life because of transport limitations.
- Lack of information.
- Lack of understanding of the roles of occupational therapists among residents in the affected areas.

In summary, key emergency response strategies that occupational therapists can potentially and usefully engage in are:

- Dispensing simple triage and rapid treatment (START) and providing basic first aid.
- Helping to evacuate older people and people with disabilities who have movement difficulties and delivering information to people with visual and hearing difficulties.

- Assisting in administration of the delivery of water, food and essential commodities of life and hygiene management while conducting needs assessments.

DISASTER RECOVERY STRATEGIES – PAKISTAN

SUMMARIZED FROM A PRESENTATION BY MIHO YOSHIDA, JAPAN, ON EXPERIENCE IN PAKISTAN, WITH REFERENCE TO A POSTER PRESENTED AT THE CONFERENCE (FURUGORI & YOSHIDA 2011)

Pakistan is a disaster hotspot, experiencing earthquakes, floods and conflict. On 8 October 2005 a magnitude 7.6 earthquake in northern Pakistan on the Kashmir border killed at least 75 000 people, injured more than 69 000 and generally affected 3 million. It is a region where people built their houses by stacking stones and dirt, and the houses simply collapsed. Enormous numbers of people were trapped under the rubble. Many who survived had fractures, injuries leading to amputations, spinal cord injury and head injury. Emergency aid service helicopters carried severely injured people to city hospitals.

Six months after the earthquake, in April 2006, Japan International Cooperation Agency (JICA) dispatched a team comprising an occupational therapist, physiotherapist, nurse and project coordinator to the National Institute for Handicapped (NIHd) in response to a request from the Pakistan Government. The five-month project targeted 220 disaster victims who had suffered spinal cord injury; 150 were female, 70 were male. The project supported women preferentially because it considered that women with disability faced a more difficult life compared with men with disability in Pakistan.

The project goal was to enable those targeted to lead a quality life, including spinal cord injury patients returning to the area in which they lived and having the support of family or the community. The project activities focused on providing medical rehabilitation and activities of daily living (ADL), and ADL training on cultural adaptive context, including training 20 community-based rehabilitation (CBR) workers, as well as the patients themselves and their families.

In 2010, five years after the earthquake and four years after the end of the rehabilitation project, we conducted a follow-up survey to find out what had happened.

Almost all the patients had returned to their homes. Generally they seemed to be healthy, with no pressure sores. They had primary education and could read and write. Their economic conditions were not very low. They were involved in CBR work in their community.

In contrast, although NIHd had officially closed the spinal cord injury ward, 20 women were still there; they had severe bed sores and complications, most were illiterate and survived on charitable gifts, and they were under pressure of displacement from NIHd.

Some insights and lessons arising from the post-project outcome study:

- Inadequate family understanding of a spinal injured person's everyday life was a major factor in why some women were unable to return home. In some cases, the person can care for themselves independently, but family poverty and environmental conditions (e.g. stoves) result in pressure sores and burns.
  Lessons: Rehabilitation personnel need to engage families better and to a greater extent, and home visits are vital.
- Conversely, those who were able to return to their home town and had informed family members experienced better outcomes, including access to clinics when required. Those women who had some education tended to have a higher level of health and wellbeing, regardless of the level of injury. The difference in quality of life for those living in urban and rural areas is unclear.
- The Pakistan Government provides social security benefits for disabled victims for three years including welfare support and free medical treatment. However, in the absence of government welfare assistance, community-based and nongovernmental organizations can sometimes provide support.
  Challenge: In the absence of any social security or welfare, our team approach could not be effective. How can we, as rehabilitation professionals, support people with significant disabilities to achieve positive living outcomes in the absence of social and economic support?

In summary, effective long-term disaster recovery strategies require us to work across a hierarchy of levels from the individual to family, community and various levels of government (Figures 28-5, 28-6, 28-7 and 28-8). As indicated in Figure 28-5, the activities and

- Individual Level   } - Occupational therapists work as practitioners
- Family Level   } - Providing medical rehab for injured people
- Community Level } - Empowering disabled people and vulnerable people, especially women

- District Level   }
- Provincial Level   } - Coordinating projects and services
- National Level   } - Policy development

Think broadly and innovatively for interventions that are relevant to the context and sustainable

Mechanisms for coordination, cooperation and information sharing across stakeholders

FIGURE 28-5 ■ Hierarchy of disaster recovery strategies.

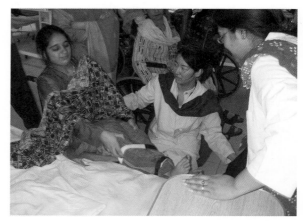

FIGURE 28-6 ■ Family member experiencing disability.

roles vary at each level. In support of these tasks, mechanisms need to be developed or engaged for coordination, cooperation and information sharing among government and nongovernmental organizations (international and national) and disabled people's organizations (DPOs).

DISASTER PREPAREDNESS STRATEGIES – GLOBAL

ADAPTED FROM A PRESENTATION BY KIT SINCLAIR, WFOT DISASTER PREPAREDNESS AND RESPONSE TEAM LEADER

Elaboration of these and related strategies is provided in Chapter 29.

Key elements:

- Risk reduction and preparedness planning.
- Involvement with key stakeholders.
- Education for emerging roles.

Key lessons learned to date:

- Local, national and global level involvements.

Points for good practice:

- Raising awareness of the role of occupational therapists in the disaster management arena.

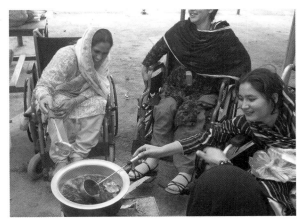

FIGURE 28-7 ■ Developing living skills (Courtesy of M Furugori; NIRM).

- Being actively involved as occupational therapists at all levels, including one's own community.
- Educating practitioners – providing education modules and learning resources.

ACCOUNTING FOR OCCUPATIONAL THERAPY PERFORMANCE AND CONTRIBUTION IN DISASTER MANAGEMENT – GLOBAL

ADAPTED FROM A PRESENTATION BY KERRY THOMAS, CONSULTANT, AND ADVISOR WITH THE WFOT DISASTER PREPAREDNESS AND RESPONSE TEAM

- As a profession, occupational therapists have an interest in developing evidence-based practice and a responsibility to account for the conduct and results of interventions.
- In disaster management contexts there are increasing formal and ethical requirements to evaluate and report on programmes and activities.
- As an emerging profession in the field of DPRR, it is necessary for occupational therapy to demonstrate its potential roles and effectively communicate these across community, government and other stakeholders.

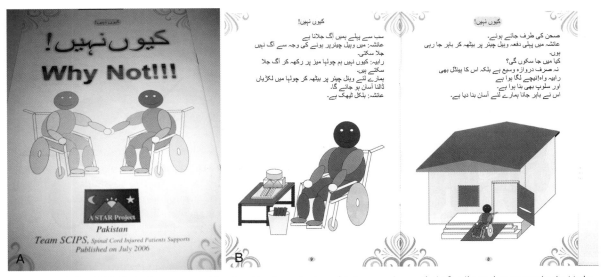

FIGURE 28-8A AND B ■ Awareness-raising booklet for spinal cord injury survivors, their family and community in Urdu.

- DPRR is a complex and challenging endeavour that engages professionals in both the technical and managerial aspects of programmes/services; both require particular capabilities, and both need to be monitored and evaluated.
- In particular, even with the best of intentions, it can be easy to inadvertently exacerbate the vulnerability of survivors; reflective practices can serve professional development and performance well in enabling appropriate, effective and efficient practice.
- Occupation and many DPRR tasks are not profession-specific; what is the added or unique value that occupational therapy can bring? How can we determine and account for this?
- There is a need to develop monitoring, evaluation, reporting/communication and improvement (MERI) strategies to serve the above functions. Evidence is needed across the input–activity–output–outcome–impact continuum. Participatory methods that involve survivors can be especially powerful – for professionals as well as survivors (Figure 28-9).

PARTICIPANT DISCUSSIONS

As a step towards enhancing symposium participants' capacity to consider the potential contribution of occupational therapy to disaster management and how capability to do this successfully could best be developed, a series of small group discussions were convened. Facilitated by panel members and others with disaster experience, approximately 60 symposium participants reflected on the presentations and shared experience in addressing the four aspects of DPRR outlined in Box 28-1.

Symposium participants included people with practical experience as both survivors and responders, be it in a volunteer or professional capacity or as service coordinators. Many others joined the symposium with a desire to gain insights and learn about preparing for engagement in the disaster management arena. Discussion in mixed groups generated stimulating conversation, networking and the responses in Box 28-1, which are valuable in guiding future preparedness and response actions. The reflections and insights arising from this and other similar symposiums have informed ongoing

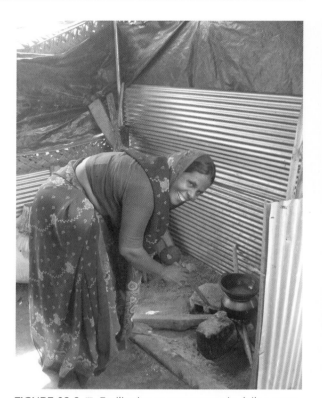

FIGURE 28-9 ■ Facilitating re-engagement in daily occupations – accounting for our contribution. Disaster and development professionals with an occupational therapy or occupational science background have potential to assist in making general response and recovery processes, interventions and outcomes significantly more appropriate, meaningful, effective, efficient and sustainable, but we need to be able to demonstrate evidence and communicate our contribution across local, programme, policy and funding levels. Engagement of suitably experienced occupational therapists from the outset of disaster management efforts can bring benefits to all stakeholders and reduce the need to reorientate poorly designed responses partway through, as can often occur in rebuilding initiatives.

practice, policy, education and research developments, at various levels from the local to the global. Chapter 32 provides further detail of considerations for ongoing development of occupational therapy engagement in the disaster management field.

CONCLUSION

Enhancing participation in occupation for all persons, as reflected in the WFOT's Position Statement on

BOX 28-1
SYMPOSIUM PARTICIPANT GROUP WORK REFLECTIONS

KEY POINTS FOR GOOD PRACTICE

- Planning for disaster events
- Early response
- Needs assessment → immediate priorities and longer-term plans for reconstruction
- Gathering selves and volunteering/offering help
- Offering support for vulnerable people
- Team up with the Health Ministry
- Coordinate with others, e.g. treatment provision, nursing services
- Working with community, e.g. people with disability and caregivers (profiling and strategizing)
- Organizing temporary shelters
- Enriching facilities (e.g. centres, camps)
- Empowering through education (e.g. ADL)
- Sharing information

WHAT SHAPES OCCUPATIONAL EXPERIENCES IN/ OF DISASTER?

- *Not their usual life situation*
- Helplessness/uselessness ... 'disuse' syndrome
- Tsunami rehabilitation team in Indonesia – working with children, adults, people with disability who needed psychosocial support
- Ability to work and study after disaster

WAYS IN WHICH HUMAN RIGHTS CAN BE CONSIDERED

- Basic needs
- Work, study
- Information

KEY PROFESSIONAL DEVELOPMENT NEEDS

- How to start – knowing where and how to go to affected areas, to ask what survivors need
- Technical capacities, for example:
  - Psychosocial support provision programme: support team, problem solving, stress mix activities for survivors with physical and psychological effects, and for different groups (e.g. children)
  - Accessibility, home modifications, universal design in rebuilding
- Community-based rehabilitation
- Support resources – for orientation and preparedness training, for field use
- Communication – mechanisms and arrangements during a disaster

---

Human Rights, requires occupational therapists to expand their roles and responsibilities into disaster response, recovery and preparedness. But we need to do this carefully and responsibly. This symposium was a step towards enhancing participants' capacity to consider our contribution and how we can develop capability to do this successfully. The reflections and insights arising from this and other similar workshops have and continue to inform ongoing practice, policy, education and research developments, at various levels from the local to the global.

REFERENCES

Furugori, M., Yoshida, W.M., 2011. The situation of earthquake victims in Pakistan five years later and long-term support for disaster victims. Poster, Asia-Pacific Occupational Therapy Congress, Chiang Mai, Thailand.

Watanabe, M., Muraoka, T., Endo H., 2011. Volunteer work for residents in the stricken area of the East Japan great earthquake. Paper, Asia-Pacific Occupational Therapy Congress, Chiang Mai, Thailand.

29

MOBILIZING OCCUPATIONAL THERAPY THROUGH POLICY, PLANNING AND EDUCATION

KIT SINCLAIR ■ MARILYN PATTISON

INTRODUCTION

The Beginning of a Major Project

I just felt overwhelmed … wanted to know what to do – my family, my friends; I'm an OT … but what to do? … where to start? …

An Indonesian occupational therapist
post 2004 Indian Ocean tsunami

When the most devastating tsunami in recorded history swept across the Indian Ocean in December 2004, the World Federation of Occupational Therapy (WFOT) was inundated with emails from occupational therapists (OTs) around the globe asking for guidance on how they could help, many wanting to know how their skills as OTs could be best utilized in the context of disaster. The WFOT responded immediately with an action plan communicated via the internet, resources to assist therapists who wanted to volunteer and a dedicated contact mechanism to respond to the numerous requests for information and offers of help. From this beginning, WFOT has continued to support the development and implementation of long-term assistance to occupational therapists wishing to respond to disasters. This has been achieved through its Disaster Preparedness and Response (DP&R) project. This chapter highlights how the DP&R project's multipronged strategy encompassing policy, planning and education is helping to support engagement in an enlarging area of professional practice. In portraying how the World Federation is tackling this task, from supporting global responses to

catastrophic events through to working with national members of the 350 000-strong Federation, insights and implications are explored for how occupational therapists can better prepare for and support the recovery of people affected by disasters.

OCCUPATIONAL THERAPY'S UNIQUE PERSPECTIVE

In the increasingly complex and challenging context of disaster and development, there is a continuing need for improving coordination and use of existing competencies to address disability and health priorities. For occupational therapists it is important to realize that much of their current skill base is applicable in these situations and the application of that skill base must occur through existing disaster response and coordination mechanisms and in collaboration with the range of stakeholders involved.

Occupational therapists bring a unique and holistic perspective to the field that potentially contributes to human development and the social vision of just and inclusive societies, where all persons have access to immediate humanitarian and development aid as needed to recover from disaster and to move forward in life, maximizing their capabilities towards reaching their full potential.

Despite significant gains in the international community towards inclusive development and increasing awareness of the need to mainstream cross-cutting issues such as gender and disability into disaster response, recovery and preparation, there remains a significant gap between policy and practice. Occupational therapists, as part of a multidisciplinary team, can help address many of these issues, but their occupational perspective and approach needs to be adapted to disaster contexts.

The WFOT plays a key role in stimulating learning and development on this front, originating with its 2005 Tsunami Project titled 'Action Learning in Practice'. It continues to play a significant global role in promoting understanding and learning, working collaboratively with international organizations to improve preparedness and response to the increasing numbers of disasters happening around the world. It continues to offer a foundation for local, national and international disaster related activities.

Action learning is an educational process where participants learn through their actions and reflections versus traditional instruction (Kramer 2007). This form of learning served as the cornerstone of the Tsunami Project as illustrated below.

THE 2005 TSUNAMI PROJECT: ACTION LEARNING IN PRACTICE

Establishing a WFOT DP&R Response Group

The WFOT established a response group and task force to manage this major project of the Indian Ocean tsunami response. The strategies developed as part of this project continue to be deployed and promoted and include collaboration with the World Health Organization (WHO) and international nongovernmental organizations (NGOs), conducting workshops, developing resources and training materials, and establishing communication networks for liaison, collaboration and capacity building. Many of these strategies grew out of an action learning and action planning process that began with a situational assessment in the tsunami-affected region in early 2005.

Situational Analysis

A situational analysis was undertaken shortly after the Indian Ocean tsunami to inform the strategic WFOT response to the disaster both locally and internationally. It involved on-site appraisal coupled with review of reports and discussions with WFOT stakeholders including WHO (Figures 29-1 and 29-2). The intent of the appraisal was to inform ways of supporting local

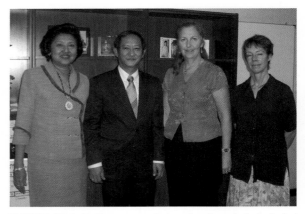

FIGURE 29-1 ■ Post-tsunami situational analysis included official meetings with government health representatives. In Thailand: Kit Sinclair and Kerry Thomas with Suchada Sakornsation, Occupational Therapist, Mental Health Technical Development Bureau (left) and Ministry of Health staff.

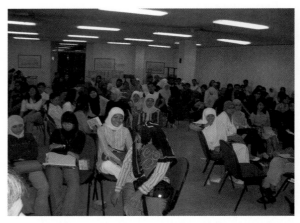

FIGURE 29-2 ■ Indonesian occupational therapists during situational analysis discussions in Jakarta.

therapists to cope within their local context and provide a framework for international support for local action. It would also lay the foundations to build ongoing worldwide occupational therapy capacity to respond to disasters in the future.

With this project, WFOT and occupational therapists were introduced more formally into the international disaster response domain, identifying implications for WFOT and occupational therapists while also identifying opportunities where appropriately experienced occupational therapists (international and national) could feasibly and meaningfully contribute to the rehabilitation and recovery phases of this disaster.

A need was acknowledged for occupational therapists in the region to shift knowledge and use of their existing skills into a new context in the occupational therapy perspective of community-based rehabilitation (CBR) and community development. This could be done through workshops on role development and practice models (adapting community approaches). Such skill development would better place occupational therapists to respond to disaster situations as well as meet wider community needs in ways that are consistent with Ministry of Health/government policy and priorities. Included in this were implications for role clarification and development and then undergraduate, post-graduate and professional development education as well as employment strategy development in the government and private/NGO sectors.

Regional and National Workshops

Recommendations from the situational analysis included conducting a regional workshop to commence building capacity, identify and build networks and partnerships, develop guidelines for emergency response, develop national action plans and identify regional support requirements. Funding was sought from major international donors, local funding agencies and WHO.

Subsequent national workshops in Indonesia, Thailand and Sri Lanka (Figure 29-3), and an e-based

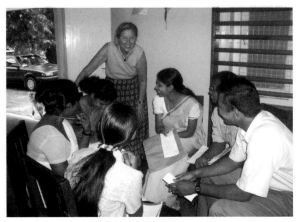

FIGURE 29-3 ▪ Kit Sinclair with an occupational therapy group in Sri Lanka.

workshop in India provided a forum where draft plans and capacities developed at the regional workshop were further advanced and contextualized at national levels.

From these workshops occupational therapists gained a gradual awakening, understanding and growing enthusiasm for the new roles and opportunities that existed for national occupational therapists in outreach, CBR and DP&R contexts. They gained an understanding of the role that pilot activities and projects can play in the process of testing and adapting occupational therapy interventions in community settings and in building community practice competencies. This included the simultaneous need for and potential offered to occupational therapists in establishing partnerships with other stakeholders, including government personnel, local and international NGOs, and community groups. It enabled the development of an appreciation for how these relationships could be developed combined with endorsement to progress development of partnership mechanisms. An example of this collaboration development took place in Sri Lanka soon after the DP&R regional workshop where NEST, a non-profit organization established to promote understanding in the area of mental health, gave a presentation on their work. The offer of opportunities for fieldwork placement for occupational therapy students was taken up by the occupational therapy education programme, opening another avenue for liaison and expanded experiences for students.

Each national group developed national DP&R plans for occupational therapy services and established task forces to progress these. Comprehensive workshop reports incorporated what was done, lessons, materials, outputs, participants, evaluations and recommendations. Pilot projects were initiated in three countries, and in Indonesia and Thailand occupational therapists have also undertaken emergency response actions in relation to further disasters and conflict situations. The emergence of new or enhanced partnerships with government bodies and NGOs by occupational therapists occurred in Indonesia, Thailand and Sri Lanka.

Other Actions

Complementary activities being undertaken by and through the WFOT network were identified and linked with the DP&R project with other actions. These included ongoing development of the WFOT website, the Occupational Therapy International Outreach Network (OTION), targeted resource development including country-specific guidelines (e.g. USA) and the development of and work on a DP&R information package. Opportunities also existed to promote valuable links between WFOT's DP&R and CBR initiatives. They highlight the way in which small initiatives to a massive disaster have galvanized the global occupational therapy community and spearheaded WFOT's ability to effectively progress the profession in this and related domains (WFOT 2007).

Tools and resources were developed and refined to guide occupational therapy engagement in DP&R policy, planning and practice, many of which were compiled into an extensive DP&R information and resource package (2007). A forum was developed on OTION with the view of potential use by people in low resource countries. The information package on CD ROM was made available through the WFOT website (www.wfot.org) for purchase by those in well resourced countries and free for those from less well resourced countries or who had been affected by disaster, thus offering a balance of sophisticated online activities with those who cannot regularly access online resources. This information package was updated in 2010.

WFOT, through its DP&R project team, is in liaison with key stakeholders, e.g. Health in Action (HAC) in WHO, Disability and Rehabilitation Team (DAR) in WHO and other stakeholders such as the international NGO, Motivation, which focuses on mobility and access, and the International Society for Physical and Rehabilitation Medicine (ISPRM). WFOT has to date offered guidance through its DP&R project reports, workshops at a range of conferences, information package and email exchanges. The WFOT Executive Team responds regularly to queries and offers networking opportunities to support local actions, including sending out the DP&R information package as a reference and foundation for further action.

OUTCOMES AND DEVELOPMENTS

A number of outcomes and new developments continue to emerge both from the initial work undertaken by WFOT in 2004/5 and from disasters that have occurred since the tsunami where OTs have played a role, reflecting changes in policy, planning, education and practice. An example of this development is shown in the work that has been undertaken in a number of countries around the world to respond to disasters as they happen (Boxes 29-1 and 29-2).

International Development

In 2005 the American Occupational Therapy Association (AOTA), in collaboration with WFOT and the American Occupational Therapy Foundation (AOTF), developed a concept paper (The Role of Occupational Therapy in Disaster Preparedness, Response and Recovery) to clarify and advocate for the profession's role and participation as members of disaster preparedness and response teams at all geographic levels in the USA on DP&R (American Occupational Therapy

---

BOX 29-1

EXTRACTS FROM EMAILS FROM BUDI, INDONESIA, TO WFOT – 30 MAY 2006 AND 6 JUNE 2006

'All hospitals are filled with survivors and there are not enough doctors and nurses in the hospitals so we sent students (OT, Nursing, PT students) to hospitals to help hospital staff to deal with the workload. Today we sent another team (Faculty members, nursing, PT, OT students) to another location, Klaten, which was also seriously damaged. I am one of Surarta Health Polytechnic (SHP) emergency task force to respond to this earthquake and we must work quickly.'

'Thousands of survivors both in Jogja and Klaten need food, clothes, tents, water, and medicines immediately and some of them have not eaten for two days. I am also going to mobilize 50 OT students (third year students) to go to Klaten to help survivors next week for the duration of two weeks.'

'These are the real lessons and challenges that we initially discussed in the WFOT tsunami workshop in Sri Lanka and here in Jakarta. We did situational analysis (on site visit) on Monday and found many people with post traumatic stress disorder (PTSD). They do not want to eat, keep quiet and remain very sensitive.'

'The program in Klaten is still going on every day. We serve approximately 50 clients with different conditions and do home visits for 10 clients with fractures, stroke & cerebral palsy (CP) (not caused by disaster). Besides serving in the health post, we were also running play therapy for children (30 children) and are now expanding to another village in the afternoon (15.00–17.30 PM). The kids start showing happy faces after participating in play.'

BOX 29-2

THE PHILIPPINES WAS HIT WITH TWO MAJOR DISASTERS IN A THREE-WEEK PERIOD – AN EARTHQUAKE IN BOHOL ON 15 OCTOBER 2013 AND SUPER TYPHOON HAIYAN ON 8 NOVEMBER 2013

From Penny Ching, 23 November 2013

'We are thinking of setting up long term goals in communities we visit ... usually because of limited resources and the enormous tasks, I refer them to NGOs or local leaders that share the same heart and would ensure the continuity of our efforts.

Right now, there is an OT in one of the affected areas in the Panay Island and I am currently coordinating with her on furthering our efforts in some communities that are affected but seem to have been receiving less help. We are looking into facilitating the return of students to school as well as helping SPED programs there.

We have just finished this phase with Bohol (the province affected by the earthquake 3 weeks before the Haiyan typhoon and related tsunami). There are still a lot of island villages that need to be visited. We visited several vulnerable individuals – mostly the elderly. Three cases stood out to me as very interesting – the elderly woman with severe open wounds that impeded her mobility and self care; a person with progressive dystonia ... and a lady who was bed-bound for 3 weeks after a hip surgery (after a cabinet fell on her during the earthquake) ... we stood her up for the first time and the whole family was very pleased. They said that they do have instructions to see a therapist but do not know where the therapists are ... they just feel blessed that someone visited them in their own home in that island village.

You should see the wide eyes of the kids who received their learning kits ... and the teachers saying, "Now you don't have any excuse for not doing your homework". The kids lost notebooks, writing implements, and of course, their parents save whatever funds they have for basic needs, so that school supplies become secondary to them. As OTs, we do look into their participation in school activities and feel that these will facilitate their return to routines. The teachers have been given teaching kits as well. We distributed a total of 550 kits to one public elementary school.

With the donations, we also managed to give tarpaulins for temporary shelter as it will definitely take a while for them to rebuild homes. Around 30 families benefited from this, especially for the partially damaged to completely damaged homes. I learned that it will cost 10k pesos (around 300 dollars) to build a simple structure per family. Medicines were also donated to island villages as we learned that only 1 midwife (who in our health system is in charge of the village health center) is in charge of 8 villages!

Our small team also managed to do psychological debriefing for kids and the well elderly group.

We are currently planning our visits to the Haiyan affected areas and gathering support and donations there. I will be shipping some of the tarpaulins to Busuanga (Palawan) and Roxas (Panay Island) for the island villages there. I also received another request to help people with disabilities and the elderly in Iloilo.

As the activities increased, a list of actions emerged. Through the month of December these included:

Capacity Building 1 for volunteers (25 people): Psychosocial and occupational debriefing activities for new OT and other allied health volunteers for Visayas

Team 1 (3 people) Community visit and needs assessment of a remote town in Busuanga, Palawan (one of the major islands affected by Typhoon Haiyan)

Capacity Building 2 for volunteers (20 people): Workshop on the use of MNRI Post-traumatic Stress Protocol

Team A (8 people) Community visit and psychosocial and occupational debriefing of orphans and house parents in Bohol (center of the 7.2 magnitude earthquake last October 2013); Training of house parents; Distribution of learning kits to the orphan children and teens. Team B (8 people) community visit and psychosocial debriefing in Roxas, Panay Islands (one of the major islands affected by Typhoon Haiyan); Distribution of needed supplies and learning kits.

Joint team of OT, PT and SP associations (composed of 9 people) Community visit and psychosocial activities for children and adult survivors of Ormoc and Tanuan Leyte. We also had exploratory talks with Tacloban-based organizations for our next mission.'

Association 2011). Most disaster response activities are at state government level in the USA, so the plan had to be modified to reflect the local context. With a number of recent hurricanes, occupational therapists have offered specific post-disaster services (Speicher 2013). Other national associations have followed a similar route.

In Latin America, following the Peruvian earthquake in 2007, the formation of a DP&R network was called

for that would enable engagement of occupational therapists. As a result, the group 'Terapeutas Ocupacionales en Alerta' (Occupational Therapists on Alert) was formed with the objective to plan for future action in relationship with disasters (Lagos & Zegers 2011). Since that time this group has continued to grow and develop and has been actively involved throughout Latin America, including the aftermath of the earthquake and tsunami in Chile in February 2010 and the floods and landslides of Venezuela in November 2010 (Gonzalez 2012).

An integral part of the WFOT's DP&R project involves meeting and collaborating with government officials at local and national levels in order to increase awareness of the profession or establish mechanisms for responses that include OT. For example, in Australia the professional association collaborated with the state and national governments following the bush fires in Victoria in 2009 to coordinate OTs wishing to volunteer, and again with the state and national governments following the 2011 floods in Queensland. WFOT supported the initiatives by providing DP&R resource materials to the state and national associations as well as individual OTs working or volunteering in the affected areas.

Since the commencement of the WFOT DP&R project, OTs are increasingly intrinsically involved in response activities (Box 29-3). Numerous other developments have occurred including the development of local education modules, presentations, seminars, workshops and think tank activities in various countries of the world; for example, the national workshop was delivered in Malaysia by Indonesian OTs (WFOT 2012).

TOWARDS THE FUTURE: NEEDS, CHALLENGES AND OPPORTUNITIES

The WFOT DP&R project has certainly taken on a life of its own; however, national action continues to revolve around response following disaster rather than preparedness prior to disaster.

Planning and Development – Facing Challenges and Creating Opportunities

There are many challenges for occupational therapy involvement in both disaster preparedness and response and the development of capacity building. There is a general lack of information and resources on occupational therapy practice in DP&R: many occupational therapists do not know where to start in this emerging field of practice, despite their willingness. We experience overloaded curricula in most occupational therapy programmes with an emphasis on the immediate needs of the present client population. Professionals are engrossed in their own work/workplace issues and development and already feel overstretched with the demands for evidence-based practice and research publication requirements for job promotion. Furthermore in many countries there is still a strong emphasis on the 'medical model', which does not view individuals within their context but rather within their 'disease process'.

DP&R is not a diagnostic model but a contextual one and interfaces completely with the person–environment–occupation (PEO) model of practice. However, DP&R is one field of practice and of course there are many others to choose from. It is not an area of practice for all occupational therapists. Nevertheless, in the current global climate of disasters increasing both in frequency and intensity, more and more

---

BOX 29-3
EXTRACT FROM WFOT E-NEWSLETTER ARTICLE (JUNE 2011) FROM NORIKO TOMIOKA, WFOT DELEGATE – JAPAN, FOLLOWING THE DISASTER OF THE TOHOKU EARTHQUAKE, THE TSUNAMI AND THE FUKUSHIMA NUCLEAR POWER PLANT ACCIDENT

Disaster Recovery Support Activities by Occupational Therapists

The recovery support activities initiated by the three Prefectural Associations of Occupational Therapists have been implemented since the early part of April. JAOT supports and assists their activities logistically by funding and recruiting volunteer applicants from all over Japan (57 were sent to Miyagi and 25 to Iwate in these 3 months, not including locally recruited volunteers).

Activities in the afflicted areas include support for the elderly and fragile people with or without disability who tend to be reserved and isolated at evacuation centres, temporary housing, or their partially destroyed homes; the prevention of 'inactivity syndrome'; and the maintenance of barrier-free environments as much as possible. Our experiences over these three months strongly suggest that occupational therapists are effective empowerment agents, and we will keep promoting sustainable support activities for the on-going recovery of communities and people's lives.

OTs will find themselves questioning what they can do – not only to assist in response and recovery efforts but very importantly in preparation and risk reduction in the contexts of their own communities and the clients they presently serve.

In overcoming challenges and developing opportunities, there are a number of strategies that can be used, including capacity building, strategic planning, networking with NGOs and local governments and forging relationships. DP&R plans need to link with existing disaster coordination mechanisms at local and national levels outside the profession.

The Broader Context

Occupational therapists at local, national and international level need to liaise with the broader audience in order to play an effective, relevant and meaningful role in the field.

- *Engage at policy level/strategic planning* at international, national and local levels across the continuum of health, social and occupational spectrums.
- *Engage proactively with key external organizations and decision makers* to assert occupational therapy leadership in essential areas of societal need (American Occupational Therapy Association 2011).
- *Promote stronger linkages and collaboration among the occupational therapy research, education and practice communities* and facilitate dissemination of occupational therapy knowledge to foster innovation in research, education and practice.

Articulating National DP&R Plans

Following disaster, national associations and groups are challenged to act on national DP&R plans. It is often, in fact, individuals who personally take up this kind of activity. There is a need in many affected countries for building capacity (understanding and skills) among national occupational therapy organizations and therapists of how national DP&R task forces and plan documents can be used practically to leverage strategic and operational developments within the profession and to attract resources to achieve these. The Philippines, for example, ran a national strategic planning workshop in 2012 (Figure 29-4) to determine

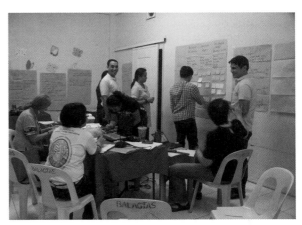

FIGURE 29-4 ■ National workshop in Manila, Philippines, with Anthony Grecia.

BOX 29-4
ROLES OF OT IN DISASTER MANAGEMENT (WFOT 2007)

Occupational therapists should be involved in all stages of planning and preparation at local district and national level for disaster management. Specific roles *post disaster* may include, but are not limited to, the following:

- Ensuring accessible environments post disaster at all stages of recovery (e.g. in displaced persons camps) and reconstruction (in rebuilding homes and community facilities).
- Organization of daily routines in displaced persons camps and surviving communities to include persons with disabilities, women, older people and children.
- Liaison with and encouragement of community leaders and others to reorganize community supports and routines.
- Use of everyday occupations including play and sports to facilitate recovery.
- Assessment of mental health status of survivors for depression and suicidal tendencies, with subsequent counselling and occupation-based activities.
- Training of volunteers to carry out 'quick mental health assessment' and counselling, thus providing more immediate services for greater numbers.

---

actions relevant to their own disaster-prone country and when Typhoon Haiyan hit Tacloban in 2013 they were ready to respond. The profession globally must stay vital and relevant within changing policy, programming and community contexts. It requires articulating roles and responsibilities, management and operational structures.

Skill development can occur through action learning workshops and sessions, at national, regional and international levels, with field-based and experienced professionals. It can include peer support and dialogue networks, secondments and attachments to existing projects, locations or organizations, exchanges of personnel, ideas, further development and dissemination of resource materials and inclusion of DP&R into undergraduate and graduate curricula.

Local action for disaster preparedness might include contacting community-based NGOs and offering technical expertise in assessing facility emergency preparation, particularly for persons with disabilities. Needs and gap analyses, as well as mapping of capacities for response in different circumstances could be undertaken in relation to the kind of disaster that the area might be affected by, e.g. bush fires in Australia or floods in Argentina. A database of key experienced occupational therapists would provide a good resource for education as well as response activities.

Linking into WFOT Strategic Plan – Policy and Planning

The WFOT is building on its accomplishments and lessons learned to continually increase its effectiveness in this area of practice. Continuing opportunities are being sought to identify, educate and prepare occupational therapists. For example, a DP&R workshop and a broad range of presentations on disaster management were presented at the WFOT 2010 Congress in Chile and again at the WFOT 2014 Congress in Japan. In addition, delegates and national associations were surveyed in 2011 on their involvement in activities that have been taking place in countries and member associations around the world. The survey showed that a majority of respondent countries were affected by natural and manmade disasters. Emerging issues were related to coping with steadily decreasing health care resources, establishing a role for occupational therapists in health teams dealing with emergencies and the inclusion of occupational therapy in national policy related to disaster management. At various levels, occupational therapy associations noted that they promote awareness through journals and newsletters and provide introductory workshops as continuing education and some capacity building.

Top priorities for capacity building as noted by respondents include protocols for action and social commitment by associations, policy development inclusion of occupational therapists as having significant roles in disaster management and rehabilitation, skills in community building and community-based programmes for trauma management, both physical and mental.

To ensure that occupational therapists have access to resources for developing capacity and best practice, the WFOT DP&R project team is presently developing an online interactive education module series. Alternative options will be made available for those who are not able to access the online modules.

WFOT Documents

The WFOT continues to develop documents and position statements related to key areas of interest supported by relevant strategies for implementation.

WFOT documents that are particularly useful reference points include the Guiding Principles on Diversity and Culture (WFOT 2009) as well as the Position Statement on Community Based Rehabilitation (CBR), the Position Statement on Human Rights (WFOT 2006) and the Position Statement on Diversity and Culture (2010). The WFOT document Guiding Principles on Diversity and Culture promotes and advocates an inclusive policy in human rights, which is reinforced by the WFOT statement that 'people have the right to participate in a range of occupations that enable them to flourish, fulfil their potential and experience satisfaction in a way consistent with their culture and beliefs' (WFOT 2010).

The WFOT Position Statement on CBR (WFOT 2004) notes that 'Occupational therapists are committed to advance the right of all people – including people with disabilities – to develop their capacity and power to construct their own destiny through occupation.'

As an emerging field of occupational therapy practice, DP&R should be incorporating human rights and CBR policy at all levels – local, national, and international – with consideration for occupation-based and community-based practice.

As noted in the WFOT Position on Disaster Preparedness and Response (2014), occupational therapists are challenged to raise awareness of the benefits of occupational therapy and occupation-based community involvement to both government and community leaders. Capacity building is necessary to ensure that occupational therapy volunteers are prepared to undertake disaster response.

CONCLUSION

If occupational therapists are to overcome these challenges they need to take their rightful places as social entrepreneurs:

What business entrepreneurs are to the economy, social entrepreneurs are to social change. They are the driven, creative individuals who question the status quo, exploit new opportunities and refuse to give up – and remake the world for the better.

Bornstein 2004, quoted in Drayton et al 2006

Emergencies create a wide range of problems experienced at the individual, family, community and societal levels (IASC 2007). At every level, emergencies erode normally protective supports, increase the risks of diverse problems and tend to amplify preexisting problems of social injustice and inequality. The position statement on CBR addresses this by stating that 'occupational therapists also have a role and responsibility to develop and synthesise knowledge to support participation; to identify and raise issues of occupational barriers and injustices; and to work with groups, communities and societies to enhance participation in occupation for all persons. Achieving this is to achieve an occupationally just society.' Challenges for occupational therapists and occupational therapy associations lie in 'accepting professional responsibility to identify and address occupational injustices and limit the impact of such injustices experienced by individuals, raising collective awareness of the broader view of occupation and participation in society as a right, learning to work collaboratively with individuals, organisations, communities and societies, to promote participation through meaningful occupation' (WFOT 2004).

Occupational therapists have a unique knowledge and skill set to identify a person's or community's needs and build upon available strengths and resources in a manner that strengthens resilience and supports long-term recovery. Furthermore, occupational therapists have an appreciation of the accessibility issues of an environment and the skills to enable participation in a variety of contexts. This is especially relevant to formulating authentic emergency evacuation and preparedness plans as well as long-term development involving vulnerable groups such as people with disabilities. The challenge for occupational therapy is in defining avenues and developing strategies for involvement and engagement at multiple levels. Through interdisciplinary engagement and collaboration we collectively learn and new possibilities emerge. As an occupational therapist from the Philippines said in an email to WFOT following her experiences of working in Sri Lanka post 2004 tsunami: 'The tsunami taught me a lot professionally – taught me to COME OUT FROM THE BOX.'

Opportunities exist to promote valuable links between WFOT programmes, further liaison with other organizations, and further competencies to work in this field. There are integrative, scaling-up and value-adding benefits to be gained through exploring and developing linkages between various WFOT and other international programmes. Occupational therapists, through engagement with local, district and national government and nongovernmental organizations, can be promoting the utilization of our unique occupational perspectives to carve out roles and approaches that offer value to these organizations and ultimately to the communities and populations affected by disaster – both natural and manmade.

The future is not some place we are going to, but one we are creating. The paths are not to be found, but made, and the activity of making them, changes both the maker and the destination.

Schaar 2004

REFERENCES

American Occupational Therapy Association, 2011. The role of occupational therapy in disaster preparedness, response and recovery. AJOT 65 (suppl.), S11–S25.

Bornstein, D., 2004. How to Change the World – Social Entrepreneurs and the Power of New Ideas. Oxford University Press, New York.

Drayton, W., Brown, C., Hillhouse, K., 2006. Integrating social entrepreneurs into the "health for all" formula. Bull. World Health Organ. 84 (8), 589–684.

Gonzalez, A., 2012. Emergency situation in Venezuela – were we prepared? WFOT Bulletin 65, 57–61.

IASC, 2007. IASC Guidelines on Mental Health and Psychosocial Support in Emergency Settings. <http://www.humanitarianinfo.org/IASC> (accessed 6 April 2014).

Kramer, R., 2007. Leading change through action learning. TPM 36 (3), 38–44.

Lagos, A., Zegers, B., 2011. T.O. en alerta Chile: contribuyendo a la preparacion y respuesta ante catastrophes. WFOT Bulletin 63, 61–62.

Schaar, J., 2004. Quote. <http://en.thinkexist.com/quotes/John_Schaar> (accessed 6 April 2014).

Speicher, S., 2013. Disaster response after-action report: occupational therapy in the wake of Hurricane Isaac. OT Practice/AOTA 18, 3, 13–17.

WFOT, 2004. Position Statement on Community Based Rehabilitation. WFOT, Perth, Australia.

WFOT, 2006. Position Statement on Human Rights. WFOT, Perth, Australia.

WFOT, 2007. Disaster preparedness and response project: phase 2 report, national workshops. WFOT, Perth, Australia.

WFOT, 2009. Guiding Principles on Diversity and Culture. WFOT, Perth, Australia.

WFOT, 2010. Position Statement on Diversity and Culture. WFOT, Perth, Australia.

WFOT, 2012. WFOT Council Meeting Report, Taipei, Taiwan. WFOT, Perth Australia.

PART III

An Occupational Perspective on Disaster and Development

■ ■ ■ ■ ■ ■ ■ ■ ■ ■ ■ ■ ■ ■ ■ ■ ■ ■

Part III draws upon the collective knowledge and experience contained in the case series, cross-disciplinary literature and practice in the field. Based on this analysis we have articulated the disaster and development occupational perspective framework (DDOP), a framework that conceptually links occupation to the field of disaster and development. Six key principles of occupation are embedded within the DDOP framework. These principles reveal the symbolic value and transformative potential of occupation and position it for change within a dynamic, emergent and socio-ecological system. Further to this, we outline a process for transforming interactions and building relationships through occupation, towards more resilient, equitable and sustainable relationships and communities (the model of occupational stewardship and collaborative engagement (mOSCE)). Considerations for policy, practice and professional development are discussed.

30

AN OCCUPATIONAL PERSPECTIVE ON DISASTER AND DEVELOPMENT AND A CONCEPTUAL FRAMEWORK

NANCY RUSHFORD ■ KERRY THOMAS

The purpose of this chapter is to elucidate an occupational perspective in the field of disaster and development by drawing upon the collective knowledge and experiences contained within the case series and the literature, as it falls under the global umbrella of disaster risk reduction, resilience and sustainability. Through this process we have articulated principles of occupation in disaster and development that represent the 'occupational context'. These principles inform the disaster and development occupational perspective (DDOP) framework and the development of guidelines (Chapter 32) to support occupational-based practice in the field. The principles, framework and guidelines conceptually link occupation to the field of disaster and development and are evolving constructs to be continuously shaped by dialogue, experience, cross-disciplinary debate and developments in the field.

AN EMERGENT OCCUPATIONAL PERSPECTIVE

Disaster tells a story about people and their relationships with each other and the world around them that is characterized by patterns of engagement, or, in other words, the occupations or activities of everyday life, as they emerge and evolve through relationships. At the beginning of this book we positioned occupation at the nexus between society and the natural world, and the critical juncture where transformative potential lies. The current global narrative on disaster calls for collective action and social change at the point of everyday activities, where natural hazards, social relations and individual choice converge (Blaikie 1994). The case series has provided a rich opportunity to explore the transformative potential of occupation and position it in the field, ultimately articulating an occupational perspective on disaster and development that would strengthen the profession's contribution to a collective and interdisciplinary global response.

Njelesani et al (2014) delineate individual and societal aspects of an occupational perspective. Microlevel aspects include, for example, subjective experiences of meaning, identity, autonomy, self-determination and empowerment; macrolevel aspects relate to everyday activities (e.g. organization, routines, choices), collective identity and social systems of support in terms of how they inhibit or promote health through participation in occupations. The stories that comprise the case series form a 'narrative-in-action' (Alasker et al 2013), where individual and community experiences and actions in the field take their meaning by belonging and contributing to the story or bigger picture about occupation and disaster.

INSIGHTS FROM EMERGENCY RESPONSE

In the emergency response and early recovery phase of the disaster management cycle, contributors described experiences of disaster in terms of how it impacted upon the activities of everyday life. Moreover, they captured the transformative potential of occupation through their descriptions of how occupation promotes disaster recovery and healing. In makeshift hospitals and displaced persons camps, people who had survived disaster were seen to engage in occupations in various forms. They tenaciously held onto familiar routines and used occupation as a means to connect them to the past, to distract them from pain, to build strength, and to occupy time. Occupations such as art and music helped survivors to express themselves, connect with one another and cope. Through collaborative occupations that enabled expressions of reciprocity and cultivated a sense of community, survivors experienced solidarity and hope. Practitioners in the case series spoke about their efforts to mobilize people both physically and figuratively towards health and recovery immediately following the traumatic event. They helped survivors to take stock of what was lost, yet shift their attention to what remained and build upon remaining capacities, through the lens of occupation. In these early stages their efforts were largely concentrated on re-establishing the routines of everyday life and recreating a sense of normalcy amid chaos and confusion.

INSIGHTS FROM DISASTER RECOVERY

Stories of disaster recovery centred largely upon the social and psychological dimensions of experiences of disaster, including social inequality and psychological trauma. Practitioners focused on re-engagement in the occupations of everyday life following disaster and recovery from trauma. This involved establishing safe 'occupational' spaces within which people could find respite and begin to (re)build routines, roles and relationships. People with disabilities, refugees, older people, women and children and people from ethnic minorities were among the most socially disadvantaged groups who faced barriers to accessing relief and resources to promote healing and recovery. Engagement, inclusion and empowerment moved beyond rhetoric and ideals in this section and began to take shape in real-life experiences. The transformative potential of occupation came to life in the manner in which the focus on everyday occupations and activities served as a tool to examine and ultimately change patterns of thinking, doing or interacting in the broader contexts of rehabilitation and reconstruction. Practitioners worked alongside traumatized individuals and socially disadvantaged groups towards empowerment, capacity building, (re)engagement and participation in the social and economic aspects of life.

INSIGHTS FROM DEVELOPMENT

The stories that involved 'development' centred upon social vulnerability and risk. Development was presented as a long-term and often complicated process that involved addressing the underlying social factors that shape vulnerability and contribute to disaster risk and the capacity for recovery. Development processes were seen in the practitioners' efforts to galvanize the work of disabled people's organizations and mainstream disability, transform the built environment, and mobilize and empower local communities and particularly vulnerable groups. Practitioners endeavoured to translate the value of occupation into social action and change by using occupation as a transformative medium or tool. Through engagement in occupations, people built relationships with each other and the world around them and created new meaning and opportunities to carry them into the future.

INSIGHTS FROM ENTERING THE FIELD

Key insights from 'entering the field' centred upon the challenges that practitioners faced in their efforts to understand and adapt their approach to the disaster-affected context. Hunt (2011) has examined the moral landscape of humanitarian and development assistance from the perspective of health professionals' experience of ethics in the field. He identified several themes that are reflected in the case series including: (1) tension between respecting local customs and values, and acting in ways that are consistent with one's core moral convictions; (2) divergent understandings and experiences of health and illness; and (3) questions of identity as a professional, humanitarian and moral person. The importance of viewing occupation in the context was illuminated in this section, coupled with ongoing critical reflection. Failure to do so risked doing more harm than good, a phenomenon that is well documented in the field (Anderson 1999, De Waal 1997, Hunt 2011).

DISASTER AND OCCUPATION: THE STORY TOLD

The case series has told a story about disaster and occupation – one where occupation is deeply embedded in the socio-ecological context and is used as a transformative medium in change processes associated with resilience and recovery. In this story the practitioner draws upon occupation to support (re) engagement in life in a manner that is stronger and more inclusive, equitable and sustainable. We believe that the insights garnered from the case series have relevance beyond the field of disaster and development in that they inform a socio-ecological practice and offer further opportunity to advance the profession's social vision of health, wellbeing and justice through occupation. Along these lines, we have developed six key principles of occupation in disaster and development based on reflections on the case series, the literature and our own experiences. The principles are embraced by and encompass four common core values: equity, participation, capability and resilience. The principles and core values are outlined in Figure 30-1 and are intended to guide occupation-based interventions within a dynamic emergent socio-ecological context.

PRINCIPLES IN PRACTICE: THE DDOP FRAMEWORK

Collectively the principles of occupation in disaster and development contribute to an occupational perspective on disaster and development, as represented by the DDOP framework that is depicted in Figure 30-2. At the heart of the DDOP framework lies occupation, as it is deeply embedded in the context. The context refers to: (1) the occupational context, including the principles of occupation in disaster and development and common assumptions of the occupational therapy profession, including that occupation has a transactional relationship with the contex, contains form, function, and meaning across individual and societal levels, is connected to health and well being, and has therapeutic value (Hammell 2009); (2) the disaster management cycle as it integrates occupation into pre- and post-disaster activities; (3) the sustainable development and resilience context and its core

principles, related to prevention and early warning, protection and relief, human rights and equity, participation, capacity-building and sustainability; (4) the complex sociocultural, political and economic forces that characterize society; and (5) the environment and ecological systems, as they pertain to the physical/built environment and the ecosystems that shape and support life on the planet.

The DDOP framework is based on the premise that people co-produce the context they inhabit through their interaction (Blumer 1969, Holstein & Gubrium 2004), which is mediated through their engagement in occupations. As such, occupation can be seen to emerge and evolve through a complex web of relationships, and in turn shapes and mirrors the qualities of these relationships. This position illuminates the symbolic value and transformative potential of occupation. The implication is that by examining 'occupation in context' and using 'occupation as a medium' we can better understand the fit between people, the environment, occupations and the natural world.

In particular, occupation can function as a conduit through which individuals and societies can emerge from disaster, mitigating its impact, adapting and building resilience; conversely, occupation can be a source of their demise, depending on the circumstances or conditions within which it unfolds. Furthermore, when occupation is viewed in the context of relationships it can be stewarded in such a way as to transform patterns of interactions and activities towards more resilient, equitable and sustainable systems, structures and relationships that ultimately protect the ecological integrity of the planet and build resilience to disaster. As such, the concept of 'occupational stewardship' is positioned at heart of the DDOP framework. The DDOP framework effectively reconceptualizes occupation and repositions it for change within our increasingly complex and interdependent global society.

RECONCEPTUALIZING OCCUPATION AND REPOSITIONING IT FOR CHANGE

Historically, the scope of occupational therapy practice has been limited by the profession's orientation to the individual sphere of occupation, based on the

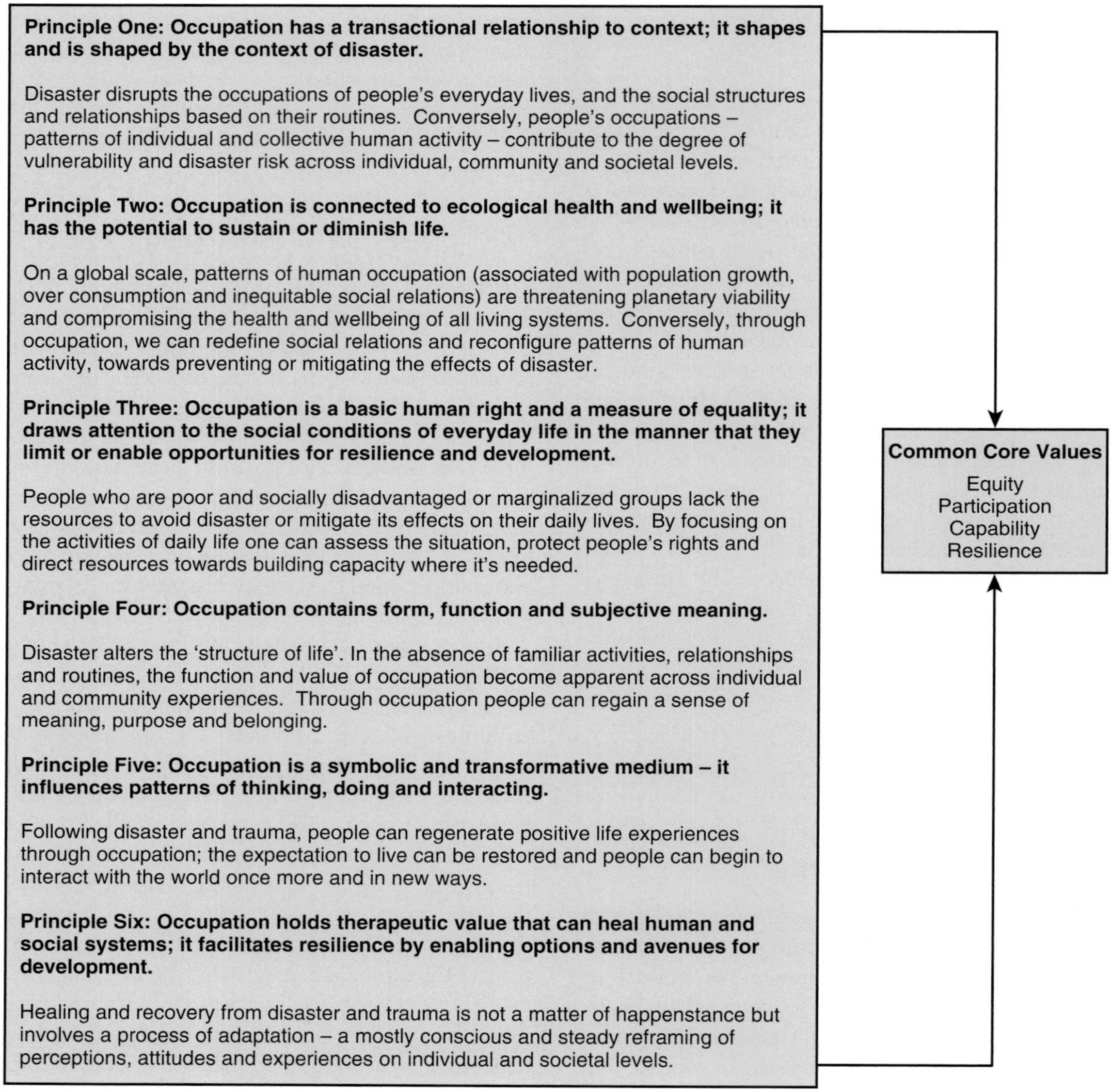

Principle One: Occupation has a transactional relationship to context; it shapes and is shaped by the context of disaster.

Disaster disrupts the occupations of people's everyday lives, and the social structures and relationships based on their routines. Conversely, people's occupations – patterns of individual and collective human activity – contribute to the degree of vulnerability and disaster risk across individual, community and societal levels.

Principle Two: Occupation is connected to ecological health and wellbeing; it has the potential to sustain or diminish life.

On a global scale, patterns of human occupation (associated with population growth, over consumption and inequitable social relations) are threatening planetary viability and compromising the health and wellbeing of all living systems. Conversely, through occupation, we can redefine social relations and reconfigure patterns of human activity, towards preventing or mitigating the effects of disaster.

Principle Three: Occupation is a basic human right and a measure of equality; it draws attention to the social conditions of everyday life in the manner that they limit or enable opportunities for resilience and development.

People who are poor and socially disadvantaged or marginalized groups lack the resources to avoid disaster or mitigate its effects on their daily lives. By focusing on the activities of daily life one can assess the situation, protect people's rights and direct resources towards building capacity where it's needed.

Principle Four: Occupation contains form, function and subjective meaning.

Disaster alters the 'structure of life'. In the absence of familiar activities, relationships and routines, the function and value of occupation become apparent across individual and community experiences. Through occupation people can regain a sense of meaning, purpose and belonging.

Principle Five: Occupation is a symbolic and transformative medium – it influences patterns of thinking, doing and interacting.

Following disaster and trauma, people can regenerate positive life experiences through occupation; the expectation to live can be restored and people can begin to interact with the world once more and in new ways.

Principle Six: Occupation holds therapeutic value that can heal human and social systems; it facilitates resilience by enabling options and avenues for development.

Healing and recovery from disaster and trauma is not a matter of happenstance but involves a process of adaptation – a mostly conscious and steady reframing of perceptions, attitudes and experiences on individual and societal levels.

Common Core Values

Equity
Participation
Capability
Resilience

FIGURE 30-1 ■ Principles of occupation in disaster and development.

premise that occupation resides in the individual and primary value given to independence and individual experience (Dickie et al 2006). Models of occupation (e.g. person–environment–occupation (PEO), model of human occupation (MOHO) and person–environment–occupation–performance (PEOP)) are generally concerned with the dynamic and interdependent relationships between the person, the environment and occupation, and delimit person–environment interactions to the form, function and subjective meaning of occupation, as it involves individuals or independent entities (e.g. an institution, a group, a population). Within this context, occupation is used both as a means and an end to facilitate interactions among the client, the environments or contexts, and the activities or occupations, in order to help the client (typically an

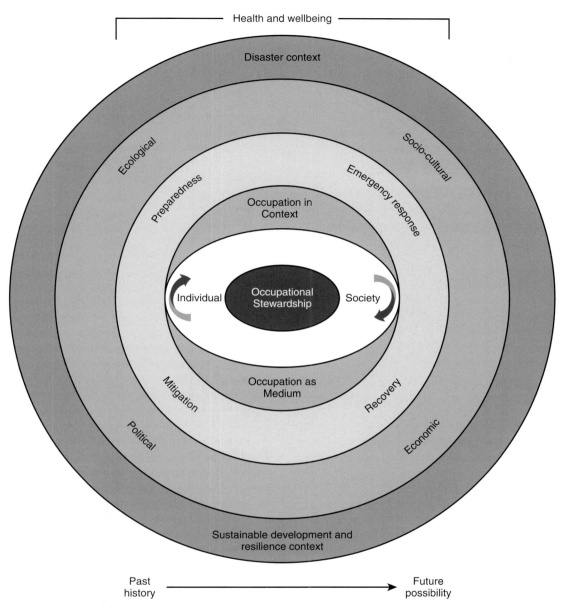

FIGURE 30-2 ■ The disaster and development – occupational perspective (DDOP) framework.

individual) to reach the desired outcomes that support health and participation in life (Trombly 1995).

Increasingly, occupational therapists and occupational scientists are considering the occupational context and are looking more broadly at the client's health and wellbeing in terms of equity and justice involving people's equal right to have opportunity, choice, participation, empowerment and balance in everyday life (Townsend & Polatajko 2007). This critical social perspective is taking occupational therapy practice beyond issues of individual performance, impairment and disability from a medical perspective to occupational engagement[1] and enablement that is orientated to cultivating the conditions for change to support participation in occupations (Polatajko et al 2007). Practitioners aim to *create possibilities and build the capacity for people to be or do something* by enabling individual and social change (Townsend et al 2007)[2]. Consequently there is increasing interest in the role of occupation in community development practices and population health needs within the broader context of human rights, sustainability and lifestyle choices. This resonates with an emergent transactional perspective on occupation within occupational science which views occupation as an important mode through which human beings, as organisms-in-environment-as-a-whole, function in their complex totality (Cutchin & Dickie 2013). Along these lines, occupational therapists and occupational scientists (Ramugondo & Kronenberg 2013, Thibeault 2013) have expanded the study of the relational dimension of occupation with attention to the notion of 'collective occupations' as they reflect intention towards social cohesion or dysfunction, advancement or aversion to a common good. Their perspective highlights the interconnectedness between individuals in context and calls for a social practice.

The field of disaster and development has much to add to a transactional perspective of occupation and the development of a social practice in occupational therapy. This is largely because disaster resilience and recovery extends beyond the sole functioning of an individual or an individual aspect of a system to reflect relationships and the ecological systems that support life on the planet, as discussed in Chapter 3. The global imperative of disaster risk reduction and sustainable development indicates that there is a critical need to heal the entire system through collective action and interdisciplinary collaboration. Ultimately, this depends upon our ability to cultivate and nurture the qualities of interactions and relationships that will enable systems continuously to adapt and thrive. An occupational perspective on disaster and development illuminates the symbolic and transformative potential of occupation as it lies within the web of relationships that characterize human occupation and activity and ultimately support life on the planet.

SUMMARY

This chapter has integrated insights from the case series into key principles and foundations for occupational therapy practice in disaster and development, as depicted in the DDOP framework. The emergent framework, with occupational stewardship at its core, illuminates the symbolic and transformative potential of occupation as it lies within a web of relationships. Essentially, DDOP reconceptualizes occupation and repositions it for change within a dynamic, emergent and socio-ecological context. This perspective holds the potential to strengthen the contribution of the profession to the global imperative of reducing disaster risk and promoting sustainable development within the broader context of health, wellbeing and planetary viability.

---

[1]Occupational engagement refers to 'all that people do to involve themselves or become occupied; to participate; to occupy themselves or others' (Townsend & Polatajko 2007, p. 24; dictionary definition).

[2]*Enabling* is the basis of occupational therapy's client-centred practice and is a foundation for client empowerment and justice (Townsend & Polatajko 2007, p. 99). When human occupation is limited, occupational therapists work collaboratively with the client to find solutions to support engagement in the occupations of everyday living. They are guided by enablement foundations (Townsend et al 2007) and the enablement process, as depicted in the Canadian Model of Client-Centred Enablement (CMCE) (Townsend et al 2007). In addition to the CMCE, there are other models and insights from the occupational therapy and occupational science literature that help practitioners to navigate the social realm of practice. These include, for example, the Kawa Model of Occupation which articulates a collective orientated and interdependent view of occupation (Iwama 2005), Thibeault's (2013) occupation-based community-building process for occupational justice, Watson & Swartz's Transformation through Occupation model (2004) and the emergent transactional perspective on occupation (Cutchin & Dickie 2013).

REFERENCES

Alasker, S., Josephson, S., Dickie, V.A., 2013. Exploring the transactional quality of everyday occupations through narrative-in-action. Meaning-making among women living with chronic conditions. In: Cutchin, M.P., Dickie, V.A. (Eds.), Transactional Perspectives on Occupation. Springer, Chapel Hill, USA.

Anderson, M.B., 1999. Do No Harm. How Aid Can Support Peace – or War. Lynne Rienner Publishers, Boulder, CO.

Blaikie, P., Cannon, T., Davis, I., Wisner, B., 1994. At Risk: Natural Hazards, People's Vulnerability, and Disasters. Routledge, London, UK.

Blumer, H., 1969. Symbolic Interactionism. Prentice-Hall, Englewood Cliffs, NJ.

Cutchin, M.P., Dickie, V.A., 2013. Transactional Perspectives on Occupation. Springer, Chapel Hill, MC.

De Waal, A., 1997. Famine Crimes: Politics and the Disaster Relief Industry. International African Institute North America: Indiana University Press, London, UK.

Dickie, V., Cutchin, M., Humphry, R., 2006. Occupation as transactional experience: a critique of individualism in occupational science. J. Occup. Sci. 13 (1), 83–93.

Hammell, K., 2009. Sacred texts: a sceptical exploration of the assumptions underpinning theories of occupation. Can. J. Occup. Ther. 76 (1), 6–13.

Holstein, J.A., Gubrium, J.F., 2004. Context: working it up, down and across. In: Seale, C., Gobo, G., Gubrium, J.F., Silverman, D. (Eds.), Qualitative Research Practice. Sage Publications, London, UK.

Hunt, M.R., 2011. Establishing moral bearings: ethics and expatriate health care professionals in humanitarian work. Disasters 35 (3), 606–622.

Iwama, M., 2005. The Kawa (river) model: nature, life flow and the power of culturally relevant occupational therapy. In: Kronenberg, F., Algado, S.S., Pollard, N. (Eds.), Occupational Therapy without Borders – Learning from the Spirit of Survivors. Churchill Livingstone, London, pp. 219–227.

Njelesani, J., Tang, A., Jonsson, H., Polatajko, H., 2014. Articulating an occupational perspective. J. Occup. Sci. 21 (2), 226–235.

Polatajko, H.J., Craik, J., Davis, J., Townsend, E.A., 2007. Canadian Practice Process Framework (CPPF). In: Townsend, E.A., Polatajko, H.J. (Eds.), Enabling Occupation II: Advancing an Occupational Vision of Health, Wellbeing, and Justice through Occupation. CAOT Publications ACE, Ottawa, ON, p. 233.

Ramugondo, E., Kronenberg, F., 2013. Explaining collective occupations from a human relations perspective: bridging the individual-collective dichotomy. J. Occup. Sci. doi:10.1080/14427591.2013.781920.

Suzuki, D., McConnell, A., 1997. The Sacred Balance. Rediscovering Our Place in Nature. Allen & Unwin, Sydney, Australia.

Thibeault, R., 2013. Occupational justice's intents and impacts: from personal choices to community consequence. In: Cutchin, M.P., Dickie, V.A. (Eds.), Transactional Perspectives on Occupation. Springer, Chapel Hill, MC, pp. 245–256.

Townsend, E.A., Polatajko, H.J., 2007. Enabling Occupation II: Advancing an Occupational Therapy Vision for Health, Wellbeing, and Justice through Occupation. CAOT Publications ACE, Ottawa, ON.

Townsend, E.A., Polatajko, H.J., Craig, J., Davis, J., 2007. Canadian Model of Client-Centred Enablement (CMCE). In: Townsend, E.A., Polatajko, H.J. (Eds.), Enabling Occupation II: Advancing an Occupational Therapy Vision for Health, Wellbeing, and Justice through Occupation. CAOT Publications ACE, Ottawa, ON, p. 101.

Trombly, C.A., 1995. Occupation: purposefulness and meaningfulness as therapeutic mechanisms. 1995 Eleanor Clarke Slagle Lecture. AJOT 40 (10), 960–972.

Watson, R., Swartz, L. (Eds.), 2004. Transformation through Occupation. Whurr, London, UK.

31

OCCUPATIONAL STEWARDSHIP AND COLLABORATIVE ENGAGEMENT: A PRACTICE MODEL

NANCY RUSHFORD

INTRODUCTION

This chapter elaborates upon the concept of occupational stewardship as introduced in Chapter 30 and translates the concept into a practice model – the model of occupational stewardship and collaborative engagement (mOSCE). Occupational stewardship, which we have placed at the centre of the disaster and development occupational perspective (DDOP) framework, involves cultivating resilience, health and wellbeing through the use of occupation as it lies within the social or relational sphere. Ultimately, it leads to stronger, more inclusive and sustainable relationships and systems. The origins, dimensions and implications of the model are discussed in terms of relevant research and practice in the field.

OCCUPATIONAL STEWARDSHIP: ORIGINS OF THE CONCEPT

Occupational stewardship is both a concept and a practice that stems from research that I conducted between 2009 and 2012 through the University of Sydney, Australia, as a part of my doctoral studies. The research sought to explore the relationship between disaster and occupation as it pertained to change processes associated with disaster resilience and recovery and involved a series of in-depth interviews with occupational therapists (Rushford 2014). Participants in the study represented a diversity of roles in the field of disaster and crossed a range of cultural contexts (i.e. India, Africa, Indonesia, China, Bangladesh,

the Caribbean). Drawing upon grounded theory as a methodology (Charmaz 2006), I developed a theory out of the stories that participants told me about their experiences. This theory is represented by the concept of occupational stewardship and the model of occupational stewardship and collaborative engagement.

Stewardship, as it is typically defined in terms of the careful and responsible planning and use of resources (Alvarez-Rosete et al 2013, Travis et al 2002), reflects an ethic that is commonly associated with environmental protection, preservation and natural resource management. The concept is reflected in aboriginal cultures that have a deep respect for nature and the creator. Stewardship is also embedded in Judaeo-Christian tradition and is captured in biblical stories and metaphors about creation that describe humanity's relationship to God and the natural world (Sanguin 2007). The concept has also been applied to disciplines such as economics, information technology and health. Within the context of health, stewardship refers to the 'careful and responsible management of the wellbeing of the population' (Travis et al 2002, p. 1) and embeds health within broader society (Alvarez-Rosete et al 2013). Relatively recently the idea of stewardship has emerged in global health governance debates and has been identified as one of the core functions of all health systems. Within the health sector a key aspect of the stewardship role involves influencing policies and actors within collaborative systems (Alvarez-Rosete et al 2013, Travis et al 2002).

Sanguin (2007) argues that the depiction of stewardship as a management function, as it is commonly represented in contemporary discourse, has limited usefulness in a world where humans are part of an intricate ecosystem. He likens people's relationships with each other and the natural world, including all living organisms and systems, as a dynamic 'dance', and asserts that our primary task is to 'find our place in the fit and flow of reality' (p. 38) rather than stand over and above nature, creation or social systems as 'managers'.

> ... *what we're involved with is a relationship with different modes of consciousness – divine, plant, animal and human. It is a communion of subjects, a dance. Precisely because we possess a unique power to shape the future of life on earth, it's imperative that we learn the steps.*
>
> *Sanguin 2007, p. 38*

The concept of 'occupational stewardship' echoes Sanguin's ecological perspective and emphasis on dynamic, collaborative engagement but positions occupation as a potential change agent or transformative medium in this process. Occupational stewardship refers to a *social process of engagement* or 'socio-ecological practice' that is embedded within natural systems, health systems and wider society. The process is grounded in the experiences of the practitioners in the field of disaster who were part of my research. These practitioners drew upon occupation to facilitate new patterns of behaviour and interaction within complex socio-ecological systems. They cultivated connections between people and endeavoured to influence relationships and systems (actors, policies) that would ultimately build resilience and promote

health and wellbeing across individual and social spheres of practice. The model of occupational stewardship and collaborative engagement (mOSCE) outlines this process of engagement and offers an emergent perspective and practice that elaborates on the symbolic and relational dimensions of occupation. In doing so, the model potentially helps occupational therapists to translate the value of occupation into social action and change, in keeping with the profession's social vision of health, wellbeing and justice through occupation.

OCCUPATIONAL STEWARDSHIP: A TWO-FOLD PROCESS

Occupational stewardship is a twofold process that involves (1) 'working within context' and (2) 'creating occupational space for engagement', towards cultivating the quality of connections that build resilience and promote health and wellbeing over the long term (Figure 31-1). The process hinges upon the analysis of occupation and activity (as a subset of occupation) and its use as a *medium* to influence how people engage with each other and the environment around them. Occupation is the primary medium through which practitioners work within context, create occupational space and guide interactions towards more resilient, inclusive and sustainable relationships and systems.

Working within Context

Working within context refers to the practitioner's ability to connect with and adapt to the context (its various aspects, elements and people). The

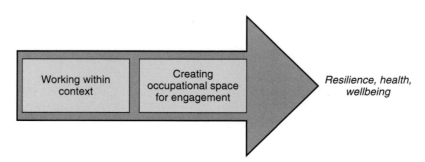

FIGURE 31-1 ■ A social process of engagement.

practitioner works within context by adopting an holistic and ecological perspective from which they seek to understand or appreciate the interrelationships between people (with each other), occupations and the environment. Occupation serves as a bridge that enables the practitioner to elicit, interpret and better understand the context in terms of its impact upon everyday life and activities. This helps practitioners to guide and adapt their intervention within the relational or social sphere according to emergent context and evolving needs.

Illustrative example:

Looking at people more holistically or in their context helps you to not only look at what was happening prior, but also the effects of actions as well on the systems around and the people around and relationships.

                                         Research participant

Creating Occupational Space

Creating occupational space refers to the practitioner's deliberate efforts to establish connections and build relationships through occupation and activity. The practitioners 'make room' or 'hold space' to guide interactions within the relational or social sphere. By creating occupational space they open up possibilities for new behaviours and patterns of interaction to emerge through the specialized use of occupation.

Illustrative example:

I always start with creating a safe space … and again, that space is created, a lot, through not necessarily dialogue but through shared occupation.

                                         Research participant

THE CONTINUUM OF ENGAGEMENT

Within the occupational spaces the practitioner draws upon occupation and activity to facilitate engagement along a continuum from 'passive' or 'divisive' engagement, reflecting disconnect or disequilibrium between actors and elements within a given system or occupation space, to 'active' and 'collaborative' engagement as associated with equilibrium, social cohesion or unity (Figure 31-2).

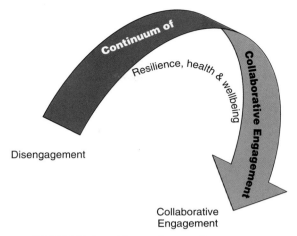

FIGURE 31-2 ■ The continuum of engagement.

Illustrative example:

I think there is a lot of trauma following any kind of disaster and there is all these groups, people need to share what has happened to them, people need to recreate links. Often people are displaced out of their original place and often also they are not within their existing community … (they) have to form a group again, as a community again. But there is also this whole relationship building between different members of the community which is new, which didn't exist before and then even gathering people who are in conflict and they need to rebuild things. So as an occupational therapist you could really work through activity building with clear objectives and an aim on choosing the activity, what form, what you want to build up, where you want to go …

                                         Research participant

Specific objectives for the practitioner's intervention within the occupational spaces vary. They may reflect typical occupational therapy concerns – such as physical or psychosocial rehabilitation (e.g. injuries, trauma) and/or social issues (e.g. inequality, conflict) as they pertain to individual health and wellbeing – or, more broadly, community development, advocacy and social change. Cross-cutting both realms of practice is the practitioner's consistent attention to the social fabric of engagement and the symbolic and relational dimensions of occupation. This is characterized by efforts to unite people through occupation and build a common purpose or collective sense of identity that in turn strengthens individual resilience and reaffirms an individual's position within the social world and an intricate ecosystem. Within these spaces individual rehabilitative goals merge with community and social development goals.

DIMENSIONS OF OCCUPATION

[Occupational stewardship] is powerful in my view because it creates a collective identity that transcends or reconciles differences, and reconnects all involved at a very deep level, to the sense of belonging to the same web of life.

Research participant

Occupational stewardship draws upon the symbolic and relational dimensions of occupation to influence new behaviours and patterns of interaction associated with resilience, health and wellbeing. Similar to the therapeutic use of activity to assess function and dysfunction and design intervention on an individual level (Polatajko et al 2007), occupation and activities can be used in the social sphere to assess and strengthen interpersonal relationships – to elicit behaviours such as

reciprocity, cooperation, trust and collaboration that effectively build community and create opportunities for integration, inclusion and social development.

The practitioners in the study used occupation across three symbolic and relational dimensions, including its use as: (1) a functional bridge; (2) a unit of analysis; and (3) a transformative tool (Figure 31-3). As a *functional bridge* occupation connects people through their everyday activities and roles and filters information in terms of everyday experience. As a *unit of analysis* it provides a means for assessing the context – people and their interactions with each other and the world around them. As a *transformative tool*, occupation is used to shift people's positions and perspectives, literally and figuratively, towards new patterns of doing, thinking and interacting. Positioned as such, occupation holds the potential to facilitate collaborative engagement and plays a role in strengthening the social fabric upon which health, wellbeing and ecological integrity lie.

OCCUPATIONAL STEWARDSHIP AND COLLABORATIVE ENGAGEMENT: ILLUSTRATIVE EXAMPLES

I have chosen three stories from the field research to provide a snapshot of occupational stewardship across individual and social spheres of practice.

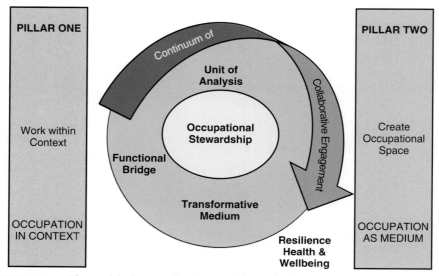

FIGURE 31-3 ■ The model of occupational stewardship and collaborative engagement (mOSCE).

Story One: Building Community from the Inside Out

Cecilia works at the local level in a community in South East Asia that has been affected by conflict and natural disaster. Under the umbrella of community-based rehabilitation (CBR), she stewards occupation in her efforts to link individual physical rehabilitation with broader goals of peace-building and community development. Occupation serves as the avenue through which she 'creates the space' for individual healing and development. Injured men engage in parallel therapeutic activities within these spaces (exercises in parallel bars) that are designed to improve their physical function. Simultaneously Cecilia creates opportunities to build relationships between the men and foster peace through the specialized use of occupation and activity. Cecilia establishes safe boundaries by grading the activities of the men from waiting alongside one another, to acting in parallel, to interacting by offering the men an incentive to communicate (microfinance opportunity). New perspectives potentially emerge from facilitated experiences and interactions on common ground. Occupation serves as a functional bridge by connecting the men through parallel activity. It acts as a transformative tool in the manner in which it is used to facilitate their interactions, create opportunities for expressions of reciprocity and build trust. The men are essentially guided by activity along a continuum of engagement, from passive or divisive[1] to active and/or collaborative, in a manner that supports individual health and wellbeing and builds relationships and potentially community.

Excerpt:

I've worked on a contract in the Southern East and, initially, it was just to have them (ex-combatants) come to the clinic at the same time, so to be in the waiting room together. No expectation to communicate. Then they would be put, let's say, at the parallel bars at the same time. But ultimately, I do microfinance and the guys would get loans only if they agreed to work together. But this process,

through all of the other exposure in occupations, was for them to get to build the common identity. They were no longer ex-combatants from different political factions. They were men needing to feed their families.

Research participant

Story Two: Enabling Opportunities for Change

Radina works with marginalized women and children in a displaced persons camp. Along with her team she partners with the women and children to create a safe 'occupational space' to inspire interaction and collaborative engagement and begin to redress social stigma within the camp. Through collaborative and playful engagement in occupations within these spaces (i.e. through cricket, a market), new perspectives emerge from the experience, potentially leading to broader social change (e.g. how a community treats widowed women and orphaned children). In this example, occupation serves as a functional bridge that connects the women and children to other members of the community. It acts as a transformative tool by creating opportunities for new positive experiences that potentially shift the communities' perceptions of the women and children.

Excerpt:

So, having that space for kids to be able to play [was important], but what we were really trying to do too was, because there was I guess, stigmas around being a widow, we wanted something to, like, bring other people that weren't part, you know living in this community, to the community – so the cricket pitch and the marketplace was kind of the idea. The activities bring in some exchanges ... and interactions between the two groups ... and then it leads also ... it was a mediator between the two groups ...

Research participant

Story Three: Towards Disability Inclusion and System Transformation

Victoria works for an international nongovernmental organization that focuses on people with disabilities in disaster and development contexts. She stewards occupation to promote disability inclusion in the

---

[1]'Passive' engagement refers to an individual's lack of active response to what happens/what others are doing around them; 'divisive' refers to separation, isolation, alienation or conflict involving two or more people.

field. In particular, Victoria uses occupation as a unit of analysis to measure inclusivity and the level of integration across sectors. She gathers information and data on how the policies and practices of the organizations impact upon disabled people's access to food, shelter, medical care and their daily occupations. Occupation serves as a functional bridge in the manner that it translates policy into the local context and illuminates any gaps and areas for improvement. Through this process Victoria connects stakeholders to the local context as it pertains to the experiences of people with disabilities. In doing so she creates the space to influence policies and actors within the system.

These three illustrations of occupational stewardship have provided a snapshot of how occupational therapists working in the field of disaster and development used occupation to cultivate resilience, health and wellbeing. In particular, their interventions highlight the interconnectedness between individuals in context and reveal the transformative potential of occupation as it lies within a web of relationships. Their stories reflect the principles of occupation in disaster and development as represented in the DDOP framework and echo the reflections on the case series.

SUMMARY

The concept of occupational stewardship, which is at the heart of the disaster and development occupational perspective (DDOP) framework, is grounded in research that drew upon the experiences of occupational therapists involved in the field of disaster. Occupational stewardship offers an ecological perspective on resilience, health and wellbeing and positions occupation as a vehicle for social change. The model of occupational stewardship and collaborative engagement describes this change process in terms of a socioecological practice that involves working within context and creating occupational space. Within these spaces the practitioner draws upon the symbolic and relational dimensions of occupation to cultivate connections between people, build relationships and influence systems. Positioned as such, occupation potentially strengthens the social fabric upon which health, wellbeing and ecological integrity lie.

REFERENCES

Alvarez-Rosete, A., Hawkins, B., Parkhurst, J., 2013. Health System Stewardship and Evidence Informed Health Policy. Working Paper #1, London School of Hygiene and Tropical Medicine. Available online: <http://www.lshtm.ac.uk/groups/griphealth/resources/health_system_stewardship_and_evidence_informed_health_policy.pdf>.

Charmaz, K., 2006. Constructing Grounded Theory. A Practical Guide through Qualitative Analysis. Sage Publications Ltd, Thousand Oaks, CA.

Polatajko, H.J., Cantin, N., Amoroso, B., McKee, P., Rivard, A., Kirsh, B., et al., 2007. Occupation-based enablement: a practice mosaic. In: Townsend, E.A., Polatajko, H.J. (Eds.), Enabling Occupation II: Advancing an Occupational Therapy Vision for Health Wellbeing and Justice through Occupation. CAOT publications ACE, Ottawa, ON, pp. 177–203.

Rushford, N., 2014. Collaborative Occupation and Transformation. A Theory Grounded in the Experiences of Disaster. University of Sydney, Australia.

Sanguin, B., 2007. Darwin, Divinity, and the Dance of the Cosmos. An Ecological Christianity. CopperHouse, Kelowna, BC, Canada.

Travis, P., Egger, D., Davies, P., Mechbal, A., 2002. Towards Better Stewardship. Concepts and Critical Issues. WHO, Geneva. Available online: <http://www.who.int/healthinfo/paper48.pdf>.

32

DISASTER AND DEVELOPMENT: PRACTICAL CONSIDERATIONS IN PROMOTING AN OCCUPATIONAL PERSPECTIVE

KERRY THOMAS ■ NANCY RUSHFORD

INTRODUCTION

This book has served to highlight three main things: (1) the nature and scale of the challenges facing humanity and the planet; (2) the character and complexity of disaster and development; and (3) the potential of occupation to illuminate pathways that can promote resilience, adaptability and transformation towards sustainability.

The case series has provided rich insight into the experience and understanding of occupational therapists and other practitioners, from which lessons and implications for future development have emerged. Drawing on these, and with reference to the disaster and development occupational perspective (DDOP) framework and the model of occupational stewardship and collaborative engagement (mOSCE), this chapter outlines a range of practical considerations to assist practitioners in confidently engaging in disaster preparedness, response, recovery and ongoing development and resilience-building activities.

The chapter is structured in three parts. First, we summarize four operational functions that have been revealed to be critical to achieving effective disaster and development outcomes. Second, we present a set of four guidelines and associated strategies that should inform all engagement in disaster and development. These guidelines operationalize the six principles of occupation in disaster and development that were introduced in Chapter 30 and are meant to express the core values of equity, participation, capability and resilience. Third, we outline some general considerations

for the profession of occupational therapy as it moves to strengthen its engagement in the field of disaster and development. Finally, a range of very practical strategies and actions are listed against each phase of the disaster management cycle.

DDOP – FROM THEORY TO PRACTICE

Figure 32-1 provides a diagrammatic representation of the relationship between the DDOP values, occupational principles, guidelines and strategies, and operational functions. Within the realm of socio-ecological interdependence as it relates to disaster and development, values inform the principles, and are expressed by them; the principles in turn inform the guidelines and associated strategies; and operational functions are carried out in accordance with these.

DDOP – KEY OPERATIONAL FUNCTIONS

At the heart of the task of operationalizing DDOP lie the functions of planning, coordination, monitoring and evaluation, and improvement. These are reflected in the disaster and development project cycle (Figure 3-3) that was introduced in Chapter 3.

Planning is central to any engagement. All interventions *must* be carefully considered and planned; already vulnerable people and communities cannot afford well-intentioned but poorly considered actions that may undermine existing capabilities or exacerbate vulnerabilities. The disaster and development arena is

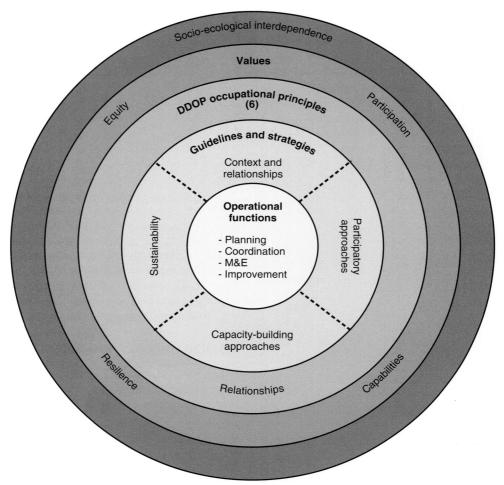

FIGURE 32-1 ■ Relationship between the DDOP framework, guidelines and key operational functions. M&E, monitoring and evaluation.

littered with good intentions that have made already dire situations even worse. Professional engagement, even in the emergency response phase, requires rapid but astute situational, context, needs and capacity assessments, and careful planning and consideration of the key values that are enshrined in international humanitarian and development mandates, as well as the occupational principles for disaster and development. As such, planning functions will necessarily span strategic and operational levels, encompass grassroots and international best practice perspectives, and be participatory – engaging survivors, other

stakeholders, disaster and development actors. But as this book has expounded, it is the voice (perspectives, needs) of survivors and local communities that must provide the foundation on which plans are developed.

Coordination is consistently identified as both a major issue and need in disaster and development. In designing and implementing disaster management and development initiatives, coordination of activities is imperative to enable effective, efficient and equitable services and programmes – that is, to ensure coverage, continuity and inclusion while preventing overlaps and wastage of scarce resources. Lack of coordination has contributed to exclusion, exacerbation of power and resource inequities and conflict, as well as corruption and misuse of donated funds and material. Importantly, operations must comply with mandates, policies and governance instruments, as set out in international and national guidelines. Coordination occurs in many ways, including through formal disaster management arrangements (e.g. clusters and coordinating committees) and climate change adaptation planning systems, as well as informal and opportunistic processes that emerge, such as facilitating networking between community people and groups. Planning, decision-making, resource allocation and communication strategies are among the functions that require coordination.

Monitoring and evaluation (M&E) involves the ongoing tracking of progress and performance, and periodic review of outcomes. It is about accounting for change – especially from a community's perspective, but also for donors and governments. M&E itself requires careful planning, implementation and management, from the outset of any programme or intervention. Information needs to be gathered that goes beyond accounting for outputs and expenditure, although these are critical to transparency and results. Importantly, and from an occupational perspective, there is an increasing desire and expectation across stakeholder groups to identify and share what the 'so what' outcomes of investment and effort have been. This requires gathering and analysing both quantitative data and qualitative information, including the lived experience of survivors and workers. These considerations compel the adoption of participatory monitoring and evaluation (PME) approaches. Key evaluative questions include, for example:

- How have the lives of survivors been impacted?
- Who has benefitted and in what way?
- How, and to what extent, has resilience to future shocks been cultivated?
- What strategies were particularly effective and efficient, and why?
- What were the challenges, shortfalls, failed strategies, and how were these addressed?
- What outcomes will be sustained, and continue to grow and adapt to changing circumstances?

Furthermore, M&E is also important in supporting development of evidence-based practice. As professionals we *can* make a difference but it is incumbent on us to critique and demonstrate what this is and how we enable it … to identify and account for the contribution and added value that occupational therapy brings to disaster and development.

Improvement occurs through learning, sharing, communication and utilization of results emerging from M&E and other sources, including research studies. At an operational level, mechanisms need to be established that allow for continual review of progress, processes and performance, to ensure that activities are addressing priority needs and continually adapting to the emerging issues, circumstances and opportunities. At a strategic level, results and lessons need to be critically appraised to extrapolate priorities and directions for refining policies, strategic plans and for advocacy development purposes. From a practice perspective, critical reflection on experience informs programme refinements and development, and contributes to evidence-based practice. But of greatest import, improvement should be focused on supporting and enabling survivors and communities to continue building their capacities and resilience in ways that are relevant and contextualized to their unique circumstances – as they exist now and might transpire in the future.

DDOP – GUIDELINES AND STRATEGIES

The guidelines and strategies presented here operate across all phases of the disaster and development continuum (as outlined in Figure 1-3 and Table 2-1) and through all stages of a disaster or development project cycle (Figure 3-3). They embody the essence of the DDOP framework (Figure 30-2) as explained in Chapters 30 and 31, and embrace the core values and DDOP principles of occupation in disaster and development as described in Figure 30-1.

Guideline 1: Understand the Context and Work through Relationships

The importance of context cannot be underestimated, for successful processes and outcomes depend upon a sound understanding of and respect for the dynamic variables of each unique disaster and development situation. Just as effective clinical results are reliant on accurate medical and therapeutic assessment, so too, disaster and development outcomes are dependent upon the quality of situational assessments. In the emergency phase, where rapid response is demanded, the strength of preparedness strategies – of affected people and communities, and of responders – becomes evident. During recovery and development, the adage of 'think global, act local' (Brower 1990, Geddes 1915, Dubos 1972) remains highly relevant as a guide in recognizing that successful strategies will reflect the unique diversity of local socioeconomic and ecological characteristics while appreciating globalization and finite planetary systems. As such, situational assessments that capture current local dynamics, needs and resources must be balanced with appreciation for the wider context and future scenarios. This demands a concerted appreciation of the complexity of interdependent and intergenerational relationships that bind these factors together.

The complexity of contexts, interdependence and resilience is increasingly understood as a myriad of dynamic relationships and as such we are witnessing increasing multisectoralization of the disaster and development arena. This is perhaps most evident in policies and approaches geared towards addressing climate change but is also a feature of sustainable development that endeavours to integrate social, economic and environmental considerations. Practitioners, including occupational therapists, will thus increasingly engage in a broadening range of multidisciplinary disaster and development initiatives that are at the cutting-edge interface between sectors.

From an occupation perspective, relationships are also the medium through which an understanding of context is achieved and through which occupational interventions occur – be it at an individual, family, community or societal level. At a very local operational level, in working with survivors, the rule of thumb is to 'listen, listen, listen … in order to respond with care, compassion and professionalism' (Figure 32-2).

Guideline 2: Adopt a Participatory Approach

Participation is both a right and a requirement within the context of disaster and development. Effective participation allows programme personnel to tap into

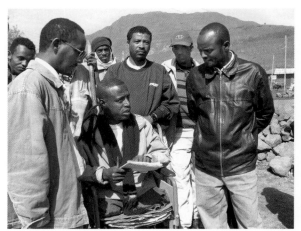

FIGURE 32-2 ■ Take time to visit, ask and listen. Go to where the people are, especially those who may be marginalized, at risk or vulnerable. Look and see. Ask about the story. And *listen* ... Seek to understand the context, the issues, dynamics and needs, existing coping strategies, capabilities and possibilities. Be culturally and gender sensitive. Participatory situational assessments and needs analyses are the foundation upon which to build effective disaster and development programmes, and to identify the people who can make it happen. Here, male team members are speaking with a disabled fighter in post-conflict Ethiopia – a strong intelligent person, ready to become part of a network of development leaders.

diverse perspectives, experience, options and strategies to improve the relevance and quality of disaster management and development activities, most particularly those of survivors and other local stakeholders (Figures 32-3 and 32-4). Effective participation also enables individuals and communities to better understand the processes and capabilities of humanitarian and development organizations and their potential programmes. Participatory approaches inherently build participants' capacity to engage in decision-making processes through development of knowledge, skills, confidence and experience; professionals' capacities are also enhanced through such collaborative engagement.

Active participation is more than provision of information, communication and consultation (Arnstein 1969). While each of these is appropriate in particular circumstances and may be required in support of effective engagement, active participation recognizes and acknowledges a central role for individuals and communities in shaping plans, programmes,

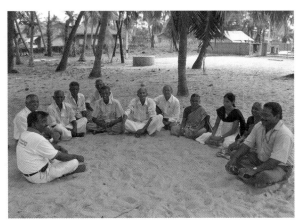

FIGURE 32-3 ■ Participatory planning starts with community leaders and government and other stakeholder representatives. Here, representatives from an international and local NGO meet with male and female community leaders to discuss post-tsunami recovery and future preparedness plans in eastern Sri Lanka.

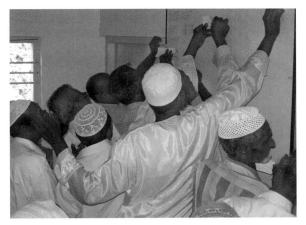

FIGURE 32-4 ■ Participatory planning and decision-making in post-tsunami Sri Lanka. Techniques that generate ideas, promote discussion and allow for equitable and transparent ranking/voting not only build capacity, community and ownership, but elicit meaningful and potentially more viable options. Methods such as this can be adapted, including drawing pictures where literacy is a consideration, and using recycled paper and the floor where notepads and boards are not available.

services and policies, and in implementing activities and monitoring and evaluating their performance.

Active participation processes enable people and communities to raise issues and needs of concern to them and encourage participants to take responsibility in contributing to plans and decisions. Importantly, such processes, if properly managed, can be empowering for people who have lost power through the disaster or who may not previously have had power; these are opportunities to (re)gain a sense of control over one's life and the prevailing circumstances.

Collaborative approaches and partnerships are among the strategies through which participation between disaster and development organizations, community groups and government authorities can occur. The effectiveness of such arrangements is dependent upon mutual respect, reciprocity, shared responsibility and accountability. Equality between partners and mutual learning underpin successful collaborations and partnerships and can pave the way for long-term relationships, contributing to wellbeing and community and resilience building.

Facilitating effective participation and engagement in complex situations characterized by trauma, and diverse and very often competing interests, requires consideration and expertise; occupational therapists have potential to contribute in this realm, particularly with respect to enabling the participation of vulnerable people and groups.

Guideline 3: Utilize Capacity-Building Approaches

Capacity building encompasses a range of processes and methods that aim to strengthen individual and community capacities and assets to improve the impact and sustainability of disaster and development efforts. Within this context, 'capacity' can be defined as the ability to perform functions and realize potential, effectively, efficiently and in a sustainable manner. Occupation is the fundamental mechanism by which people build and utilize capacity.

Communities can be considered to possess five interrelated types of capacity (adapted from Flora 1997):

- human (e.g. skills, abilities, history and experience of community members);
- social (e.g. levels of trust and reciprocity, social networks, cultural and political competencies, leadership, approaches in managing difference and diversity);

- economic (e.g. financial, livelihood and enterprise capability);
- physical (e.g. infrastructure, public facilities, transport, housing and equipment); and
- environmental (e.g. spaces, biodiversity, air and water quality).

Traditionally, capacity-building approaches were based on the presumption that there was something missing or deficient in disadvantaged and vulnerable communities, thereby reinforcing and perpetuating reliance on external resources and expertise that may not be culturally or contextually relevant. While a deficit perspective may be partially appropriate in disaster contexts, from both development and occupational perspectives, approaches that recognize and build on existing capabilities and resources are substantially more empowering and sustainable.

While 'capacity building' is becoming a commonplace term in disaster and development policies, plans, proposals and programmes, it continues to defy a shared definition of what it means in practice. Some describe it as an *approach* or *process* (e.g. a way of working ... towards reducing poverty), while others see it as an *objective* (e.g. specific components and/or activities ... targeting community group capabilities). Many definitions fall somewhere between these two *means* and *ends* perspectives (Bolger 2000, Eade 1997, Thomas 2002). Within disaster and development contexts, capacity building should exhibit broad-based participation and be locally driven, build on lived experience and reflect diversity and contextual characteristics, embody ongoing learning (Figures 32-5, 32-6, 32-7 and 32-8) and adaptation and integrate activities at various levels to address complex challenges (Kaplan 2000).

There are three interrelated levels and associated approaches through which development of capacity can occur, each of which is characterized by a different level of community participation and impact regarding sustainability (adapted from O'Gorman 1992 and CDRA 2001):

1. *'Training'* people in specific knowledge and skills, which is quick but has low sustainability impact.
2. *'Enabling'* people to better plan and manage their own projects and change processes, which

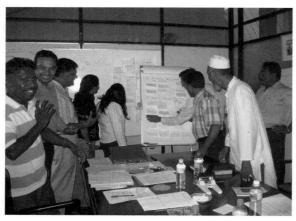

FIGURE 32-5 ■ Participatory 'action learning – action planning' in practice. Here a team comprising community leaders and local NGO staff worked with the author to design, implement and analyse an evaluation of tsunami response activities in Sri Lanka. This process involved pre-training, simultaneous guidance and mentoring during site visits and participatory evaluative activities with beneficiaries and other stakeholders, and collective debriefing to reflect on both evaluation results and learning about M&E. Not only did the process allow for deeper, richer information gathering and triangulation of results across different cultural groups, it also built capacity for ongoing evaluation and planning.

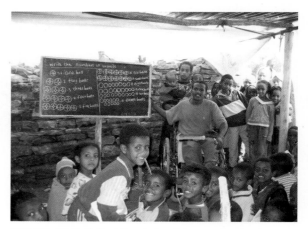

FIGURE 32-6 ■ Enabling 'win-win' capacity development and occupational engagement. In post-conflict, drought-affected northern Ethiopia, creative approaches to disaster and development included helping ex-fighters with disabilities into meaningful occupations, such as teaching orphaned and local children at a makeshift school.

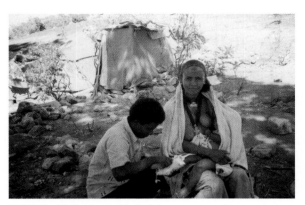

FIGURE 32-7 ■ Disabled fighters were also trained to become community-based rehabilitation workers, providing the only disability services available in remote communities. A number of blind ex-fighters were trained in therapeutic massage to assist with postoperative recovery and contracture management. Some of the disabled CBR workers were subsequently supported to become qualified physiotherapists and continue to provide hospital and rehabilitation services. They have employment and also break down barriers and stigma about people with disability.

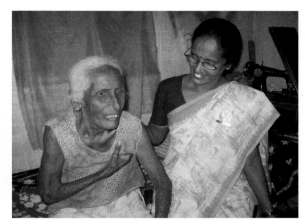

FIGURE 32-8 ■ Survivors recovering together. Training local survivors in community care and basic rehabilitation provides them with a role and small stipend and expands a network of monitoring and support to especially vulnerable and often hidden people who may otherwise fall through the gaps of health and rehabilitation services. Research shows that older women, with life experience and a desire to remain in the local community, tend to comprise the most reliable, effective and enduring cadre.

is more time consuming but achieves moderate sustainability impact.

3. *'Empowering'* people to understand and address the underlying causes and structures of discriminatory practices, which is a long-term process but generates high sustainability impact in the form of enduring, reflexive transformation.

Occupational therapists need to be cognizant of the spectrum of conceptualizations and definitions that characterize the domain of community capacity building in order to clearly locate and define its perspective and practice in this area. As a profession and as individual practitioners this is crucial in establishing a meaningful, credible role.

Guideline 4: Promote Sustainability

Sustainability is about facilitating processes and giving priority to initiatives that encourage self-reliance, that develop the capacity of people and communities to deal with issues as they arise, and that generate outcomes that can be maintained and extended after support and programmes wind up.

Within the context of disaster and development, sustainability is more deeply concerned with facilitating

the health and wellbeing of individuals and communities in ways that do not deplete the earth's capacity to provide for future generations (Bruntland 1987). However, as we discussed in Chapter 3, human activity is a major contributor to the conditions that are wreaking havoc, creating disasters and changing patterns of wellbeing and survival. As such, disaster and development interventions increasingly need to use disaster and disaster response programmes as an opportunity to transform patterns of human occupation to redress factors contributing to risks and future disaster, climate change being the most significant. This involves working with survivors and communities to engage in complex and challenging decision-making about how to balance enabling current survival and wellbeing with choices that address future landscapes and planetary survival, and build resilience to the inevitable shocks that will characterize a world in transition.

Sustainability thus gives consideration to (adapted from Goldie et al 2005):

■ Integrating economic, social and ecological factors, seeking mutually supportive benefits.

- Engaging people through access to information, knowledge and transparent updates, to inform options and decision-making.
- Applying the precautionary principle.
- Promoting equity and human rights, including equitable access to and distribution of common earth resources.
- Protecting biodiversity and ecological integrity.
- Reducing our ecological footprint through changing patterns of resource use and occupational activity while simultaneously reframing and improving quality of life.
- Recognizing the significance and diversity of communities for the management of the earth and the critical importance of 'sense of place' and heritage in planning for the future.
- Building resilience through designing for surprise and managing for adaptation.
- Promoting a new vision and nurturing hope through innovative and creative occupations.

When presented in this way, the potential of occupation and occupational therapy to promote sustainability in both disaster and development contexts begins to emerge and offers exciting opportunities (Figure 32-9).

Table 32-1 outlines indicative strategies through which the guidelines and DDOP occupational principles are expressed.

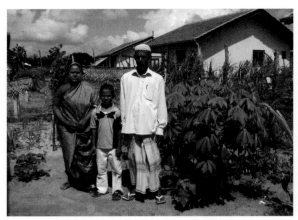

FIGURE 32-9 ■ Building back better. Post-tsunami recovery efforts have involved resettling survivors into new housing areas, and providing support to reestablish gardens for food and nutrition and for sale. A mix of species, including low-water-requirement and trusted 'old' varieties, have been promoted, supported by access to extension workers, installation of rainwater harvesting tanks, and workshops on nonchemical, organic methods such as permaculture, in an aim to enhance ecological sustainability. Economic resilience is promoted through micro-loan and savings schemes, while opportunities for value adding such as drying excess product for extended storage and market times, have been promoted. Family reunification and intergenerational considerations, and establishment of self-help groups and community cooperatives are also key occupational actions that aim to strengthen recovery, sustain outcomes and build resilience and adaptive capacity to future shocks.

DDOP – GENERAL CONSIDERATIONS IN STRENGTHENING OCCUPATIONAL ENGAGEMENT

The case series and frameworks have illuminated potential roles for occupation in promoting resilience within a dynamic, emergent and socio-ecological context. Through the case stories, a wide range of experience and learning has been elaborated about engagement across the disaster continuum. Arising from these are implications for the profession of occupational therapy in terms of policy, practice, education and research.

It is widely acknowledged that the profession is in its infancy with respect to engagement in the disaster and development arena, and that more needs to be done to strengthen capacity to operate effectively and

meaningfully in the field. There are already initiatives underway at international and national level, primarily through the World Federation of Occupational Therapists and national associations (Chapter 29), as well as at regional and local levels, which are frequently in response to disastrous events. In Japan and New Zealand, for example, concerted policy and planning action has arisen from review of the profession's involvement in the earthquake disasters affecting their respective countries, while in India a recent research study by Nair & Tyagi (2014) has focused on identifying strategies to increase occupational therapy involvement in disaster preparedness, response and recovery. The considerations outlined in Box 32-1 are thus presented as a stimulus to support ongoing thinking and further development.

TABLE 32-1	
DDOP – Key Guidelines and Indicative Strategies	
Guideline	**Indicative Strategies**
1. Understand the context and work through relationships	■ Promote, protect and ensure the rights and dignity of vulnerable and marginalized groups.
	■ Enable equitable access to planning and services for all people, especially vulnerable and marginalized groups.
	■ Ensure activities are consistent with international mandates and national policies.
	■ Consider social, occupational and ecological justice factors in undertaking situational and needs assessments, planning, implementation, monitoring and evaluation.
2. Adopt a participatory approach	■ Utilize participatory and partnership strategies across the project and disaster cycles, from start to finish; refer to freely available international and community development resource materials for practical guidance.
	■ Adopt a people-centred approach, expanding on client-centred philosophy.
	■ Enable inclusion of poor, vulnerable, marginalized groups through demonstration, facilitation and advocacy.
	■ Consider ways to promote a 'triple-track'* approach: mainstreaming, specialized support and self-help.
	■ Use the 'ladder of participation' as a tool to consider methods and evaluate levels of participation and empowerment.
3. Utilize capacity-building approaches	■ Consider whose capacity is being built and for what purpose.
	■ Harness existing assets, skills and capabilities and build on these.
	■ Identify capacity-building strategies that simultaneously: assist personal recovery and promote community healing; address immediate needs while promoting adaptability and future resilience; provide compassionate care yet build independence.
	■ Embrace 'protection, prevention, promotion'.
	■ Utilize a combination of capacity-building methods, e.g. training, counterparting, information, education, systems strengthening, networking.
	■ Mix and match/coordinate capacity-building strategies across all stakeholders – survivors, local personnel, agency and government organizations, coordination networks.
	■ Enable occupational engagement.
4. Promote sustainability	■ Consider ways to embrace the three pillars of sustainability – social, environmental, economic – in the design and conduct of disaster preparedness, response and recovery.
	■ Balance enablement with sustainable choices and activities: be smart in addressing short-term needs that can also promote long-term self-reliance, socio-ecological and economic resilience against future shocks.
	■ Encompass three interacting 'streams' of activity in designing for sustainable initiatives: community/people, agencies/organizations, and advocacy/influence/networking; effort is required across all three if desired outcomes are to be sustained.
	■ Utilize participatory and capacity-building approaches.
	■ Role model social and environmental sustainability principles: e.g. recycle, reuse, use locally available 'renewable' resources.
	■ *When you leave ... what will continue?* Consider the 'absorptive capacity' and resources of people and organizations to take on and continue initiatives – good *basic* services/functions that can be maintained with limited resources will have a positive lasting legacy.

*The 'triple-track' approach was first proposed by Helen Pitt and Kerry Thomas, *inter*PART, in 2005, in developing an Integrated Regional Disability Strategy for Tigray in Ethiopia. This disaster-affected, resource-poor area is indicative of contexts where the 'twin-track' approach of mainstreaming combined with specialized services has significant limitations, and self-help strategies are very often the most effective in promoting resilience, sustainability and empowerment.

BOX 32-1
PROMOTING OCCUPATIONAL THERAPY ENGAGEMENT IN DISASTER AND DEVELOPMENT – CONSIDERATIONS FOR POLICY, PRACTICE, EDUCATION AND RESEARCH

POLICY

- National policies and strategic plans – that provide a coherent, contextually relevant professional framework for involvement in the disaster management and sustainable development (climate change) sectors, identify priorities for development and are able to leverage resources, including expertise and funds.
- Networking and engagement with the disaster management and sustainable development (climate change) sectors – in order to carve out meaningful roles and to integrate effectively with disaster preparedness, response and recovery systems and efforts to build community resilience and capacity to adapt to climate change scenarios.
- Coordination – including the establishment of clear roles and responsibilities, communication processes, and activation and management procedures in responding to an emergency, including coordination between the profession and disaster management systems.
- Organizational policies and plans – within our own organizations, engagement in development of contextually relevant disaster management processes and manuals, and promotion of ecologically sustainable practices.
- Partnerships – developing cooperative arrangements with mainstream disaster and development organizations, through which to build mutual capacities in disaster management and sustainable development.
- Recognition and accreditation – developing criteria against which to acknowledge, assess and support development of appropriate practitioner expertise in disaster management.
- Accounting for engagement, performance and improvement – establishing mechanisms to adequately monitor, evaluate and report and communicate on professional engagement and performance in disaster management and sustainable development as it relates to climate change action, and the use of results and learning to improve policies and practices.

PRACTICE

- Recruitment and engagement – processes and procedures to facilitate timely and appropriate engagement of professionals to disaster management efforts, including those mobilized by governments and non-governmental organizations; establishment of human resource databases including pre-accredited professionals; screening for disaster tourism.

- Orientation – consistent with professional practice in the wider disaster and development field, establishment of pre-accredited training, orientation training and briefings relevant to disaster and development contexts and systems; critical self-reflection on one's own values, capacities (including ability to manage stress) and competencies.
- Work competencies – develop or strengthen professional capacities including the ability: to work from the voice of survivors and the unique characteristics of the local environment; to work effectively and efficiently within the disaster and development system; to design and implement initiatives for participation, inclusion, capacity building, resilience and sustainability including socio-ecological imperatives; to translate the value of occupation into practice across individual and social realms (bridge the gap between discourse and practice within the profession); to work cross-culturally and with translators where appropriate; to demonstrate therapeutic competence, adapted to contexts.
- Support and supervision – arrangements for providing personal–professional support, assistance and supervision, particularly for those on disaster response assignments.
- Debriefing – arrangements by which professionals returning from disaster response assignments are debriefed and, where appropriate, provided with access to follow-up support or post-traumatic stress management options.

EDUCATION

- Professional development – a portfolio of options and resources that align with 'accredited' practice standards and lend themselves to being readily adapted and contextualized to national and local situations and languages; modules to support different levels and types of expertise building.
- Undergraduate and graduate education – including disaster management and sustainable development in curricula in some way that is appropriate to local and national contexts but supports consistent professional practice in international roles.
- Educating others – about what occupational therapy can bring to the disaster management and sustainable development sectors – government authorities, non-governmental organizations and community stakeholders; providing technical training to mainstream

PRACTICAL GUIDELINES TO SUPPORT OCCUPATIONAL THERAPY ENGAGEMENT ACROSS THE DISASTER AND DEVELOPMENT CONTINUUM

While the practical guidelines that follow in Table 32-2 have relevance to the general population, there is a focus on strategies that support vulnerable people and groups in particular.

In the context of disaster and development, vulnerable people are identified as being people with disabilities, older people, children and unaccompanied minors, pregnant women, malnourished people, and those who are ill or immunocompromised. Marginalized or minority groups, including for example ethnic and religious minorities and asylum seekers, are also vulnerable in disasters. Those living in poverty are also considered to be vulnerable, given that common consequences of poverty such as malnutrition, homelessness, poor housing and destitution may be exacerbated in times of disaster.

Furthermore, in recognition of the fact that most practitioners will probably be engaged in working with individuals, families and communities, strategies that particularly support these levels of intervention are highlighted in Table 32-2.

It is tempting to provide a 'toolkit' of resources and materials in support of the roles, functions and strategies outlined in this chapter. We have refrained from doing so for both philosophical and pragmatic reasons. Every situation and context is unique, so menu-based approaches are to be avoided. In a diverse and rapidly changing world, some resources are quickly outdated. As we have highlighted, it is processes and relationships that are critical to learning, engagement, the nurturing of adaptability, self-reliance and resilience – and these begin with our own preparedness and involvement in the field of disaster and development. In a web-connected global world, it is increasingly easy to link into networks and to access useful resource materials in languages and formats to suit almost any context. We encourage you to explore some of the many websites and references listed in this book – they are rich with freely available manuals, guidelines, policies and handbooks!

SUMMARY

This chapter has brought together the main themes emerging from disaster and development experience and our occupational framework to summarize a range of practical considerations for successful engagement in this field. Four critical operational functions that underpin any professional endeavour – planning, coordination, monitoring and evaluation, and improvement – were outlined. In support of the process to achieve desired outcomes, a set of four guidelines and associated strategies to facilitate engagement during and across all

TABLE 32-2
Disaster Preparedness, Response, Recovery and Development – Indicative Roles for Occupational Therapy

Key Activities	Indicative Roles for Occupational Therapy
Preparedness ■ Risk assessment and vulnerability reduction, including capacity assessment ■ Preparedness planning ■ Engagement and coordination with key stakeholders ■ Training for emerging roles ■ Early warning methods	■ Personal and professional preparedness – individually and as a professional community. ■ Engage and coordinate with disaster preparedness authorities and other stakeholder organizations. ■ Facilitate active participation of vulnerable and marginalized people in local risk assessment, vulnerability reduction, mapping, capacity identification and utilization, preparedness and early warning planning, and evacuation processes and exercises (e.g. people with disability, older people, migrants). ■ Promote accessibility – early warning, evacuation – universal design, communication formats and methods for people with different disabilities. ■ Promote resilience, and contingency planning. ■ Train others in how to interact with vulnerable groups in planning, and first responders in how to help vulnerable groups in emergency situations. ■ Educate others, including authorities, about the contribution of occupational therapy in disaster management. ■ Ensure your own organization and professional association have preparedness and response plans.
Emergency Response ■ Search, rescue, evacuation, first aid ■ Registration ■ Relief: shelter, water, food, medicine ■ Trauma care ■ Coordination	■ Coordinate with emergency response authorities and implementing organizations (government, NGOs, disabled people's organizations, etc.). ■ Help to evacuate children, older people and people with disabilities who have mobility difficulties and provide information to people with visual and hearing difficulties. ■ Provide basic first aid and triage. ■ Help deliver emergency provisions (water, food, essential items to sustain life and hygiene) while conducting needs assessment. ■ Ensure that older people and people with disabilities are included on registers, e.g. disaggregated data; type of disability, special requirements. ■ Help vulnerable groups get access to relief: physical accessibility and design; facilitating special provisions (e.g. separate lines for people with disability/older people at distribution points). ■ Ensure information and communication is in accessible formats and methods (e.g. visual, hearing impaired). ■ Facilitate access to eye glasses, mobility aids, medications for those who need them. ■ Assist in trauma care, emergency surgery and recovery, medical rehabilitation, prevention of disabling conditions, *appropriate* psychosocial support. ■ Enable survivor participation in decision-making and activity; regaining control is vital to recovery, as is 'doing'. ■ Ensure vulnerable people have a voice on camp/relocation committees and in making decisions that affect them. ■ Make toilets and washing places accessible, private but safe for vulnerable people – they are at higher risk of abuse. ■ Create child friendly spaces and activities for all children, including art and school, and help ensure the safety of those who are separated or orphaned while family tracing is carried out. ■ Create spaces for survivors to talk and do things together (to regain some control over their lives, for psychosocial benefits), e.g. plan and implement religious ceremonies, make food, share meals – normalizing routines and daily activities. ■ Facilitate reunification – for healing and for carer support. ■ Train emergency and relief personnel, e.g. how to communicate with and assist people with disability/older people. ■ Look after yourself – have your own basic survival kit.

TABLE 32-2
Disaster Preparedness, Response, Recovery and Development – Indicative Roles for Occupational Therapy (Continued)

Key Activities	Indicative Roles for Occupational Therapy
Recovery	
■ Health ■ Livelihoods ■ Education ■ Home and community care ■ Infrastructure ■ Services	■ Coordinate with disaster recovery authorities, health and social development networks, NGOs, etc. ■ Work with individuals, families, groups, communities – in clinical, rehabilitation, social development roles. ■ Facilitate survivor participation in decision-making and programmes. ■ Facilitate (re)establishment of 'occupational' routines and programmes – self-care, food, social, healing. ■ Facilitate education for children. ■ Provide post-trauma clinical and rehabilitation services – recovery from emergency surgery and injuries, as well as longer-term rehabilitation for those with longlasting impairments. ■ Help prevent disability. ■ Mobilize community-based rehabilitation approaches, working with volunteers and community health workers in camps/community/resettlement areas. ■ Establish self-help groups for people with disability and for older people through which to assist/ channel longer-term recovery efforts. ■ Facilitate livelihoods and access to small income-generating activities, especially for vulnerable people. ■ Contribute to design of rebuilding efforts – promote universal design and accessibility codes. ■ Consider ways in which recovery efforts/activities/processes can enhance longer-term development and resilience building.
Development	
■ Community building ■ Resilience building ■ Sustainability strategies	■ In regular occupational therapy and community work, integrate risk reduction, adaptation and resilience capacity building into rehabilitation and community-related programmes. ■ Engage in cross-sectoral sustainable development and climate change planning processes to promote consideration of health implications, especially for those who are more vulnerable and at risk. ■ Promoting consideration of occupational implications in climate change planning and strategies. ■ Undertake M&E and research studies to generate evidence and support engagement in the above. ■ Ensure programme outcomes can be sustained when you leave – that is, carried on and adapted by those whose lives they affect.

phases of the disaster and development continuum were elaborated: context and relationships, participatory and capacity-building approaches, and sustainability. These guidelines operationalize the six principles of occupation in disaster and development and express the core values of equity, participation, capability and resilience. We then presented some general considerations for the profession of occupational therapy as it moves to strengthen its engagement in the field of disaster and development, for policy, practice, education and research. Finally, a range of very practical roles and strategies were provided to guide an occupational therapist in each phase of the disaster management cycle,

together with suggestions for accessing more detailed resource material.

REFERENCES

Arnstein, S., 1969. Ladder of citizen participation. J. Am. Inst. Plann. 35 (4), 216–224.

Bolger, J., 2000. Capacity development. Occasional Series: Canadian International Development Agency Policy Branch Vol 1 (1).

Brower, D., 1990. For Earth's Sake: The Life and Times of David Brower. Gibbs-Smith, Salt Lake City.

Bruntland, G., 1987. Our Common Future. Oxford University Press, Oxford.

CDRA, 2001. Community Development Resource Association Workshop Materials. Community Development Resource Association, Woodstock, South Africa.

Dubos, R., 1972. <http://www.unep.org/Documents.Multilingual/Default.asp?DocumentID=97> Report from the United Nations Conference on the Human Environment held in Stockholm. UNEP (United Nations Environment Program).

Eade, D., 1997. Capacity-Building. An Approach to People-Centred Development. Oxfam UK and Ireland, Oxford.

Flora, C., 1997. Enhancing Community Capitals: The Optimisation Equation. Rural Development News 21 (1).

Geddes, P., 1915. Cities in Evolution, Williams, London.

Goldie, J., Douglas, B., Furnass, B., 2005. In Search of Sustainability. CSIRO, Collingwood, Australia.

Kaplan, A., 2000. Capacity building: shifting the paradigms of practice. Dev. Pract. 10 (3 & 4).

Nair, P., Tyagi, N., 2014, Occupational Therapy: Metamorphosis with Vision in Public Health for Disaster Preparedness, Response and Recovery. Paper presented at the scientific session of the 51st Annual National Conference of AIOTA; Bhubaneswar.

O'Gorman, F., 1992. Charity and Change: From Bandaid to Beacon. World Vision, Melbourne.

Thomas, K., 2002. Capacity Building: Discussion Papers in support of strengthening AusAID's East Timor Programs (Australian Aid for International Development). *inter*PART, Macclesfield, South Australia.

33 CONCLUSION

Disaster exposes the interdependence of all living things, yet in this web of interdependencies relationships are not equal. Social conditions and inequities shape the choices and opportunities people have to live long, healthy and active lives, to avoid or recover from disaster and build resilience. On a global scale our choices as a human race reflect uneven patterns of growth and consumption that drive disaster risk and threaten the vitality of the ecosystems upon which all life depends. People living in poverty and socially disadvantaged groups face the most immediate risk and bear the cumulative burden of disaster and crises that are occurring around the globe. This reality calls to question the resilience of our global society to disaster. Moreover, it necessitates widespread social and ecological transformation as evidenced by new patterns of human occupation and activity that reflect the reality of shared resources and a finite planet.

The profession of occupational therapy has a contribution to make to a collective and interdisciplinary global response to disaster that is based on its capacity to transform patterns of human occupation and activity. In response to increasing disaster risk on a global scale, and the disproportionate burden of risk and loss experienced by socially disadvantaged groups, occupational therapists are compelled to align their practice with efforts to galvanize action and enable social change in the field. This involves reconceptualizing occupation, upholding the value of interdependence, and orientating practice to the socio-ecological realm. Within this realm occupational therapists are essentially 'social practitioners with an occupation-based approach'. At the point of everyday activities, where natural hazards, social relations and individual choice converge, they steward occupation in order to strengthen the social fabric and ecological integrity upon which resilience, health and wellbeing lie.

INDEX

Page numbers followed by "f" indicate figures, "t" indicate tables, and "b" indicate boxes.